Advancing Women's Health Through Medical Education

Advancing Women's Health Through Medical Education

A Systems Approach in Family Planning and Abortion

Edited by

Uta Landy
University of California, San Francisco

Philip D. Darney
University of California, San Francisco

Jody Steinauer
University of California, San Francisco

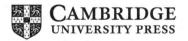
CAMBRIDGE
UNIVERSITY PRESS

CAMBRIDGE
UNIVERSITY PRESS

University Printing House, Cambridge CB2 8BS, United Kingdom

One Liberty Plaza, 20th Floor, New York, NY 10006, USA

477 Williamstown Road, Port Melbourne, VIC 3207, Australia

314–321, 3rd Floor, Plot 3, Splendor Forum, Jasola District Centre, New Delhi – 110025, India

103 Penang Road, #05–06/07, Visioncrest Commercial, Singapore 238467

Cambridge University Press is part of the University of Cambridge.

It furthers the University's mission by disseminating knowledge in the pursuit of education, learning, and research at the highest international levels of excellence.

www.cambridge.org
Information on this title: www.cambridge.org/9781108839648
DOI: 10.1017/9781108884709

First published 2021

A catalogue record for this publication is available from the British Library.

Library of Congress Cataloging-in-Publication Data
Names: Landy, Uta, editor. | Darney, Philip D., editor. | Steinauer, Jody, 1969– editor.
Title: Advancing women's health through medical education : a systems approach in family planning and abortion / edited by Uta Landy, Philip D. Darney, Jody Steinauer.
Description: Cambridge, United Kingdom ; New York, NY : Cambridge University Press, 2021. | Includes bibliographical references and index.
Identifiers: LCCN 2020053911 (print) | LCCN 2020053912 (ebook) | ISBN 9781108884709 (epub) | ISBN 9781108839648 (hardback)
Subjects: | MESH: Reproductive Health Services | Women's Health | Women's Health Services | Abortion, Induced--education | Education, Medical
Classification: LCC RG136.2 (ebook) | LCC RG136.2 (print) | NLM WQ 200.1 | DDC 613.9/4--dc23
LC record available at https://lccn.loc.gov/2020053911

ISBN 978-1-108-83964-8 Hardback

• •

This book honors all of the family planning fellows and Ryan Program faculty around the world who have dedicated their careers to reproductive justice and health through patient care based on social and clinical research and to teaching successive generations of clinicians, researchers and advocates.

Contents

Contributors

Ferid Abbas Abubeker MD
Department of Obstetrics & Gynecology,
St. Paul's Hospital Millennium Medical College,
Addis Ababa, Ethiopia

Lois V. Backus MPH
Medical Students for Choice, Philadelphia,
PA, USA

Leonel Briozzo MD
Department of Obstetrics & Gynecology,
University of the Republic, Pereira Rossell
Hospital, Montevideo, Uruguay

Joyce Cappiello PhD FNP FAANP
College of Health & Human Sciences, University
of New Hampshire, Durham, NH, USA

Wendy Chavkin MD MPH
Columbia University Mailman School of Public
Health, New York, NY, USA

Amanda Cleeve PhD MSc RNM
Department of Women's & Children's Health,
and the WHO collaborating centre in Human
Reproduction, Karolinska Institute and
Karolinska University Hospital, Stockholm,
Sweden

Vanessa K. Dalton MD MPH
Department of Obstetrics & Gynecology,
University of Michigan, Ann Arbor, MI, USA

Philip D. Darney MD MSc
Bixby Center for Global Reproductive Health,
Department of Obstetrics, Gynecology &
Reproductive Sciences, University of California,
San Francisco, San Francisco, CA, USA

Christine Dehlendorf MD MAS
Departments of Family & Community Medicine,
University of California, San Francisco,
San Francisco, CA, USA

Angela Dempsey MD MPH
Department of Obstetrics & Gynecology, Medical
University of South Carolina, Charleston,
SC, USA

Teresa DePiñeres MD
Initiatives in Reproductive Health
Miami, FL, USA

Maeve Eogan MD MRCOG FRCPI
National Maternity Hospital, Dublin, Ireland

Verónica Fiol MD
Department of Obstetrics & Gynecology,
University of the Republic, Montevideo,
Uruguay

Kristina Gemzell-Danielsson MD PhD
Department of Women's & Children's Health,
and the WHO collaborating centre in Human
Reproduction, Karolinska Institute and
Karolinska University Hospital, Stockholm,
Sweden

Laura Gil MD
Fundación Oriéntame, Bogotá, Colombia

Emily M. Godfrey MD MPH
Department of Family Medicine,
University of Washington, Seattle,
WA, USA

Alisa B. Goldberg MD MPH
Department of Obstetrics, Gynecology and
Reproductive Biology
Brigham and Women's Hospital
Harvard Medical School
Boston, MA USA

Lisa M. Goldthwaite MD MPH
Department of Obstetrics & Gynecology
Stanford University School of Medicine,
Stanford, CA, USA

Maryam Guiahi MD MSc
Department of Obstetrics & Gynecology,
University of Colorado Anschutz Medical
Campus,
Aurora, CO, USA

Mengistu Hailemariam MD
Center for International Reproductive Health
Training, Addis Ababa, Ethiopia

Lisa H. Harris MD PhD
Department of Obstetrics & Gynecology,
University of Michigan, Ann Arbor, MI, USA

Rebecca R. Henderson MA
School of Medicine, University of Florida,
Gainesville, FL, USA

Mary F. Higgins MD FRCPI FRCOG
University College Dublin Perinatal Research
Centre, National Maternity Hospital, Dublin,
Ireland

Sabrina Holmquist MD MPH
Planned Parenthood of the Rocky Mountains,
Denver, CO, USA

Carole Joffe PhD
Bixby Center for Global Reproductive Health,
Department of Obstetrics, Gynecology &
Reproductive Sciences, University of California,
San Francisco, San Francisco, CA, USA

Sirjana Khanal MBA MPH
Teaching Hospital, Maharajgunj,
Kathmandu, Nepal

Rajshree Jha Kumar MD
Mumbai, India

Uta Landy PhD
Senior Advisor Bixby Center for Global
Reproductive Health, Department of Obstetrics,
Gynecology & Reproductive Sciences, University
of California, San Francisco, San Francisco,
CA, USA

Amy J. Levi PhD CNM WHNP-BC
University of New Mexico School of Medicine,
Albuquerque, NM, USA

Patricia A. Lohr MD MPH
British Pregnancy Advisory Service, London,
UK

Carla Lupi MD
Kaiser Permanente Bernard J. Tyson School of
Medicine, Pasadena, CA, USA

Erin McCoy MPH
Department of Obstetrics & Gynecology,
University of Washington, Seattle, WA, USA

Laura MacIsaac MD MPH
Department of Obstetrics & Gynecology,
Mount Sinai Health System, New York,
NY, USA

Oscar Marroquin MD
Fundación Oriéntame, Bogotá, Colombia

Lisa A. Martin PhD
Institute for Research on Women & Gender,
University of Michigan, Dearborn, MI, USA

Rachel Masch MD MPH
Department of Obstetrics, Gynecology &
Reproductive Science, Mount Sinai Beth Israel,
New York, NY, USA

Karen R. Meckstroth MD MPH
Department of Obstetrics, Gynecology &
Reproductive Sciences, Zuckerberg San Francisco
General Hospital,
University of California, San Francisco,
San Francisco, CA, USA

Prof. Emmanuel S.K Morhe
Department of Obstetrics and Gynecology,
School of Medicine University of Health and
Allied Sciences, Ho, Ghana

Cliona Murphy MD
Coombe Women & Infants University Hospital,
Dublin, Ireland

Maria Nozar MD
Department of Obstetrics & Gynecology,
University of the Republic, Montevideo,
Uruguay

Alissa C. Perrucci PhD MPH
Women's Options Center, San Francisco General
Hospital, San Francisco, CA, USA

Sarah Ward Prager MD MAS
Department of Obstetrics & Gynecology,
University of Washington, Seattle, WA, USA

Swaraj Rajbhandari MD MPH
Department of Obstetrics & Gynaecology, Nidan Hospital, Kathmandu, Nepal

Dame Lesley Regan MD
Department of Obstetrics & Gynaecology, Imperial College School of Medicine at St Mary's Hospital, London, UK

Maria I. Rodriguez MD MPH
Department of Obstetrics & Gynecology, Oregon Health & Science University, Portland, OR, USA

Patricio Sanhueza MD
Department of Reproductive Health, Secretariat of Health of Mexico City, Mexico City, Mexico

Raffaela Schiavon MD
IPAS Mexico, Mexico City, Mexico

Courtney A. Schreiber MD MPH
Department of Obstetrics & Gynecology, University of Pennsylvania School of Medicine, Philadelphia, PA, USA

Meghan Seewald MA
Department of Obstetrics & Gynecology, University of Michigan, Ann Arbor, MI, USA

Katherine Simmonds, PhD, MPH, WHNP-BC
MGH Institute of Health Professions, Boston, MA, USA

Jody Steinauer MD PhD
Department of Obstetrics, Gynecology & Reproductive Sciences, University of California, San Francisco, San Francisco, CA, USA

Diana Taylor PhD, MS, RNP
School of Nursing, University of California, San Francisco, San Francisco, CA, USA

Jema K. Turk PhD MA MPA
Department of Obstetrics, Gynecology, & Reproductive Sciences, University of California, San Francisco, San Francisco, CA, USA

David Turok MD MPH
Dpeartment of Obstetrics and Gynecology, University of Utah Hospital, Salt Lake City, UT, USA

Maria Vivas MD MPH
Fundación Oriéntame, Bogotá, Colombia

Katharine O'Connell White MD MPH
Department of Obstetrics & Gynecology, Boston University School of Medicine, Boston, MA, USA

Preface

While this book's focus is on integrating training after contraception and abortion become legal, many, if not all, of the systems and approaches described in this book are equally applicable in countries where abortion is illegal or access to abortion and contraception is limited. Our educational concepts and approaches may seem too complex, expensive or impractical for resource-poor countries where family planning services, no matter how poorly delivered, are judged adequate or are so controversial that ignoring them is the safest course. In fact, this attitude perpetuates the status quo, prevents progress or leads to a deterioration of health care. In the context of family planning, this view is particularly detrimental. It reinforces the perception that family planning and reproductive health have little status or value in health-care delivery and therefore in medical education. Ensuring a scientifically informed, motivated and caring workforce not only to deliver clinical care but to drive research and policy must be the aim of every country. Education of that workforce is paramount for promoting health in general and reproductive health in particular. While legalization of abortion is an essential element in promoting women's and public health, the advocates for reform and those responsible for its implementation often do not consider the essential link: the systemic education of all involved in providing the care, for which we hope this book will offer inspiration and guidance.

Acknowledgments

The editors thank Lauren Parker of UCSF for her invaluable assistance and Nick Dunton of Cambridge University Press for his encouragement to create this book and support of our efforts.

Introduction

Uta Landy

Contraception and abortion allow women to control their reproduction. The means to accomplish reproductive control have improved over the past century as the result of revolutionary social and medical advances. The subtitle of this book refers to family planning and abortion, but our primary focus is on abortion. Contraception, while still politically embattled and not universally available, is no longer in the eye of the reactionary storm in most countries. Nevertheless, integration of all aspects of contraception into medical education is incomplete.

Termination of pregnancy ranges from simple interventions – misoprostol and mifepristone and manual or electric aspiration – to surgically complex dilation and evacuation (D&E) of the uterus. Abortion education can also be seen as a series of skills of increasing complexity taught to practitioners – nurses, medical students and residents. A book about training these practitioners could focus on these medical skills, understanding the basics of the underlying science, patient eligibility criteria, the treatment of complications and pregnancy prevention, but that is not our objective here. Instead, our vision is a systems approach: Who should be trained, and how, by whom, and where should that training be accomplished? What should it include and who defines those parameters? Who is responsible for training standards and their enforcement? What systems are in place to define and regulate training mandates? What impacts do the training of various practitioners have on health policy, on the workforce and on professionals' responsibilities as educators, researchers and social change agents?

While training represents the core of our book, its context and impact, we address the education of the medical workforce in broad health and social contexts such as maternal mortality, the politics of abortion, religion and the roles of government agencies and medical organizations in determining a country's medical workforce and practices. We address creation and implementation of the research necessary to inform policy and improve women's health. We describe the communities that have been created as components of training, both locally and globally, and their impacts, interpretations of professional responsibilities versus personal conscience and considerations of economic and social justice in access to care.

We have chosen to make training of obstetricians and gynecologists (ob-gyns) our primary focus. In the USA, it was this community, its department chairs and academic leaders and the American College of Obstetricians and Gynecologists who advocated for the legalization of abortion and, later on, for passing a training mandate and supporting abortion access despite unrelenting political interference. As one of the "core specialties," ob-gyns are responsible not only for training their own residents and fellows, but also educating all medical students in reproductive health by developing the reproductive health curriculum and organizing its implementation for most medical schools. They often participate similarly in the reproductive health aspects of training general practitioners, midwives and nurses.

We divided the book into four major sections. Section I, Abortion Training: Workforce, Leadership, Social & Political Impact, addresses major areas relevant to training, policy and access. In Chapter 1, we look at the history and reforms of the field of medical education during the past century, beginning with the Flexner Report and its impact on creating a science-based education system, published more than a century ago, leading to the 2010 Global Commission's report published by the *Lancet*, "Health Professionals for a New Century: Transforming Education to Strengthen Health Systems in an Interdependent

World." We consider workforce, professionalism and leadership in the context of the medical education systems in the USA, and the role of the Fellowship in Family Planning and the Ryan Residency Training Program in achieving a systems-integrated family planning workforce aligned with the goals of the Lancet Commission.

Chapter 2 addresses maternal mortality, a long-standing global crisis, and interventions and successes in reducing maternal deaths worldwide, highlighting the role of family planning policy, safe abortion and training of the workforce. The high rate of and the failure to reduce the maternal mortality rate (MMR) in the USA is compared to the steeply falling rates of Ethiopia and Nepal, two examples of countries whose institutionalized training programs for abortion and contraception have been pivotal in improving women's health.

The history of integrated family planning education (Chapter 3) highlights the trajectory of abortion access, service, ob-gyn educational mandates and their implementation in creating a robust and vital physician workforce to train future practitioners, conduct research, promote medical culture change and advocate for family planning, as elaborated in Chapters 4, 6 and 7. Two factors played key roles: a professional training mandate including assessment of physicians' skills and overall knowledge, and a national professional effort, in the case of the USA, two private educational initiatives, to ensure implementation.

The medical community, in particular physicians, especially ob-gyns, is uniquely positioned to advocate for abortion. In the advocacy chapter (4), we recount the history, and accomplishments of the ob-gyn academic community in promoting the legalization of and access to safe abortion during the past fifty years. A unique aspect of the national education initiatives and essential for their success was the organization of a "community of practice" (Chapter 5) that fosters learning, well-being and shared expertise in clinical care, research and advocacy.

Research is vital to evidence-based practice for improved reproductive health. The Fellowship in Family Planning's (FFP) research has built evidence for clinical practice and policy development. Chapter 6 highlights two examples of the impacts of FFP: the increase in use of long-acting reversible contraception (LARC) in the USA and

the availability and safety of second-trimester surgical abortion.

Chapter 7 offers a comprehensive look at the impacts of the FFP and the Ryan Residency Training Program on reproductive health in the USA and abroad. It describes the evidence these programs have created through research, the policy developments and the roles and leadership fostered. The first section of the book closes with a review of what continues to be a major topic of debate and controversy among physicians: the role of conscience in providing abortion and reproductive health care, acceptance of training and service mandates and the laws governing conscience clauses in US and global settings (Chapter 8).

Integration of Abortion into Medical Education

In Section II, Integration of Abortion into Graduate Medical Education, Chapter 9 begins with a review of family planning training in the USA, the extent to which it has been integrated into medical education, its outcomes and the challenges met. Further exploring implementation, Chapter 10 delineates steps for the establishment of training services in teaching hospitals, highlighting the history and current services of one of the earliest abortion training and research services at the University of California, San Francisco (UCSF) which became the first FFP site and has been used as a model for the Ryan Residency Training initiative.

Uterine evacuation skills are necessary not only for the termination of a pregnancy but also in cases of early pregnancy loss. Political and institutional restrictions can make a pregnancy loss service the only option to teach uterine evacuation (Chapter 11). A systems-based approach is used to integrate clinical services for pregnancy loss into the teaching hospitals' outpatient and emergency services to enhance trainees' competence in uterine evacuation and reinforce the broader applications of uterine evacuation in clinical practice.

Collaborations with community partners, described in Chapter 12, are essential and valued components for the success of teaching hospital services and training. They offer abortion and contraceptive training opportunities not available in the teaching hospital, introduce learners to other models of care, strengthen institutional and community partnerships, add social and political perspectives and contribute to advocacy efforts.

A special chapter is devoted to the unique challenges of providing family planning services in a Catholic hospital, obligated to follow Catholic doctrine (directives) set and enforced by Catholic bishops and hospital administration (Chapter 13). As a result, these hospitals fail to offer any abortions except under the most extreme life-threatening circumstances, and hence are not able to fulfill the ob-gyn abortion training mandate or ensure contraceptive competency for their residents. The chapter describes how training can occur through collaboration with partner institutions or clinics.

The education of medical students is a crucial factor in preparing a competent workforce, particularly in countries where students are expected to practice immediately after graduation and may not have further training in essential services like contraception and uterine evacuation. Chapter 14 offers a comprehensive review of medical student education in abortion and family planning and guidelines for implementation.

Chapter 15's focus is on the efforts of family medicine physicians in promoting training and ensuring access. Although lacking an enforceable mandate for abortion training, family physicians have been in the forefront of providing services, particularly in community clinics. They have established national initiatives, in collaboration with ob-gyn services and community clinic partners. Advanced-practice clinicians (APCs), another essential group in the medical workforce, play a pivotal role in ensuring access to family planning services in the USA and abroad. Chapter 16 describes research that demonstrates the advantages of APCs providing abortions as well as approaches to the training and education of APCs.

In Section III, Family Planning Curricular Design and Implementation, we introduce comprehensive how-to guides on educating students and residents about abortion and family planning. We begin with Chapter 17 on the key practical steps of starting a family planning clinical service in a teaching hospital and making it financially sustainable. The chapter highlights challenges and pitfalls, and outlines the steps for designing a resident family planning rotation and preparing residents for abortions, including those who chose to participate only partially in training.

Chapter 18 describes a specific curriculum to enhance clinical teaching including the larger context of abortion care, the public health implications for safe abortion, established evidence for elements of practice and the psychosocial aspects of the provider and patient interaction. Educators can use this process for curricular design, implementation of learning assessments and program evaluation.

Chapter 19 addresses defining, implementing and assessing milestones – an integral part of medical education. The FFP created milestones for its fellows, which entailed a complex process of defining clinical skills and learning outcomes and their measurement. These milestones for advanced fellow training can be adapted to the resident curriculum.

Chapter 20 concerns the integration of family planning in the education of the 154 US medical schools that, despite professional advocacy efforts, has been inconsistent, in part as a result of traditional approaches to medical education. Reforms toward competency- and outcomes-based learning offer opportunities for innovation in teaching methods, curricular content and mentorship.

While medical school faculty worked toward reproductive health-relevant education content and systems, medical students themselves formed their own advocacy body through Medical Students for Choice, described in Chapter 21. Founded at UCSF in 1993, it now supports more than 200 medical school chapters worldwide. Students advocate for curricular reform and have created an active and influential national and global community.

Simulation has become a valued tool in medical education, as shown in Chapter 22, and is particularly useful to enhance training in family planning clinical skills. Simulation promotes interactive learning, acquisition of skills and competence before the learner begins to interact with a patient. Simulation techniques include simple, inexpensive approaches such as the "Papaya Workshops," which have been used around the world to introduce first-trimester uterine evacuation, long-acting reversible contraceptives, dilation and evacuation for advanced gestations, team-based communication skills and management of emergencies, such as uterine hemorrhage.

Chapter 23 addresses an important challenge of integrated family planning resident rotations; when residents choose to "partially participate in" or "opt out" of some or all aspects of the family planning rotation, patient care and staff scheduling and relationships are affected. Gauging residents' personal, moral or religious perspectives while accomplishing the learning objectives mandated by the Accreditation Council for Graduate Medical Education (ACGME) and Residency Review Committees (RRCs) is a complex task for the faculty mentor. The evaluation team of the Ryan Residency Training Program conducted studies during the past twenty years to explore residents' and faculty members' experiences with partial participation.

The stigma surrounding abortion has a profound effect on everyone involved in abortion care: learners, faculty, clinic staff and the women they serve. Chapter 24 describes the impact of stigma on the work and life of family planning providers and offers approaches to relieve the burden of stigma. Special attention paid to the emotional realm of abortion work for physicians and trainees through dedicated workshops in "values clarification" and "providers share," created by one of the chapter authors, can help to counteract and reduce stigma.

Further exploring the emotional aspects of abortion training, Chapter 25 describes the emotional, social and economic contexts patients bring to their abortion experience and the importance of acknowledging them. Skills such as active listening, refraining from making assumptions and self-reflection are necessary in pregnancy options counseling. Emotional support is also essential for the entire clinic team, including staff, and physicians, and particularly the students and residents who need to come to terms with their own emotional and professional perspectives in addition to those of their patients.

Section IV of the book, Reproductive Health Services & Abortion Training: Global Examples, looks at reproductive health services and education from a global perspective. Country studies from Nepal, Ghana, Ethiopia, Columbia, Uruguay and Mexico, and three European examples, Sweden, the United Kingdom and Ireland, describe the systems, models and considerations that inform training and services. The section begins with Chapter 26's global perspective on creating a workforce in sexual and reproductive health, its central role in improving population health outcomes and the need for making it an urgent public health priority. The author summarizes national and global workforce considerations made by the United Nations (UN), World Health Organization (WHO), the Lancet Commission and the US Health Force Commission, the complexities and difficulties in defining and achieving a competent workforce in reproductive health and the progress that has been made in a number of countries, including the USA.

Finally, in Chapters 27 through 35 we present descriptions of systems integration of abortion and reproductive health education. We chose the country examples because many of their efforts are connected to those in the USA through the Fellowship in Family Planning and the Ryan Residency Training Program. Each country's approach is uniquely informed by parameters of legality, the health-care and medical education systems, physician attitudes and leadership and culture.

Family Planning and the COVID 19 Pandemic

During the final editing of this book, COVID 19 spread around the world with devastating effects, particularly on pregnant women. The physicians who care for them, whose training is the subject of the book, could not prepare for the unknown effects of the disease on their patients or on pregnancies. Obstetricians know that respiratory disease, the primary cause of death from COVID 19, takes a particularly grim toll on pregnant women. It is the third most common cause of indirect maternal mortalities. Viral pneumonias are difficult to treat: the case fatality rate (CFR) for pregnant women in the pandemic influenza of 1918 was 27%; for the pandemic flu in 1958 it was twice as high (10%) in pregnancy than for non-pregnant women. The most common obstetrical effects of pneumonia in pregnancy are prematurity, intrauterine fetal growth restriction and demise, and neonatal death. Severe acute respiratory syndrome (SARS), the closest relative of the virus causing COVID 19, took a particularly grim toll on pregnant women. The Zika epidemic showed that new infectious diseases sometimes cause terrible fetal deformities. These past experiences suggest that family planning services are critically important for women during viral epidemics in order to prevent maternal deaths and avoid bad obstetrical outcomes.

In response to the pandemic, the family planning physicians described in this book cared for a wide range of patients. Some of these physicians became infected themselves and, in turn, infected their families and, subsequently, lost elderly parents. Throughout the course of the pandemic, they struggled to maintain abortion services for all women, particularly those whose lives or pregnancies could be threatened by the infection. They advocated and succeeded in declaring abortion to be an "essential service" in their hospitals and clinics. In some states, for example, Texas, Iowa, Ohio, Louisiana, Oklahoma, Tennessee, Arkansas and Alabama, politicians sought to exploit the pandemic by closing freestanding clinics that were not associated with hospital care, claiming that these abortions consumed medical resources and forcing some women to continue an unwanted pregnancy, risking COVID infection and their own and fetal health. The community of experts supported each other across the country in making contraceptive care available with telemedicine and expediting approval for self- or pharmacy-administered medroxyprogesterone acetate. They exchanged clinical care and protocols in response to the new COVID demands on hospitals and published a *New England Journal of Medicine* Perspective: "Abortion during the Covid-19 Pandemic – Ensuring Access to an Essential Health Service."

This book offers a comprehensive historical review and practical guide for anyone interested in family planning: historians, current family planning providers, educators, researchers or policy makers. By describing the growth and impact of two landmark educational initiatives and the enormous changes they led to along with the experiences in countries on every continent, the reader learns:

- the impact on the education and practice of physicians, particularly ob-gyns, students and nurses
- the policy, institutional and organizational changes necessary to integrate family planning into medical education
- the cultural and political hurdles encountered and practical guidelines and considerations to address them, both in the USA and abroad
- the essential roles of community and systems changes, regardless of the legal parameters, but particularly after legalization, on reproduction
- the impact on women's health by increased access to care through research and advocacy
- the recognition by all medical professionals, societies and governments that family planning care, standards for training and education are an essential part of women's health

Chapter

1

A Systems Approach to Medical Education

Uta Landy

1.1 Historical Background of Health Education

The first reforms in health education occurred in response to the publication of the Flexner Report in 1910, more than a hundred years ago [1]. The reforms, sparked by the discovery of the germ theory in Europe and other scientific advances, led to the integration of early developments in medical science into the academic education of physicians. Ten years ago, the *Lancet* published a report, "Health Professionals for a New Century: Transforming Education to Strengthen Health Systems in an Interdependent World," based on the findings of a global independent commission to address the inequities in health, despite enormous scientific advances in medicine [2]. In this report, twenty professional and academic leaders representing the perspective of diverse countries defined an educational strategy for medicine, nursing and public health. Its intention was to consider the relationship between health systems and education and recommend strategies to produce a workforce that addresses the health needs of a particular country.

According to the report, the initial reforms following the Flexner Report led to a radical transformation of medical education based on scientific evidence. This shift to a scientific foundation into the education of health professionals made such enormous differences as doubling the

life span during the twentieth century [2]. The authors of the *Lancet* report summarized three levels of learning: informative learning of skills acquisition, formative learning of values and professionalism and transformative learning to prepare for leadership (Figure 1.1). Transformative learning is considered the highest level, which, following the acquisition of skills to establish expertise and acquiring values and professionalism, develops leadership attributes to "produce enlightened change agents."

The Fellowship in Family Planning's educational vision and implementation are aligned with all three objectives: it defines and imparts clinical skills, fosters ethics and professionalism and, finally, produces leaders who change medical education, service delivery and health policy. (See Chapters 3 and 7.)

1.2 Health Systems: Preparing the Workforce

According to the World Health Organization (WHO), health systems have six components: leadership and governance, health information systems, health financing, human resources, essential medicines and technologies and delivery of health services (Figure 1.2).

The education of professionals is affected by and in turn impacts all components of the health system. Most important, health services and their

	Objectives	Outcome
Informative	Information, skills	Experts
Formative	Socialization, values	Professionals
Transformative	Leadership attributes	Change agents

Figure 1.1 Levels of learning [2]

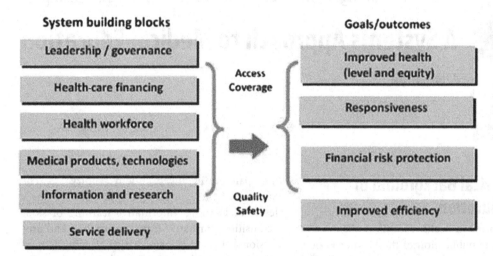

Figure 1.2 WHO health systems components [3]

delivery directly depend on the education of professionals to create the needed workforce. Professionals, in turn, because of the time-consuming and financial investment in their training, bear special responsibilities to become competent beyond the basic technical skills to be effective in teamwork, critical analyses, coping with uncertainty, conducting themselves ethically and becoming leaders in effective health systems [2, p1951]. It is the professional who is capable of focusing on innovations for learning and institutional change.

Professional education in turn depends on a number of factors:

1. Who has the authority to create mandates?
2. How transparent is the system?
3. What are the roles of governments, professional organizations and other bodies in ensuring the education of the workforce?
4. How accountable is the process?
5. What function does accreditation play?

1.2.1 Educating a New Workforce in Family Planning through Integration into the Educational Systems

When a formerly illegal medical intervention becomes legal, there is an immediate need to prepare a new workforce. The 100 professors who published their statement in anticipation of the legalization of abortion attempted to describe the anticipated service delivery in hospital wards that formerly treated women suffering from medical complications from illegally induced abortion [4]. They did not address specifically the demands and challenges of integrating this new aspect of women's health into education and training of obstetrician-gynecologists (ob-gyns). Likely they assumed that by providing the services, the residents would be trained as they are trained in all other clinical interactions and procedures taking place in the teaching hospital.

While some hospitals did initiate abortion services, most ceded to the newly created outpatient clinics, creating a serious gap in educating physicians needed to build a solid family planning workforce of physicians, nurses and other health-care workers. (See Chapter 3.)

Systems integration of family planning into medical education requires many changes, including institutional attitudes and practice. A number of important questions need to be asked:

1. What institutions are responsible for medical education?

For example, in the USA, there are 1,100 teaching hospitals. They might be academic, private, public and/or religiously affiliated institutions. There are 120 such hospitals directly affiliated with a medical school, and these are typically tertiary care hospitals, which take care of patients with complex medical problems and engage in research.

2. Who pays for the training of the workforce?

The primary financial source of resident education in the USA is the federal government, through Medicaid and Medicare funds allocated to teaching hospitals in a complex arrangement

[5]. Additional training funds come from the state governments for state-affiliated, sometimes also private teaching hospitals, and public or private insurance payments for clinical services. Faculty are typically paid through clinical revenues, research grants and contracts. They may be paid a small proportion of their salaries by the medical school itself depending on their clinical, research and administrative responsibilities.

3. Who is responsible for setting and enforcing training standards?

1.2.2 The US Systems Responsible for Post-Graduate Medical Education

Instead of a ministry or other governmental body, US physicians have created their own transparent systems of evaluation through professional medical organizations that set educational post-graduate standards and systems of enforcing them, both for the individual residents and fellows as well as the training sites.

1.2.2.1 The American Board of Medical Specialties (ABMS)

The American Board of Medical Specialties (ABMS) was formed in 1933 to create national standards for the education and practice of specialist practitioners [6]. In the past, the process of certification relied on occasional continuing medical educational courses and periodic assessment. It has evolved into a continuous cycle of assessment, learning and evaluation. It now places greater emphases on professionalism, patient safety and performance improvement.

In this system,

physicians become active participants in the evaluation of their own practices. They can see how their practice compares to those of their peers, how it differs from published best practices, and how their own practice evolves over time, progressing toward the ideal practice. [6]

ABMS is responsible for approving medical specialties and subspecialties and certifying its members through member boards. Twenty-four specialties are currently represented on the ABMS board. The American Board of Obstetrics and Gynecology (ABOG) serves on the board on behalf of obstetrics and gynecology (obgyn). Obgyn subspecialties were created in the early 1970s in response to a "biological revolution in

the reproductive sciences" to address, for example, the rapidly growing scientific understanding of hormonal action, conduct further research into maternal and fetal health and translate these findings into clinical practice and innovations [7]. More specific, in-depth study beyond generalist training was necessary to pursue research and expand scientific knowledge [8,9].

1.2.2.2 American Board of Obstetrics and Gynecology (ABOG)

ABOG was one of the founding members of ABMS, the third board of medical specialties in 1930 following the College of Surgeons and the American Board of Ophthalmology, which established the first system of certification.

ABOG is a not-for-profit professional medical organization representing the ob-gyn specialist areas and subspecialist divisions of reproductive endocrinology and infertility, maternal and fetal medicine, gynecologic oncology and female pelvic medicine and reproductive surgery. Its mission is "to define standards, certify obstetricians and gynecologists, and facilitate continuous learning to advance knowledge, practice, and professionalism in women's health" [10].

ABOG, as ABMS's specialty board, is responsible for the certification of ob-gyns and, until recently, the certification of ob-gyn subspecialties. The board creates and administers both oral and written exams that ob-gyn residents are eligible to take after four years of training. The board's examinations are based on a rigorous system of case lists and subject-specific questions indicating clinical experience, competence and knowledge of the current evidence of practice and its underlying scientific principles. (See Chapter 19.) After passing the exams, a graduated resident becomes certified to practice in the field. Board certification confers "Diplomate" status that has to be reviewed periodically. Although ABOG certification is voluntary, it is required to practice in hospitals and other institutions as well as for membership as a fellow in ACOG.

Certification is also required for hospitals' credentialing systems. To practice in a hospital, the physician must undergo a process of credentialing, which may, for example, include specific operations. The performance of a later second-trimester abortion, for example, may require the licensed physician to be proctored and credentialed before given permission to practice.

ABOG also administers written and oral exams in the four ABMS-approved subspecialties that now include family planning as the Fellowship in Complex Family Planning. Once a practice area achieves recognition as a subspecialty, ABOG selects representatives from the subspecialty community to inform the design of questions for the written and oral exams in a transparent, complex sequence of reviews of the depth and breadth of practice and roles of the subspecialist. In addition, ABOG creates a new division and appoints the members of the division based on the recommendation of, in the case of Complex Family Planning, ACOG, the Society of Family Planning and the National Office of the Fellowship. Each division is headed by a division chair who represents the division on the ABOG board.

1.2.2.3 Accreditation Council for Graduate Medical Education (ACGME)

The Accreditation Council for Graduate Medical Education (ACGME) is a nonprofit professional organization that was established in 1981, preceded by the Liaison Committee for Graduate Medical Education formed in 1972. ACGME is the accreditation organization that sets and maintains the educational standards of graduate medical education programs to ensure they meet the institutional and program requirements for which they prepare their graduates [11].

It currently oversees the post-graduate education and training (residents and fellows) in 830 teaching hospitals for all US medical doctors and doctors of osteopathy. As of 2020, it accredits 180 specialties and subspecialties through its current 28 Residency Review Committees (RRCs). Its mission is "to improve the quality of health care by ensuring and continually improving the quality of graduate medical education for residents by establishing graduate medical education standards, assessing training programs continually through a process of accreditation, and promoting high-quality educational programs for trainees" [11].

"We accomplish our Mission guided by our commitment to the Public Trust and the ACGME values of:

- Honesty and Integrity
- Excellence and Innovation
- Accountability and Transparency
- Fairness and Equity
- Stewardship and Service
- Engagement of Stakeholders
- Leadership and Collaboration" [11]

Site visits are conducted at the time of the initial accreditation request, two years after initial accreditation, and later if the yearly Accreditation Data System information prompts concern or needs follow-up. They involve a complex process of gathering information from the residency program director, department chairperson, faculty members, current residents as well as chairpersons of other clinical departments or hospital administrators involved in residency training.

Programs can be put on probation at the discretion of the Review Committee.

All sponsoring institutions and programs undergo a full accreditation site visit every 10 years. This is preceded by a comprehensive self-study process that includes a description of how the sponsoring institution or program creates an effective learning and working environment leading to the desired educational outcomes. For the self-study, programs are also asked to review their aims and conduct an analysis of strengths and areas for improvement and to formulate and document plans for improvement.

Practice and training standards are periodically revised.

It was the ACGME that issued the first US abortion training mandate in 1995.

1.2.2.4 The Residency Review Committee (RRC)

The RRC represents each specialty (currently twenty-eight) under the ACGME and is responsible for defining and enforcing training standards for residents and subspecialists. Members of the RRC are nominated by the American Medical Association's Council on Medical Education; the specialty board that certifies physicians within the specialty (ABOG); and by the professional college or another professional organization or society associated with the specialty [12].

Committee members are expected to be actively involved in graduate medical education; experienced in administration and/or teaching in the specialty, that is, as a Residency Program Director; be familiar with the accreditation process; and be part of an institution or program in good standing with the ACGME. The committee's chair is elected by the committee membership.

The purpose of the RRC is to assess whether an institution or program is in substantial compliance with the institutional requirements and to confer an accreditation or recognition status. Programs with serious shortcomings and deficiencies will receive citations, which may lead to a shorter ACGME accreditation period or probationary status. For example, if residents do not perform a minimum number of a particular surgery, the department may receive a citation. Several citations and overall quality concerns can lead to probationary status. Departments have received citations for lack of abortion training.

Training expectations for subspecialty fellows in Family Planning and their sponsoring sites are defined and published in the *Guide to Learning* and the *General Requirements* [13,14]. While these guidelines were produced by the Fellowship's National Office and Fellowship in Family Planning (FFP) directors previously during a period of twenty years of programmatic growth, ACGME will define new learning objectives with the recognition of subspecialty status.

1.2.3 The Teaching Hospital Prepares the Workforce

As the Lancet Commission report states:

> Recognition the teaching hospital is a critical component of the Health Care System as it delivers services and trains the future health care worker.
>
> We see educational institutions as crucial to transform health systems. ... Through their educational function, they produce professionals who can implement change in the organisations in which they work. [2, p1928]

Successful institutional changes in service delivery and training depend on a comprehensive understanding of the components of the system: the agencies that deliver care, those that finance it and the regulatory bodies that ensure that both workforce and care adhere to agreed-upon standards.

The health-care workforce educated in the teaching hospital includes physicians, nurses and other health-care providers. The physician workforce depends on the teaching hospital for core training of students, residents and fellows. Each teaching hospital, whether private or public, associated with a medical school or religiously affiliated, community-based or part of a hospital chain, is a component of the health system.

While revenue streams may vary, patient care and overall training objectives are similar. Operating rooms, outpatient clinics, emergency departments, labor and delivery wards, pharmacy and specialty departments all make up the hospital system, each with its own particular service-delivery structures and culture and driven by the economics that determine its survival.

Recognition of family planning as an essential aspect of women's health sets the stage for integrating family planning into the curriculum and services with expert faculty who provide care, teach, mentor, do research and are capable of leadership.

Integration requires familiarity with what roles the specialist will play within the system, interaction with other departments and their leadership and gaining their support.

1.2.3.1 Changing Hospital Services to Ensure Family Planning Training

Most FFP graduates join teaching hospitals as junior faculty members. To be an effective participant in a teaching hospital, particularly when attempting to change systems and services, requires understanding the domains of authority and the complex interactions among a multitude of stakeholders and decision makers: deans; hospital and nursing administrators; labor and delivery and outpatient clinic nurses; operating room (OR) staff, including anesthesiologists, nurses and technicians; leaders in central supply to ensure appropriate equipment, particularly for the OR; and directors of the emergency department (ED) as well as pharmacy. Every hospital unit and staff may be directly or indirectly part of abortion or contraceptive services. Establishing collaborations with pharmacy, for example, is necessary to ensure stocks of contraceptives and distribution of mifepristone.

Teamwork with departments and hospital units is essential to forge successful collaborations for the integration of family planning services. The authors of the *Lancet* Report observed that "Professionals are falling short on appropriate competencies for effective teamwork, and they are not exercising effective leadership to transform health systems" [2, p1926].

The priorities of each hospital player must be taken into consideration when introducing new technologies and services.

The head of the obgyn department plays a significant role in facilitating institutional support. While some may be focused primarily on department finances, others may stress their departments' educational mission. Family planning requires the introduction of new approaches and interventions in many points of service and departments and collaboration with various teams in order to gain the endorsement of the leadership. Nursing and anesthesia play a particularly decisive role in supporting and participating in abortion. Workshops and in-service trainings, specifically in the context of abortion, can be essential to gain support and cooperation. (See Chapters 10 and 17.)

In addition to understanding and connecting with the operational side of the hospital, knowledge of its overall philosophy of patient care and the economics of practice will inform any attempts for change. It is also helpful to become familiar with the diverse roles and degree of influence of each stakeholder. When the hospital is part of a medical school, private or public, the educational and political roles of deans and heads of the school are informed, at least in part, by their relationship with hospital administration and governing bodies such as boards of regents.

Each teaching hospital has an office of Graduate Medical Education (GME) responsible for training residents and fellows, including allocating their funding. The GME leadership is responsible for upholding and facilitating the educational expectations as defined by the professional educational organizations, which in the USA are the ACGME and the RRC.

What are the demographics and payer mix of the hospital's patient population? What roles do patient numbers, access to care and patient satisfaction play in the hospital's priorities? What connections exist with the community outside of the hospital, the other health service providers and practitioners, such as abortion clinics? What is the history of any collaborations and their effectiveness? (See Chapter 12.) What are the institution's sources of pride and prestige? How much weight is given to its reputation as a teaching institution versus its technical innovation and research? How much are research grants valued? How much effort is focused on fundraising from private donors, adapting new technologies and media visibility?

A last question that can have an enormous impact on the institution and its leadership is whether it is a public or private institution. In either case, how and by whom is the relationship with the legislators carried out? To what degree are the deans and department chairs involved? Does the family planning expert provide evidence of patient care and satisfaction, the impact of family planning on the student and resident curriculum, the health impact of contraception and abortion care, particularly on vulnerable and medically complex patients? What role, if any, do training mandates, the education mission and workforce considerations play when legislators and government threaten interference? A family planning workforce prepared to engage in effective advocacy can play a pivotal educational role in contending with institutional and political interference and controversy.

And finally, what are the policies that directly affect patient care and training in family planning? What are hospital policies regarding pregnancy termination, postpartum contraceptive practices and sterilization? Even in states that have liberal laws regarding abortion care, hospital policies may be restrictive [15].

Gaining an understanding of the numerous aspects of institutional functions, interrelationships and cultures takes time, but gaining familiarity with the hospital system and becoming an engaged member will increase the likelihood of making effective and lasting changes to institutionalize family planning training.

The family planning faculty will also benefit from connecting and becoming visible in the larger institutional context:

1. presenting the evidence
2. making personal connections
3. using patient stories as an advocacy tool
4. serving on committees and in roles in the department, school, hospital or institution, even if they don't seem immediately related to family planning

With the institutionalization of services and training, the teaching hospital plays a major role in access to care:

1. as a referral site for other departments and specialists
2. in collaborations with community partners
3. in research
4. by educating future practitioners and change agents

When expert contraception and abortion services are in place, patients who are treated for other diseases can benefit from evaluation for their contraceptive needs and options for pregnancy termination. Professional collaboration among specialists within the hospital allows for optimal patient care.

1.2.4 Partnerships with the Private Sector to Enhance Training

While significant changes in the teaching hospital can be achieved, the number of abortions may be insufficient to train residents and fellows to achieve the expected clinical competence, particularly in hospitals with severe restrictions on abortion services. Under these circumstances, the teaching hospital seeks partnerships with the private sector freestanding clinics that provide the bulk of abortion care. Again, successful training outcomes depend on understanding patient care philosophy and economic demands of the clinics. Financial viability is of primary concern in most. Training may be perceived as interfering with efficient patient care, and special arrangements are made to provide incentives, either by having the academic physician mentor teach the residents while working in the clinic, offering needed equipment, or with an agreement to treat complex patients and complications. (See Chapter 17.)

1.3 The Global Realm

Unlike the US model, the education of health professionals in mid- and low-income countries is often under the purview of ministries of health or education, determining the parameters of health-care services and education of their medical workforce. Here, WHO or nongovernmental organizations (NGOs) may inform the country standards of care and their enforcement mechanisms. Colonial history is likely to impact the models for training and service, for example, in the countries formerly under British colonial rule in which the UK training model is used. Considerations for access and country health priorities, as well as the burden of disease such as maternal mortality, often determine the focus for family planning. (See Chapter 2.) Quality of care or training the future workforce may be of lesser concern.

When abortion laws are changed, again, access remains the primary, often only, concern. As the Lancet Commission states, external donors and NGOs are brought in for specific training initiatives, whereas the education of professionals is overlooked. (See Chapters 29 and 32.) As a consequence, integration of services and didactics into graduate, resident education is often missing, as are considerations of long-term workforce needs and policy leadership.

1.3.1 Impediments to Creating an Effective Workforce

The latest edition of the WHO's "Technical and Policy Guidance for Health Systems" on safe abortion (2012) reflects its priorities of workforce capacity and training midlevel practitioners [16]. The preceding guidance (2003), "Putting Services in Place," stress the need for standards including provider skills [17]. "Training programmes, both pre and in-service, should be based on a competency approach . . . to allow the health practitioner to demonstrate clinical competence" [17, p70].

The health system's responsibility is to ensure supervision and clinical competence. No consideration is given to the role that physicians and medical education must play, as described by the Lancet Commission, beyond skills acquisition to develop professionalism and ethical practice, and educate physicians for change agent leadership in research and policy making. Instead, WHO states in its Guidance that as for Certification and Licensing of Health Professionals and Facilities, "its sole purpose should be to ensure that providers meet essential criteria for the safe provision of abortion care, as with other medical procedures" [17, p73].

Typically, the ministry of health or education prescribes learning outcomes and may engage NGO partners for implementation and/or evaluation. Eventually, however, institutionalization is essential to ensure a vibrant in-country workforce that leads and moves the field ahead: creating a system that develops experts to create educational standards, encourage research and advocate for an evidence-based health policy.

A major impediment to systems integration can be the stigmatization of abortion. (See Chapter 24.) It can discourage personal engagement and leadership and may prevent institutional implementation of the law after its passage.

Effective institutionalization of family planning training may also be hindered by the traditional staffing and setting of the family planning clinic in the teaching hospital. (See Chapter 29.) For example, the location of the clinics, far from other parts of the hospital where surgeries take place and residents work, may connote low status and service priority for the trainees. In addition, a high-volume, understaffed service may leave little room for the introduction of new technical advances or a focus on quality of care and patient interactions.

Academic teaching hospitals in any country can play an essential role in transforming the health system. By institutionalizing training of a physician and nursing workforce, they can document the impact and shortcomings of new services on patient care and the parameters and approaches to educating its future medical workforce, that is, residents, students and nurses. (See Chapters 20, 23 and 16.) Findings can then be used to change practices in the organization and hospitals in which they work. By virtue of the professionalism these leaders demonstrate, they will engender trust and confidence in their institutions: "This trust is earned through a special blend of technical competence and service orientation, steered by ethical commitment and social accountability, ... [and] forms the essence of professional work" [2, p1925].

1.3.2 Institutionalizing a Global Physician Community

The *Lancet* report states:

Our vision is global rather than parochial, multiprofessional and not confined to one group, committed to building sound evidence, encompassing of both individual and population-based approaches, and focused on instructional and institutional innovations. Our goal is to encourage all health professionals, irrespective of nationality and specialty, to share a common global vision for the future. In this vision, all health professionals in all countries are educated to mobilise knowledge, and to engage in critical reasoning and ethical conduct, so that they are competent to participate in patient-centred and population-centred health systems as members of locally responsive and globally connected teams. The ultimate purpose is to assure universal coverage of high-quality comprehensive services that are essential to advancing opportunity for health equity within and

between countries. The aspiration of good health commonly shared, we believe, resonates with young professionals who seek value and meaning in their work. [2, p1951]

1.3.2.1 The Fellowship in Family Planning's Global Vision

XII. International Family Planning

Terminal Objective:
The Fellow must have knowledge of the public health, legal, and service delivery aspects of family planning, abortion, and reproductive health in less developed nations.

Enabling Objectives:
A. Fellows should complete a three- to eight-week placement in a less developed country during their two-year fellowship.
B. Fellows must have knowledge of the effects of limited resources on family planning in the country of their placement.
C. Fellows must have knowledge of the public health, legal, and service delivery aspects of family planning care in the country of their placement. [16]

From start of the Fellowship in Family Planning in 1991, its vision reflected a global perspective that foresaw many opportunities for exchange of educational and clinical perspectives, institutional implementation and research in contraception and abortion. The vision stemmed from the founder of the FFP, Dr. Philip Darney, who participated in global exchanges with governmental agencies, the Agency for International Development (AID), the Centers for Disease Control and Prevention (CDC) and NGOs. These experiences demonstrated the lasting, mutually inspiring effects that strengthened health-care delivery, leadership, advocacy and research. His global vision was institutionalized through the FFP global health rotations and the Fellowship's close collaborations with WHO.

Many of the fellows over the years pursued these opportunities to build community and experience the interdependence of individuals and institutions in bringing about system changes in family planning. Exchanges relied on already established contacts by Fellowship directors whose work connected them globally, or institutional connections already in place between academic institutions, departments and individual physicians. Visibility through presentations and posters by the national director and a growing number of Fellowship graduates, some of whom presented their research at international professional meetings, such as the International Federation of Gynecology and Obstetrics (FIGO) and the International Conference on Family Planning (ICFP), led to new interests for collaboration [18].

1.3.2.2 Impact on the Fellows

While not all fellows are inclined toward a global perspective or establishing formal connections, the experience is enriching for both fellow and host. Differing cultural perspectives on education, health-care systems, educational approaches and service delivery bring new insights about access to care, patient interactions and physician championship. Witnessing the consequences of unsafe abortions, overcrowded family planning clinics, the social injustice inflicted on women, and lack of professional, governmental or social support serves as a stark reminder and motivator to protect reproductive health and access at home. In addition, professional connections lead to further exchanges and research collaborations post-fellowship, which enhance local infrastructure and capacity. At their best, these exchanges help everyone to feel affirmed and empowered, recognizing the many similarities and opportunities to strengthen each other in the global quest for reproductive health and justice.

Fellows established global connections in Nepal where they helped institutionalize abortion and contraception training; in Vietnam, where they published a side-by-side English and Vietnamese contraceptive guide for medical students, *Managing Contraception*; and other projects in Malawi, Haiti, Thailand, Zimbabwe, Rwanda, Kenya, Uganda, India and many other countries around the world [19]. Some of the initial contacts were maintained by extended in-country stays at partner institutions to pursue research with local academic physicians, for example, or consulting visits over years with NGOs and continuing relationships through subsequent fellows.

1.3.2.3 Institutional Impact

The impact of these placements and exchanges encompass many areas: introducing new technologies and procedures offered to patients;

addressing specific aspects of service delivery, educational principles and approaches, such as the evaluations of students, residents and faculty; and the principles of professionalism and mentorship.

1.3.2.4 Research: Mulago Hospital, Makarere University, Uganda and the University of California, San Francisco

The research projects of several fellows at the Mulago Hospital in Uganda, the national teaching and referral hospital in Kampala with 30,000 deliveries per year, led to a formal collaboration between the obgyn departments of the University of California, San Francisco (UCSF) and the Mulago Hospital at Makerere University. Goals included expanding research activities that support evidence-based practice of abortion and contraception care in Uganda and strengthening capacity to conduct independent research in family planning. Previous fellows' research studies helped set in place the research infrastructure to conduct a larger randomized trial on the effect of immediate versus delayed initiation of postpartum contraceptive implants. Each study involved residents, fellows and junior and senior faculty at both institutions, enhancing training in research skills at many levels.

As a result, one Ugandan faculty member completed his PhD in reproductive science and developed an independent research program with a specific focus on postpartum contraception and contraception for women at risk for HIV and living with HIV. A Medical Students for Choice chapter at Makerere University will be supported with mentorship and teaching by the US partners who are now faculty and direct family planning fellowships at US teaching hospitals. The chair of the Mulago hospital is pursuing further clinical training, particularly in dilation and evacuation (D&E), and the Ministry of Health in Uganda lent its support for the research proposals and the results of the studies informed policy change at the national level. The collaboration led to publications in major peer-reviewed journals [20,21,22,23,24].

1.3.2.5 Research: Malawi College of Medicine and the University of North Carolina

Another example of systems building is that of the collaboration between the University of North

Carolina's (UNC) Division of Global Women's Health, the Malawi government and the Malawi College of Medicine. A graduated fellow and faculty member at UNC worked for five years in Lilongwe, Malawi, with UNC Project—Malawi to help build up obgyn clinical and research infrastructure. There, she worked with both governmental and nongovernmental organizations to advance women's health research and clinical capacity through teaching, mentoring and serving on various Malawi Ministry of Health (MoH) committees. For example, she served on the National Family Planning Sub-Committee, Safe Motherhood Sub-Committee, Population and Development Technical Working Group, and Cervical Cancer Control and Prevention Program Task Force, partnering with the MoH to implement postpartum intrauterine device (IUD) insertion throughout the country and advising the MoH on its National Cervical Cancer Control Strategy 2016–2020 [21].

In addition to her contributions to Malawi family planning policy, in her role as an Honorary Senior Lecturer at the Malawi College of Medicine, she was a founding member of the country's first obgyn Residency Program in 2013, establishing the country's first annual obgyn Scientific Meeting, developing the country's first obgyn protocols and guidelines handbook, and leading the residency's first weekly journal clubs and didactic sessions. The residency has now graduated twelve residents, with another thirteen currently in training, which will quadruple the number of Malawian ob-gyns practicing in-country within a decade. She also helped to build clinical capacity by teaching the residents and other learners while working at Lilongwe's two biggest public hospitals and by organizing trainings for hundreds of providers in family planning, long-acting reversible contraception (LARC) insertion, postpartum IUD insertion, cervical cancer screening and emergency obstetrics and neonatal care (EmONC) [25,26,27]. Four family planning fellows completed their international fellowship rotations with her in Malawi, helping to lead the postpartum IUD trainings and implementation and publishing related research [28,29]. Finally, she has mentored fourteen Malawians in research to date, including Malawian ob-gyns, residents, medical officers, nurses and social scientists, most of whom have already either published or submitted first-author manuscripts [30,31,32,33,34,35].

1.3.2.6 Education: Guyana, Kenya and Ethiopia

GUYANA: Over a period of seven years, ten fellows spent their global health rotations in Georgetown at the Georgetown Public Hospital Corporation, the teaching hospital of the University of Guyana. For some, these were training and consultation visits based on partnerships between their own academic institution and Guyana, or through an NGO. Their focus was on abortion training, leading the country's annual safe abortion workshops, including Train the Trainers workshops. The trainees were residents and nurses, physicians from other regional hospitals to encourage decentralization and widen access to safe abortion services throughout the country, who received training and proctoring, leading to certification by the Guyana Ministry of Health in manual vacuum aspiration (MVA) and D&E. Another accomplishment was the initiation of post-placental IUD insertions. Their teaching efforts led to the tripling of physicians who incorporated abortion into their practice.

Kenya and Ethiopia – recent examples of infrastructure building

KENYA: A recently graduated family planning fellow, now on the faculty at Indiana University's School of Medicine, leads an academic global health collaboration between Indiana University and Moi Teaching and Referral Hospital in Eldoret, western Kenya. Her focus is expanding access to family planning, especially among women with HIV and other chronic medical conditions. As a visiting faculty member in the Department of Reproductive Health, she teaches residents and medical students about family planning and conducts research and care projects expanding the roles of community health workers to improve linkages to reproductive health care, integrating family planning services within the hospital and outpatient chronic disease clinics, and improving reproductive health counseling for women with HIV and other chronic diseases. [36,37,38]

ETHIOPIA: A partnership was created by the Ethiopian Society of Obstetricians and Gynecologists, ACOG, the Ethiopian Federal Ministry of Health and the Center for International Reproductive Health Training (CIRHT), which is committed to improving maternal health to help build infrastructure through medical education and preparedness by transforming equity and quality of care.

Specific projects included standardization of residency training and assessment of outcomes, as residency programs recently increased from three to ten, leadership development, research infrastructure and creating a code of medical ethics, among others.

Expanding on these systems and educational infrastructure building efforts, a new Ethiopian Fellowship in Family Planning was started by CIRHT in 2017 to produce competent clinicians, trainers, researchers, advocates and leaders in family planning. (See Chapter 29.) A Fellowship graduate and director of the Fellowship Program at the University of Washington joined the faculty at the St. Paul's Hospital Millennium Medical College (SPHMMC) during a one-year sabbatical as director of this first Family Planning Fellowship in Ethiopia, building on the educational infrastructure of Ethiopian colleagues and other Fellowship graduates to strengthen capacity. The Fellowship will soon have its first three graduates, who will be able to manage the administration and training requirements of the SPHMMC fellowship and continue to train other ob-gyns in Ethiopia in contraception and abortion. In partnership with the Ethiopian and US family planning specialists, she is developing a curriculum for continued training, along with necessary exams to evaluate skills and knowledge [39].

1.4 Institutional Mandates and Prescriptions for Medical Practice after Legalizing Abortion

As countries consider legalization of abortion, the medical profession plays a pivotal role. Their support is necessary for two reasons: to emphasize the health consequences of unsafe abortion and the positive impact on patient care of safe abortion, and to ensure commitment to create the necessary systems educating the next generations of practitioners. (See Chapter 4.) Tensions over the role of conscientious objection often arise, especially in countries where religion plays an important role [40]. Should physicians, particularly gynecologists, be expected to do abortions? Feminist groups are united in their recommendation that they should, whereas physician organizations insist on physician autonomy to opt out or object.

Several factors likely affect these attitudes. While stigma surrounding illegal abortion and religion, especially in countries that are predominantly Catholic, lead to reluctance to do them once legal, many physicians lack the necessary skills and clinical competence. In addition, the stigma of illegality combined with the perception that abortion is a low level of medical practice lacking the prestige of other aspects of obgyn care likely discourage physicians to seek training. Even if physicians have been instrumental advocates for legalization (Uruguay), they do not support the demand that every physician must do abortions [41].

The focus and often controversy whether current practitioners intend to do abortions distracts from the most consequential consideration, the long view: the need for institutionalizing and mainstreaming abortion and family planning practice by setting mandates and expectations for training the future generations of practitioners. Training requirements can be institutionalized through academic medical centers, although current practice cannot, although Uruguay and Nepal are examples of institutionalizing services and training of current practitioners. (See Chapters 31 and 27.)

Establishing training mandates, implementing education and ensuring a future workforce will make legalization meaningful and sustainable. The clinical skills, acquired sense of professionalism and the understanding of the social and emotional aspects of abortion will be valuable when they decide to incorporate abortion in their future practice, without forcing them to make such a commitment. (See Chapter 23.)

"Those who conscientiously serve women seeking abortion often face stigma and discrimination from their colleagues, exacerbating other obstacles that complicate their work. Health care providers at the convening underscored the importance of comprehensive training and support for those who work in abortion care " [40].

Another advantage to institutionalizing education and training is their effects over time on attitudes and practice. (See Chapters 7 and 23.) While in the USA the ob-gyn physician leadership endorsed legalization and anticipated its ability to fulfill the demand for safe abortion once legalized, stigmatization continued, and the initial enthusiasm and structured training declined until the passage of a professional mandate and the launch of national training initiatives. (See Chapter 3.) These initiatives, the US Ryan Residency Training Program and the Fellowship in Family Planning, ensure implementation of the law and long-term patient access by teaching the necessary technical skills, fostering research and inspiring new champions who continue to transform the cultures in their institutions and beyond. (See Chapter 7.)

1.5 Medication Abortion and Institutionalization of Abortion

When legalization is under consideration, access to medication abortion outside of the legal system may hinder institutional and professional support. Misoprostol availability can lead to misleading conclusions that (1) abortions are accessible to women if they want them, without the need to legalize, and (2) the skills necessary to administer medication abortion are simple and do not require the care of a clinician. While both may be correct on the surface, they fail to acknowledge that institutionalization of physician training creates the in-country workforce necessary to serve as trainers, set standards of care, conduct research, act as change agents and inform policy makers who will promote the practice of safe legal abortion as an integral part of women's health. In turn, stigma will decline as a result of integrated training of health-care providers.

1.6 Conclusion

Medical education is an essential part of a country's health-care system. It may be governed by the county's ministries or by professional organizations. Its effectiveness depends on governmental and societal support and acknowledgment of its impacts on health. The Lancet Commission's report on "Health Professionals for a New Century" scrutinized the impact of medical education on health systems and proposed a new philosophy and vision. Family planning, contraception and abortion offer a concrete example of

the role of medical education in transforming health [2]. The Lancet Commission's report creates a guide to understanding the systems of health care and the role of medical education in creating a competent workforce empowered to lead and be responsive to the health-care needs of its community.

A systems approach to institutionalize training in abortion and contraception depends on a number of factors, all equally important for success:

1. understanding the ownership, affiliations and structures of the health-care system
2. knowing which institutional bodies define medical education standards and are responsible for their enforcement
3. setting a professional training mandate for abortion and contraception
4. understanding the systems in which training takes place
5. preparing the workforce to become

   a. expert service providers who abide by their professional and ethical responsibilities
   b. researchers and evaluators of services
   c. leaders, advocates and change agents

      i. for service and policy within teaching hospitals,
      ii. the systems in which they work,
      iii. their professional associations and
      iv. their communities and society at large

6. creating a system to ensure a community of support

Educational initiatives like the Fellowship in Family Planning and the Ryan Residency Training Program are systems-changing programs. By educating the obgyn workforce, these programs ensure access to care and the availability of services, set standards of professionalism, foster research and promote systemic institutional change within teaching hospitals and professional organizations. They work to set and enforce standards and ultimately change the professional culture.

References

1. Flexner A. Medical education in the United States and Canada. From the Carnegie Foundation for the Advancement of Teaching, Bulletin Number Four, 1910. *Bull World Health Organ.* 2002;**80**(7):594–602.

2. Frenk J, Chen L, Bhutta ZA, et al. Health professionals for a new century: transforming education to strengthen health systems in an interdependent world. *Lancet.* 2010;**376**(9756):1923–1958. doi:10.1016/S0140-6736(10)61854-5

3. Manyazewal T. Using the World Health Organization health system building blocks through survey of healthcare professionals to determine the performance of public healthcare facilities. *Arch Public Health*. 2017;**75**:50. doi:10.1186/s13690-017-0221-9

4. A statement on abortion by one hundred professors of obstetrics. *Am J Obstet Gynecol*. 1972;**112**(7):992–998. doi:10.1016/0002-9378(72)90826-5

5. *Federal Support for Graduate Medical Education: An Overview*. Congressional Research Service; 2018. https://fas.org/sgp/crs/misc/R44376.pdf.

6. ABMS | American Board of Medical Specialties. www.abms.org. Accessed April 4, 2020.

7. Ryan KJ. Historical Perspective, 1972–73 Revisited. In *Conference on Impact of Subspecialization on Residency Training and Practice of Obstetrics and Gynecology*. Chicago, IL: The American Board of Obstetrics and Gynecology; 1991:3–4.

8. Creinin MD, Darney PD. Methotrexate and misoprostol for early abortion. *Contraception*. 1993;**48**(4):339–348. doi:10.1016/0010-7824(93)90079-m

9. Goldberg AB, Greenberg MB, Darney PD. Misoprostol and pregnancy. *N Engl J Med*. 2001;**344**(1):38–47. doi:10.1056/NEJM200101043440107

10. ABOG. www.abog.org. Accessed April 4, 2020.

11. ACGME Home. www.acgme.org. Accessed April 4, 2020.

12. Committees and Members Selection Process. www.acgme.org/About-Us/Committees-and-Members-Selection-Process. Accessed April 4, 2020.

13. Fellowship in Complex Family Planning Advisory Board.

Guide to Learning in Complex Family Planning. 2019.

14. Fellowship in Complex Family Planning. *General Requirements for a Post-Graduate Program in the Subspecialty Area of Complex Family Planning*. 2019.

15. Zeldovich VB, Rocca CH, Langton C, Landy U, Ly E, Freedman L. Abortion policies in United States teaching hospitals: formal and informal parameters beyond the law. *Obstet Gynecol*. 2020;**135**(6):1296–1305.

16. *Safe Abortion: Technical and Policy Guidance for Health Systems*. 2nd ed. Geneva: World Health Organization; 2012. www.ncbi.nlm.nih.gov/books/NBK138196/. Accessed April 4, 2020.

17. *Safe Abortion: Technical and Policy Guidance for Health Systems*. Geneva: World Health Organization; 2003.

18. Landy U. Medical education in family planning in the United States: why and how. Poster presented at Cape Town, South Africa; 2009.

19. Zieman M, Hatcher RA, Allen AZ, Lathrop E, Haddad L. *Managing Contraception: For Your Pocket*. 15th ed. Managing Contraception, LLC; 2018.

20. Morse JE, Rowen TS, Steinauer J, Byamugisha J, Kakaire O. A qualitative assessment of Ugandan women's perceptions and knowledge of contraception. *Int J Gynaecol Obstet*. 2014;**124**(1):30–33. doi:10.1016/j.ijgo.2013.07.014

21. Lester F, Kakaire O, Byamugisha J, et al. Intracesarean insertion of the copper T380A versus 6 weeks postcesarean: a randomized clinical trial. *Contraception*. 2015;**91**(3):198–203. doi:10.1016/j.contraception.2014.12.002

22. Kakaire O, Byamugisha JK, Tumwesigye NM, Gemzell-

Danielsson K. Clinical versus laboratory screening for sexually transmitted infections prior to insertion of intrauterine contraception among women living with HIV/AIDS: a randomized controlled trial. *Hum Reprod Oxf Engl*. 2015;**30**(7):1573–1579. doi:10.1093/humrep/dev109

23. Averbach S, Kakaire O, McDiehl R, Dehlendorf C, Lester F, Steinauer J. The effect of immediate postpartum levonorgestrel contraceptive implant use on breastfeeding and infant growth: a randomized controlled trial. *Contraception*. 2019;**99**(2):87–93. doi:10.1016/j.contraception.2018.10.008

24. Averbach S, Kakaire O, Kayiga H, et al. Immediate versus delayed postpartum use of levonorgestrel contraceptive implants: a randomized controlled trial in Uganda. *Am J Obstet Gynecol*. 2017;**217**(5):568.e1–568.e7. doi:10.1016/j.ajog.2017.06.005

25. Lemani C, Tang JH, Kopp D, et al. Contraceptive uptake after training community health workers in couples counseling: a cluster randomized trial. *PLoS One*. 2017;**12**(4):e0175879. doi:10.1371/journal.pone.0175879

26. Lemani C, Kamtuwanje N, Phiri B, et al. Effect of family planning interventions on couple years of protection in Malawi. *Int J Gynaecol Obstet*. 2018;**141**(1):37-44. doi:10.1002/ijgo.12439

27. Tang JH, Kaliti C, Bengtson A, et al. Improvement and retention of emergency obstetrics and neonatal care knowledge and skills in a hospital mentorship program in Lilongwe, Malawi. *Int J Gynaecol Obstet*. 2016;**132**(2):240–243. doi:10.1016/j.ijgo.2015.06.062

28. Krashin JW, Lemani C, Nkambule J, et al. A comparison of breastfeeding exclusivity and duration rates between immediate postpartum levonorgestrel versus etonogestrel implant users: a prospective cohort study. *Breastfeed Med.* 2019;**14**(1):69–76. doi:10.1089/bfm.2018.0165

29. Krashin JW, Haddad LB, Tweya H, et al. Factors associated with desired fertility among HIV-positive women and men attending two urban clinics in Lilongwe, Malawi. *PloS One.* 2018;**13**(6):e0198798. doi:10.1371/journal.pone.0198798

30. Chinula L, Nelson JAE, Wiener J, et al. Effect of the depot medroxyprogesterone acetate injectable and levonorgestrel implant on HIV genital shedding: a randomized trial. *Contraception.* 2018;**98**(3):193–198. doi:10.1016/j.contraception.2018.05.001

31. Chinula L, Hicks M, Chiudzu G, et al. A tailored approach to building specialized surgical oncology capacity: early experiences and outcomes in Malawi. *Gynecol Oncol Rep.* 2018;**26**:60–65. doi:10.1016/j.gore.2018.10.001

32. Gausi B, Chagomerana MB, Tang JH, et al. Human immunodeficiency virus serodiscordance and dual contraceptive method use among human immunodeficiency virus-infected men and women in Lilongwe, Malawi. *Sex Transm Dis.* 2018;**45**(11):747–753. doi:10.1097/OLQ.0000000000000868

33. Mbichila TH, Chagomerana M, Tang JH, et al. Partnership duration and HIV serodisclosure among people living with HIV/AIDS in Lilongwe, Malawi. *Int J STD AIDS.* 2018;**29**(10):987–993. doi:10.1177/0956462418769730

34. Bula A, Kopp DM, Maman S, Chinula L, Tsidya M, Tang JH. Family planning knowledge, experiences and reproductive desires among women who had experienced a poor obstetric outcome in Lilongwe Malawi: a qualitative study. *Contracept Reprod Med.* 2018;**3**:22. doi:10.1186/s40834-018-0075-8

35. Mwafulirwa T, O'Shea MS, Hamela G, et al. Family planning providers' experiences and perceptions of long-acting reversible contraception in Lilongwe, Malawi. *Afr J Reprod Health.* 2016;**20**(2):62–71. doi:10.29063/ajrh2016/v20i2.7

36. Bernard C, Pekny C, Omukagah CO, et al. Integration of contraceptive services into anticoagulation management services improves access to long-acting reversible contraception. *Contraception.* 2018;**98**(6):486–491. doi:10.1016/j.contraception.2018.07.139

37. Patel RC, Jakait B, Thomas K, et al. Increasing body mass index or weight does not appear to influence the association between efavirenz-based antiretroviral therapy and implant effectiveness among HIV-positive women in western Kenya. *Contraception.* 2019;**100**(4):288–295. doi:10.1016/j.contraception.2019.06.011

38. Bernard C, Jakait B, Fadel W, et al. Preferences for multipurpose technology and alternative methods of antiretroviral therapy among women living with HIV in western Kenya. Poster presented at Mexico City, Mexico; 2019.

39. Negussie D, Bekele D, Curran D, et al. Ethiopian and American collaboration: process, accomplishments, and lessons learned. *Obstet Gynecol.* 2020;**135**(3):703–708. doi:10.1097/AOG.0000000000003705

40. Truong M, Wood SY. *Unconscionable: When Providers Deny Abortion Care.* International Women's Health Coalition; 2018. https://31u5ac2nrwj6247cya153vw9-wpengine.netdna-ssl.com/wp-content/uploads/2018/06/IWHC_CO_Report-Web_single_pg.pdf.

41. Stifani BM, Couto M, Lopez Gomez A. From harm reduction to legalization: the Uruguayan model for safe abortion. *Int J Gynaecol Obstet.* 2018;**143**(Suppl 4):45–51. doi:10.1002/ijgo.12677

Chapter

2

Training in Contraception and Abortion to Reduce Maternal Mortality

Philip D. Darney

2.1 Introduction

Maternal deaths are a tragedy for families and societies, and the risk of pregnancy in comparison to other threats to life is generally underestimated (see Table 2.1). The consequences of maternal deaths to families and societies are also underestimated: worldwide, the children left behind after the deaths of their mothers are 10 times more likely to die themselves than those who continue to have mothers' care. The economic welfare of families and nations is dependent on women's work. African women, for example, head the majority of businesses, produce 80% of the food, and are 70% of the workforce. One third of the world's gross domestic product (GDP) is accounted for by the unpaid work of women. Governments around the world have recognized that women are critical to national advancement and, for the past 30 years, have made reducing maternal mortality a focus of national health systems. Maternal mortality ratio (MMR; the number of maternal deaths per 10,000 live births) is recognized as among the most sensitive indicators of the performance of a government in

securing its citizens' health. The common causes of maternal deaths are shown in Table 2.2. They are remarkably consistent from country to country with some exceptions. For example, in the USA, opioid overdose is an important cause of maternal mortality, while in some sub-Saharan African nations HIV is a frequent cause.

A critical determinant of decreasing maternal mortality worldwide, as achieved by nations that reached in 2015 their UN "Millennium Development Goal 5" (MDG 5) – substantial reduction in maternal mortality ratio – was the increase in deliveries by trained birth attendants. In fact, training of birth attendants was identified by the Maternal Health Workgroup of the Global Health Policy Summit as one of the seven most cost-effective interventions for decreasing maternal mortality 25% to 75% in eleven countries achieving their 2015 MDG 5; these seven cost 0.1% of the GDP [1]. Saving women's lives is not expensive: the two most cost-effective interventions are contraception and safe abortion (see Table 2.3). The subject of this book is training of physicians and other providers of sexual and reproductive health (SRH) care in family planning. The aim of this chapter is to describe the effects of training in contraception and abortion on maternal mortality [2].

Table 2.1 Death probabilities of UK citizens' selected activities, 2012

Pregnancy	8,200 pregnancies
General anesthesia	185,000 operations
Hang gliding	116,000 flights
Scuba diving	200,000 dives
Rock climbing	320,000 climbs
Canoeing	720,000 outings
Fairground rides	834,000 rides
Rail travel	43 million journeys
Air travel	125 million flights

Source: Causes of Mortality, Vital Data, United Kingdom, 2012

Table 2.2 Causes of 358,000 maternal deaths worldwide, 2012 [2]

Hemorrhage	35%
Unsafe abortion	**14%**
Hypertension	11%
Infection	10%
HIV	7%
Obstructed labor	6%
Other causes	17%

Table 2.3 The most effective interventions to prevent maternal deaths [2]

Intervention	Women saved/year	Maternal deaths prevented (%)
Family planning	107,000	30
Safe abortion	46,000	13

2.2 The Importance of Training in Family Planning to Reduce Maternal Mortality

All around the world, as the proportion of babies delivered by trained people increased, maternal mortality decreased (see Figure 2.1). Most of those trained were not obstetricians or physicians. They were much more likely to be nurses or midwives, some with only a secondary school education. Evidence-based training in maternity care, particularly with regard to recognition of abnormalities in labor and delivery and how to treat or transfer for treatment of complications like hemorrhage, hypertension and obstructed labor, is critical in saving pregnant women's lives. Because they are the most cost-effective interventions, training in abortion and contraception is also critical to reducing maternal mortality. Most of the abortions and contraceptives worldwide are provided by non-physicians (see Chapter 26), but physicians, particularly those in academia, play a critical role in training medical students; resident and specialist physicians; and non-physician providers in maternity, abortion and contraceptive care. All are necessary to reduce maternal mortality, improve child health and ensure the economic security of families and nations.

Coordination of training in family planning and pregnancy care is important because it is often the same caregivers who provide both to their patients. In addition, postpartum contraception is critical to maternal and infant health. For example, Rodriguez et al. showed, in a record review of California births and subsequent care, that postpartum contraception was by far the most important intervention in preventing premature delivery, the primary cause worldwide of infant and childhood mortality [3,4]. (See Table 2.4.)

Even though they provide a small proportion of maternity, abortion and contraceptive care

(a)

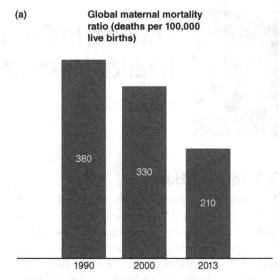

Figure 2.1a Global maternal mortality ratio (deaths per 100,000 live births) [1] The Millenium Development Goals Report 2015

(b)

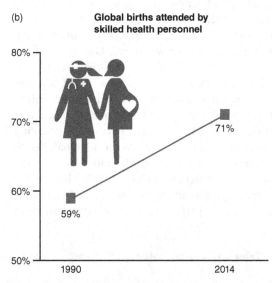

Figure 2.1b Global births attended by skilled health personnel [1] The Millenium Development Goals Report 2015

around the world – higher in rich nations with many physicians – doctors are often key leaders in health planning and training. For example, several obstetrician-gynecologists have served as ministers of health in African, Asian and Latin American nations. In these roles, they can encourage policies and programs focused on reducing maternal mortality through training of maternity care providers in emergency cesarean delivery, postpartum contraception, manual vacuum

Table 2.4 Effect of various interventions on proportion of preterm birth risk reduction achieved in California, 2005–2010 [3]

Smoking cessation	0.01%
Progesterone supplementation	0.03%
In vitro fertilization embryo transfer reduction	0.06%
Cervical cerclage	0.15%
Postpartum contraception for 1 month	1.10%
Postpartum contraception for 6 months	**6.30%**

aspiration (MVA) and medical abortion. All of these have been demonstrated as effective in reducing maternal mortality and all require the collaboration of physicians who themselves have training and confidence in these procedures and know the skills required to safely accomplish them. For example, as shown in Figure 2.1, there is a strong relationship between declining MMR and increasing proportion of deliveries attended by trained providers. The same relationship exists for MMR and training in abortion.

2.3 Importance of Physician Leaders in Training to Reduce Maternal Mortality

A women's health program must have physician leaders who recognize and support their nursing, midwifery and medical colleagues in providing contraception and safe abortion and who emphasize them as key components of reducing maternal mortality through training of providers of SRH. This support is most likely to come from academic obstetrician-gynecologists who, as residents or fellows, learned about contraception and abortion as integrated components of comprehensive care for all women and who, therefore, are dedicated to advocacy for family planning as critical to women's health and rights. (See Chapter 5.) Even though these physicians will provide a small proportion of contraceptive and abortion care themselves, they will have a broad impact by educating and inspiring the young physicians, midwives, nurses and others who pass through training institutions. This "institutionalization" of family planning as a key component of training for women's health care cannot be

accomplished simply through continuing (or "in service") education of those who are unaffiliated with training institutions. These unaffiliated practitioners usually have limited influence beyond their own patients and local area and little opportunity to inspire the next generation. Continuing reductions in maternal mortality require long-term leadership from experts who understand its causes and are skilled at implementing the most effective interventions.

This chapter will contrast the failure to reduce MMR in the USA to the steeply falling rates of Ethiopia and Nepal, two excellent examples of institutionalized training programs for abortion and contraception that have made profound contributions to reducing MMR and improving women's health in those countries. (See Chapters 29 and 27 for more details.) The failure of the USA to reduce its maternal mortality demonstrates the need for reproductive health policies that institutionalize both care and training in family planning. The decreases in MMR in Ethiopia, Nepal and other countries demonstrate effective family planning interventions led by national training programs.

2.4 Characteristics of Maternal Mortality in the USA

Figure 2.2 shows that MMR in the USA during the past twenty years has failed to improve in contrast to other wealthy countries with lower health-care expenditures, where maternal mortality has declined. Figure 2.3 summarizes MMR in the USA as a whole compared to the declining rate in California specifically. These two figures demonstrate important characteristics of the USA's MMR: the regional variations are as great as those seen in countries where health expenditures are much lower than in the USA, and the MMR variations from region to region in the USA are large even though US regional health expenditures vary little compared to global differences. For example, MMR in Texas has remained 3 to 4 times higher than in California, but per capita health-care expenditures in the two states were comparable during the period of divergence in maternal mortality.

Figure 2.4 demonstrates another remarkable characteristic of the USA's MMR: extreme racial variation. Though maternal mortality has not improved in any group with the exception of

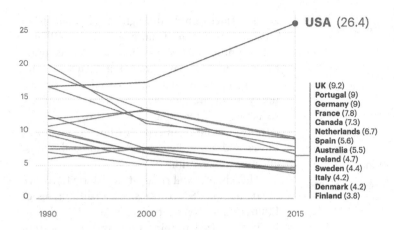

Figure 2.2 Maternal mortality is falling in other wealthy countries but not in the USA [23]

USA (26.4)

UK (9.2)
Portugal (9)
Germany (9)
France (7.8)
Canada (7.3)
Netherlands (6.7)
Spain (5.6)
Australia (5.5)
Ireland (4.7)
Sweden (4.4)
Italy (4.2)
Denmark (4.2)
Finland (3.8)

Maternal mortality rate

MATERNAL DEATHS PER 100,000 LIVE BIRTHS (1999–2013)

Health leaders in California have taken steps to reduce pregnancy-related deaths, as the maternal mortality rate in the country as a whole climbed.

Figure 2.3 Maternal deaths per 100,000 live births, USA and California, 1999–2013 [24]

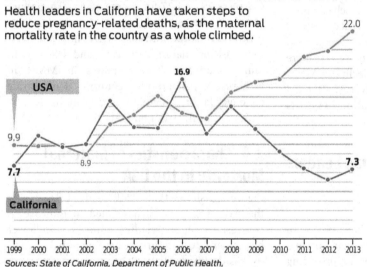

Sources: State of California, Department of Public Health, California Birth and Death Statistical Master Files, 1999-2013.

John Blanchard / The Chronicle

Asians, it has risen most among black and non-Hispanic white women [6]. Explanations for racial differences are complex and include health-care inequalities, stress experienced from long-standing racism and political restrictions on abortion and contraceptive care [7]. The UK, where, unlike the USA, maternal mortality has steadily decreased, also has great discrepancies by race [8], but places a greater public health emphasis on maternal safety as opposed to fetal survival [9].

As in most countries, cardiovascular diseases and hemorrhage are important contributors to US maternal mortality, but the USA differs from many other countries in that opioid use is the third most important contributor and HIV and unsafe abortions are not frequent causes, as they are in, for example, sub-Saharan Africa. There are racial and regional variations in the USA in the causes of maternal mortality that do not occur in most other countries. For example, opioid use is a more common cause among non-Hispanic white women in Eastern and Appalachian states than in other races and regions [10]. Explanations for high maternal mortality in the USA include many factors but their relative influence and actions required to mitigate them remain unclear [11,12].

A clear cause of maternal mortality unique to the USA among developed nations, but common in less developed ones, is undesired pregnancy.

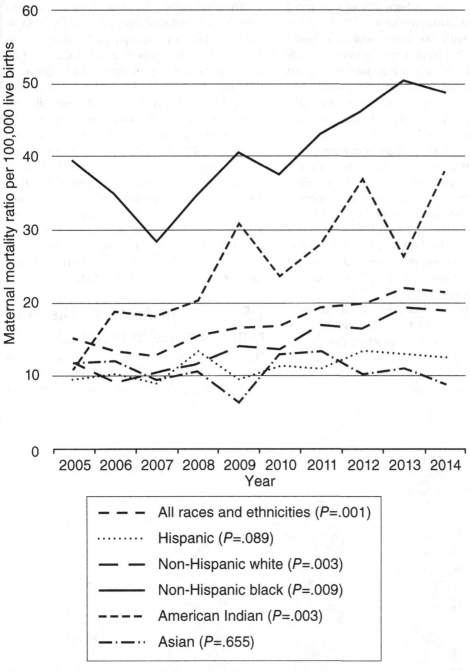

Figure 2.4 Trends in maternal mortality ratio (maternal deaths/100,000 live births by ethnic group and race: USA, 2005–2014) [25]

About 900 women die yearly in the USA from causes related directly or indirectly to pregnancy, and about half of these pregnancies are likely not intended, a much higher proportion than in other high-income countries. Prior to legalization of abortion beginning in about 1970 in the USA, there were at least 200 maternal deaths yearly from illegal abortion; there are currently fewer than 10. Many other countries have had the same experience. Among countries with large reductions in maternal mortality are Ethiopia and Nepal (described below) that, along with legalization, institutionalized abortion training. Several chapters in this book describe that process in the

USA where abortion has been almost eliminated as a cause of maternal mortality.

US states with the worst women's health services, including restrictions on access to safe abortion and abortion training, have the highest rates of maternal mortality. California and Texas provide contrasting examples; over the past 15 years California's maternal mortality steadily decreased and Texas's increased. At the same time, Texas progressively restricted access to reproductive health services (RHS), including contraception and abortion, while California increased access to these services through the Affordable Care Act's (Obama Care) Medicaid expansion and further abortion law liberalization. In the USA, contraception is often provided by non-physician clinicians, but abortion is most often done by physicians. In fact, only about a third of states permit advanced-practice women's health clinicians to provide abortions, and their training typically does not include abortion practice despite the demonstrated importance of abortion to women's health and the adverse effects of unintended obstetrical delivery.

The relationship between access to abortion services and maternal mortality in the USA is demonstrated by comparing MMRs from 1995 to 2017 in states that restricted abortion access to those that protected it. Investigators at Washington University in Saint Louis, Missouri, found that MMRs were not significantly different between restrictive or protective states in 1995, but they diverged by 2009, after restrictive states enacted legislation limiting abortion access and training. By 2017, restrictive states had much worse maternal mortality than protective ones, where MMR had decreased or remained stable for all races, while it had increased, particularly for black and Native American women, in states that had restricted abortion access. In states that neither restricted nor protected abortion access, changes in MMR were intermediate [13].

2.5 Training in Abortion to Reduce Maternal Mortality in Ethiopia

Data from Ethiopia, a nation of 100 million where MMR fell from 871 in 2000 to 412 in 2016 (Figure 2.5), illustrate the association of

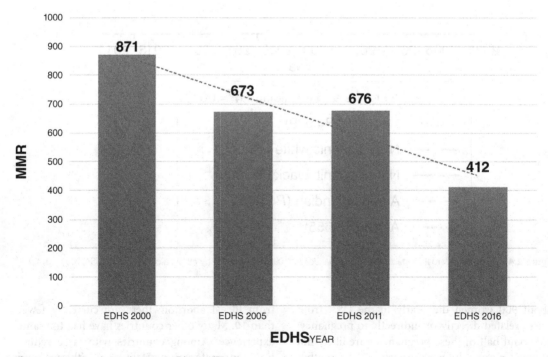

Figure 2.5 Maternal mortality ratio in Ethiopia (EDHS), magnitude and trend

improved access to safe pregnancy termination with rapidly declining maternal mortality. Ethiopia provides a good example of the importance of training in reproductive health care (see Chapter 29). Educational and economic opportunities for women, infrastructure and other social and medical progress occurred during the change to increased access to safe abortion, but were not extensive enough to explain the substantial decrease in MMR. Maternal deaths attributable to abortion decreased from 31% to 2% from 2000 to 2013 (Figure 2.6) [14]. During that period the abortion law was liberalized, public health institutions were directed to provide abortion care, lower- and mid-level health workers were educated about changes in access and directed to inform women and make referrals, contraception was offered to women after both spontaneous and elective abortion to help them avoid subsequent unintended pregnancies, and new abortion procedures (manual uterine aspiration and medical termination with mifepristone and misoprostol) were introduced on a large scale including to health professionals' training programs [15].

(a)

Yifru B, 2014

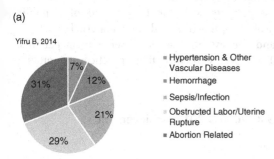

Figure 2.6a Causes of maternal mortality, Ethiopia, 1990–1999 [15]

(b)

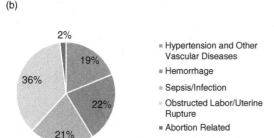

Figure 2.6b Causes of maternal mortality, Ethiopia, 2015 [15]

2.6 Training in Abortion to Reduce Maternal Mortality in Nepal

Nepal is a landlocked country, and its diverse terrain creates geographic barriers that make the equitable distribution of health services difficult (see Chapter 27). A decade-long conflict in the country and the unstable political situation posed challenges in providing health care to its population of about 28 million. Nepal reported one of the highest maternal mortality ratios (MMR) in the world, with a high proportion of maternal deaths and injuries attributable to unsafe abortion [16]. In 1998, abortion and abortion-related complications contributed to approximately 15% of maternal mortality in Nepal. Provision of safer abortion through institutionalized training is partially responsible for a reduction in MMR from 539 in 1996 to 259 by 2016 [17] (see Figure 2.7).

Nepal's progress in improved health for women is associated with legislative changes to promote their self-determination including the rights to inherit property, divorce husbands and control fertility. An abortion law that jailed women who terminated pregnancies was nullified in 2002 by this new legislation. A consequence of the new law was the Ministry of Health's (MoH) implementation of a national program to reduce maternal mortality through training physicians and nurses to provide safe abortion: at first of mostly urban physicians in manual uterine aspiration (MUA) in the first trimester, then in dilatation and evacuation (D&E) in the second trimester. Later, nurses and midwives, who serve both urban and rural women, were trained in MUA and medication abortion [18] (Table 2.5).

Legal changes and the abortion training program were strongly associated with the decline in MMR. A ten-year study by the Nepal Center for Reproductive Health, Environment and Population (CRHEPA) and the Bixby Center for Global Reproductive Health at the University of California, San Francisco, demonstrated that safe, legal abortion accounted for a significant portion of the decrease. Investigators used the approach by the US Centers for Disease Control and Prevention (CDC) to document the effects of changes in abortion laws in the USA following liberalization in 1973. They reviewed admissions to "sentinel hospitals," where most abortion complications are treated, and demonstrated a decrease in abortion admissions as MMR declined (see Figure 2.8) [19].

In addition to making abortion safer, the MoH made contraception more available, particularly in rural areas, increasing the prevalence of modern contraceptives from 35% to 43% in the decade from 2000 to 2010. This increase was associated with a decrease in total fertility rate (TFR) – the average number of births a typical woman would have in her lifetime – from 4.6 in 1996 to 2.6 in 2016, the period of rapid decline in MMR. The decrease in unintended pregnancies directly led to an accelerated decline in MMR in Nepal. Other effects of the law included increased educational and economic opportunities. For example, after enactment, the proportion of girls enrolled in secondary school increased by 48%, and extreme poverty (daily income per capita < US$1.25) fell from 68% to 25% of the population. These changes also contributed to the decline in TFR by decreasing desired family size and increasing access to health care, but improved access to both contraception and safe abortion was a primary contributor.

2.7 The Role of Family Planning Training in Decreasing Maternal Mortality

Well-trained physician leaders are critical in developing a medical school curriculum that emphasizes a public health approach to reducing maternal mortality and the family planning elements of successful programs. In the clinic they must demonstrate the specific skills required to better serve women at the level at which their students will practice. For example, many countries require medical school graduates to serve in rural areas before they continue residency training. These students should leave for their assignments with the background of a public health approach to reducing maternal mortality and the essential skills to serve their patients. These will vary with their practice assignment;

Table 2.5 Abortion method and trained services providers, Nepal, through 2018 [18]

Type of services	Trained providers		No. of listed sites
	Type	No.	
MVA	Doctors	1656	591
	Staff nurses	671	
MA	ANM	1582	825
Second-trimester services	Doctors only	58[*]	29

Source: Records; Ministry of Health/Family Welfare Division, Nepal
ANM, auxiliary nurse midwife; MA, manual aspiration; MVA, manual vacuum aspiration
[*] Though 86 were trained, only 58 are providing services at present.

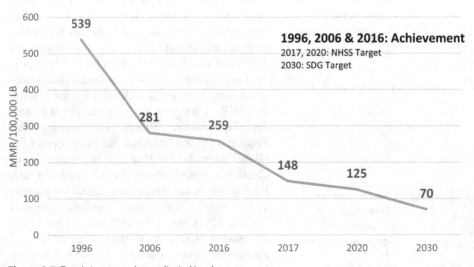

1996, 2006 & 2016: Achievement
2017, 2020: NHSS Target
2030: SDG Target

Figure 2.7 Trends in maternal mortality in Nepal

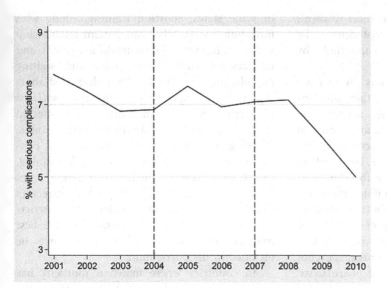

Figure 2.8 Trends in the percentage of abortion cases with serious complications presenting at four tertiary care hospitals in Nepal, 2001–2010, n = 23,493 [26]

for work in a rural area, they are likely to include estimation of gestation and assessment of pregnancy status and complications, initiation and cessation of contraceptives, including immediate postpartum intrauterine devices (IUDs) and implants, medical abortion methods and manual uterine aspiration for incomplete and elective abortions. Those who will practice in more isolated areas may require training in emergency cesarean delivery and evacuating the uterus in emergencies. In addition to specific skills appropriate to the practice situation, the physician or nurse or midwife should have had orientation to a team approach to patient care and know how to collaborate across professions. Respect for and cooperation with other members of the women's health-care team are key components of training that should come with the institutional responsibilities of women's health leaders. The best trained leaders in women's health must demonstrate to their students that "collaborative practice" is essential to good outcomes, particularly for reducing maternal mortality.

2.8 Unique Aspects of Abortion Provision

After abortion liberalization in the USA and in many other countries, only a small proportion of doctors became "abortion providers." Instead, abortion services in most countries were concentrated in specialized clinics – the Marie Stopes

clinics provide a good example. Their efficiency brought safe care at a low price, but most of them were in cities and only a few physicians did most of the abortions. In countries or regions without many physicians, abortion was not available, nor was abortion integrated into typical hospital care or into physician training programs.

Even in places with high concentrations of physicians, like the USA, the need for abortion in rural communities prompted reconsideration of laws that limited abortion and, therefore, abortion training, to physicians. When the US Food and Drug Administration (FDA) approved medical abortion, California, for example, changed its law to permit nurses to provide it so that it would be available in rural areas. There was little physician opposition. A few years later, after a demonstration project showed that nurse practitioners and midwives could use the hand-held syringe to do early abortions as safely as could physicians, the California law was further amended to permit advanced-practice clinicians to do surgical abortions. (See Chapter 26.) Other states, including, recently, Virginia, have followed, but these legal changes have not been supported by changes in the training in most nursing schools. Opposition to these changes has come not from physicians, but from those opposed to abortion for religious and political reasons. Physicians who learn in their own training about the importance of abortion for women's health recognize the value of collaborative practice to meet women's needs for abortion in the way that delivery by nurse-midwives was earlier supported by obstetricians.

Pharmacist provision is a way to increase access by allowing physicians and other clinicians simply to write a prescription for women who request abortion and is already an important source of abortion services in some countries, like Nepal [20,21]. Prescriptions can be filled in person or by mail, as is the case for almost all other drugs including those with much more serious side effects than those of abortion medications, which are very safe. A pelvic examination or sonography is not required if the woman is reasonably sure of the duration of her pregnancy, but pharmacist provision requires that pharmacists' training include abortion. Academic physician leaders, who themselves have been educated in the importance of abortion for women's health, can support training for abortion drug provision in the pharmacy schools of their universities.

2.9 Conclusion

In the USA, politicians have increased maternal mortality by restricting access to abortion services with laws targeted at abortion clinics and, in some states, abortion training. Along with intruding into the clinician–patient relationship with requirements for untruthful consent and unnecessary clinic visits, tests and waiting periods, these restrictions have decreased abortion training opportunities and are associated with rising maternal mortality in the affected states. Despite these restrictions, most trainees, knowing the importance of abortion and contraception for women's health, seek training, sometimes traveling outside their home states to receive it. In fact, training program directors from around the country, including in restrictive states, report that recruitment of the best trainees requires that abortion practice be included in the curriculum.

In countries where maternal mortality has decreased substantially (eg, Ethiopia and Nepal), institutionalized abortion training has been critical to providing access to safe abortion with its consequent effect of reducing maternal mortality. In those countries where laws restrict abortion training and access (eg, Brazil and Thailand), the component of maternal mortality attributable to abortion remains high. Further progress in reducing maternal mortality will depend on policies that promote improved training in and access to contraception and safe abortion.

References

1. The Millennium Development Goals Report 2015. New York: United Nations; 2015:75. http://mdgs.un.org/unsd/mdg/Resources/Static/Products/Progress2015/English2015.pdf.

2. Arulkumaran S, Hediger V, Manor A, May J. Saving Mothers' Lives: Transforming Strategy into Action. Imperial College, London: Global Health Policy Summit, Report of the Maternal Health Working Group; 2012:19.

3. Rodriguez MI, Chang R, Thiel de Bocanegra H. The impact of postpartum contraception on reducing preterm birth: findings from California. Am J Obstet Gynecol. 2015;213(5):703.e1–6.

4. White K, Teal SB, Potter JE. Contraception after delivery and short interpregnancy intervals among women in the United States. Obstet Gynecol. 2015;125(6):1471–1477.

5. McDorman M, Declercq E, Cabral H, Morton C. Recent Increases in the US maternal mortality rate: disentangling trends from measurement issues. Obstet Gynecol. 2016;128:447–553.

6. Moaddab A, Dildy G, Brown H, et al. Racial differences in maternal mortality in the USA. Obstet Gynecol. 2018;131(4):707–712.

7. Joseph K, Lisonkova M, Giulia M, et al. Factors underlying the temporal increase in maternal mortality in the United States. Obstet Gynecol. 2017;129(1):91–100.

8. Knight M, Bunch K, Tuffnell D, et al. (Eds.), on behalf of MBRRACE-UK. Saving Lives, Improving Mothers' Care: Lessons Learned to Inform Maternity Care from the UK and Ireland Confidential Enquiries into Maternal Deaths and Morbidity 2014–16. Oxford: National Perinatal Epidemiology Unit, University of Oxford; 2018. www.npeu.ox.ac.uk/mbrrace-uk

9. Womersley K. Why giving birth is safer in Britain than in the U.S. ProPublica; August 31, 2017.

10. Terplan M. Women and the opioid crisis: historical context and public health solutions. Fertil Steril. 2017;108:195–196.

11. Petersen EE, Davis NL, Goodman D, et al. Vital signs: pregnancy-related deaths, United States, 2011–2015, and strategies for prevention, 13 states, 2013–2017. *MMWR Morb Mortal Wkly Rep.* 2019;**68**:423–429. doi:http://dx.doi.org/10.15585/mmwr.mm6818e1

12. Chescheir, N. Drilling down on maternal mortality. *Obstet Gynecol.* 2016;**128**:427–428.

13. Addante, A, Eisenberg D, Leonard J, Hoofnagle M. The association of restricted abortion access and increasing rates of maternal mortality in the United States. *Contraception.* 2019;**100**:306.

14. Yifru, B. *National Maternal Death Surveillance and Response (MDSR) Annual Report, 2010 EFY.* Ethiopian Public Health Institute, Public Health Emergency Management System (PHEMS); 2011.

15. Yifru, B. Abortion-related mortality in Ethiopia. *Ethiop J Health Sci.* 2014;**24**(Suppl 0):15–28.

16. Pathak LR, Malla DS, Pradhan A. *Maternal Mortality and Morbidity Study.* Kathmandu: Ministry of Health; 1998.

17. Samandari G, Wolf M, Basnett I, Hyman A, Anderson C. Implementation of legal abortion in Nepal: a model for rapid scale up of high-quality care. *Reprod Health.* 2012;**9**:7.

18. Abortion Task Force. *Workshop Report – National Implementation Plan for Abortion Services.* Kathmandu: Ministry of Health, Department of Health Services, Family Health Division; November 18–19, 2002.

19. Henderson JT, Puri M, Blum M, et al. Effects of abortion legalization in Nepal, 2001–2010. *PLoS One.* 2013;**8**(5):e64775.

20. Tamang A, Puri M, Lama K, Shrestha P. Pharmacy workers in Nepal can provide the correct information about using mifepristone and misoprostol to women seeking medication to induce abortion. *Reprod Health Matters.* 2015;(Suppl 44):104–105.

21. Rocca CH, Puri M. Shrestha P, et al. Effectiveness and safety of early medication abortion provided in pharmacies by auxiliary nurse-midwives: a non-inferiority study in Nepal. *PLoS One.* 2018;**13**(1):e0191174. doi:10.1371/journal.pone.0191174

22. Darney P, Nakamura C, Regan L, Surur F, Thapa K. Maternal mortality in the USA compared to Ethiopia, Nepal, Brazil and UK: contrasts in reproductive health policies. *Obstet Gynecol.* 2020;**135**:1–6.

23. Martin N, Montagne R. The last person you'd expect to die in childbirth. ProPublica; May 12, 2017. www.propublica.org/article/die-in-childbirth-maternal-death-rate-health-care-system

24. Veklerov K. How California learned to keep pregnant women, new moms from dying. *San Francisco Chronicle*; September 4, 2018. www.sfchronicle.com/news/article/How-California-learned-to-keep-pregnant-women-and-13204352.php

25. Moaddab A, Dildy GA, Brown HL, et al. Health care disparity and pregnancy-related mortality in the United States, 2005–2014. *Obstet Gynecol.* 2018;**131**(4):707–712.

26. Henderson JT, Puri M, Blum M, et al. Effects of abortion legalization in Nepal, 2001–2010. *PLoS One.* 2013;**8**(5):e64775.

Chapter 3

The History of Integrated Training in Abortion and Contraception for Obstetrician-Gynecologists in the USA

Uta Landy

After decades-long efforts to reform the abortion laws in the USA, the US Supreme Court changed the law in all states with its *Roe* v. *Wade* decision in 1973, based on the constitutional argument of the right to privacy of the woman in consultation with her physician [1]. While many feminist and other organizations submitted friend of the court briefs, the justices' arguments relied primarily on medical evidence and the autonomy of medical practice: "the Supreme Court issued a decision that appeared mainly responsive to the arguments of the medical community. In page after page, Roe reasoned from medical science, and in its main holding affirmed the autonomy of doctors to act in what they believed to be the best interest of their patients" [2]. Two major medical organizations, the American Medical Association (AMA), the largest and most influential medical society in the USA, and the American College of Obstetricians and Gynecologists (ACOG) submitted friend of the court (amicus) briefs providing the physician perspective and support for legalization. Physicians have remained important advocates through many organizations and channels. (See Chapter 4.)

Several states legalized abortion before *Roe* in 1973, with certain restrictions. New York made abortion legal without limitations, including being a state resident. Dr. Christopher Tietze, a scientist at the Population Council in New York, began to document the health consequences of legal abortion, joined by the Centers for Disease Control and Prevention (CDC) of the US Department of Health and Human Services (HHS), the following year in the Joint Program for the Study of Abortion (JPSA) [3,4]. This study, later used as a template to study the public health effects of legal abortion worldwide (see Chapter 2), served as an important source of scientific evidence for the Supreme Court decision in *Roe* v. *Wade*.

The new law permitted abortions up to twenty-four weeks' gestation. Gestational limits and the

state's interest were more clearly defined or expanded over the years, including the initial requirement by some states that abortions at more advanced gestations be performed in a hospital against which the Supreme Court later ruled. Over the years, the Court addressed other aspects of clinical care and service enacted by states, for example, hospital requirements for second-trimester abortions, backup agreements between clinics and hospitals and other barriers to abortion access.

A year prior to the 1973 decision, a group of 100 academic obstetrician-gynecologist (ob-gyn) leaders, including department chairs at medical schools in most US states, published a statement anticipating the change of law [5]. Their focus was on meeting the new demand for services and the responsibility to ensure access to care. (See Chapter 4.)

3.1 Freestanding Clinics and Teaching Hospitals

In the USA, four states and the District of Columbia had legalized abortions before the *Roe* v. *Wade* Supreme Court decision in 1973 [3]. In response to the new laws, outpatient specialized clinics outside of the hospital were organized and began to meet the sudden demand for legal abortion [6]. For example Harry Levin, a businessman who worked with the Population Council for a time, launched several outpatient not-for-profit clinics, which became the Preterm Consortium, the first in Washington, DC, right after abortions were legalized there, followed by others in Boston, Cleveland, Pittsburgh and, later without legal sanction, in Bogota, Columbia [7,8]. (See Chapter 31.) He created the Preterm Institute and published guidelines for the clinical and administrative aspects of outpatient abortion detailing all aspects of care, and describing a newly created role of lay counselors as educators and patient advocates. He was prescient for his attention to the "... physical and spiritual environment that pervades a pregnancy termination facility" and his concern with a "warm, very human, very supportive atmosphere" [6].

The Preterm Clinic in Brookline, Massachusetts, and its manuals gave direction to the outpatient hospital teaching service at the Boston Lying-in Hospital (now Brigham and Women's), a major teaching hospital of Harvard Medical School. It was this abortion clinic, the "A Service," begun right after the 1973 *Roe* decision, that, in turn, served as a model for the training program described in this book, and after whose founder, Professor Kenneth J. Ryan, the "Ryan Residency Training Program" was named. The principles of patient-centered care, use of lay counselors and creation of an affirming and physically soothing environment served as an inspiration for a similar outpatient service seven years later, the Women's Options Center (WOC) (see Chapter 10), started by Ryan's resident at Harvard, Professor Philip Darney at the University of California, San Francisco (UCSF).

The WOC in turn served as a national model for the Kenneth J. Ryan Residency Training Program in Abortion and Family Planning. This national initiative to formally integrate family planning training into ob-gyn residencies, was founded by Dr. Uta Landy at the UCSF Bixby Center for Global Reproductive Health. Dr. Ryan, who, as chair at Boston Hospital for Women of Harvard Medical School, initiated the "A Service," agreed to lend his name to the national initiative.

A number of teaching hospitals around the USA began to provide abortions after legalization as promised in the "100 Professors" statement in states like North and South Carolina and Texas [5]. Many eventually discontinued. Their hospital-based abortion clinics generated controversy and demanded education and support from institutional officials, including department chairs and their faculty, administration and nursing and anaesthesia staffs. Unlike freestanding clinics, those associated with a hospital are required to meet standards set by the Joint Accreditation Commission for Health Care Organizations (JACHCO). Freestanding outpatient clinics could operate like physicians' offices. They were more efficient, cost less to build and operate and quickly emerged as the primary providers of abortion

services in most cities. Ownership varied and included individual physicians, business entities and non-profit groups, including Planned Parenthood and feminist health centers [9]. Care, service and cost at the clinics made those in the hospital, particularly for routine, early abortions, impractical as they took up valued hospital space and generated little revenue because of the hospital-wide staffing and equipment requirements of JACHCO [10]. Another factor in the steep decline of hospital services was the elimination of federal funding for abortion with the passage of the Hyde Amendment by the US Congress in 1976 [11]. Since both public and private hospitals in the USA serve a significant number of patients who are recipients of federal aid, many hospitals stopped abortions when federal insurance (Medicaid) no longer paid for them.

Although some states compensated for federal funding with state tax revenues, hospitals now perform only 4% of the abortions in the USA as shown in Figure 3.1 [12].

Despite the decline in hospital abortion services and lack of public funding, the rapid rise of freestanding clinics met the need of the more than 1.5 million women who sought abortion each year after *Roe*. At the same time, clinics functioned outside of the medical mainstream and became marginalized. Standards of care were questioned in exposés in the media [14]. A national professional membership organization (the National Abortion Federation, NAF) for clinics started in 1977 to provide community and define clinical and service delivery standards. However, these standards were not formulated, endorsed or enforced by the mainstream medical associations and did not change the outsider status of the abortion clinics or their practitioners. A rising antiabortion movement made the clinics targets of growing physical and legal harassment [15,16].

3.2 Medical Education and the Teaching Hospital

Medical education, particularly graduate, resident education in the USA, takes place primarily in the nation's more than one thousand teaching hospitals. Of these, 375 of the larger institutions belong to the Association of American Medical Colleges' Council of Teaching Hospitals and

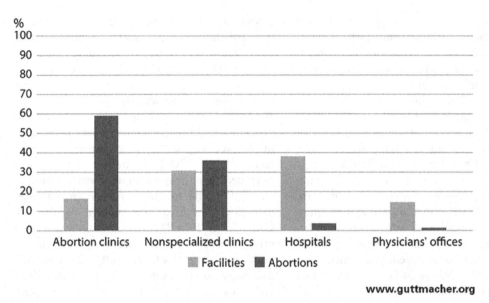

Figure 3.1 Percentage of abortion-providing facilities accounted for by each facility type, and percentage of abortions that are performed in each type of facility, 2014 [13]

Health Systems (COTH). Of those, 121 are part of a medical school or university.

US teaching hospitals are a critical part of the health-care system. They are responsible for the clinical training of future physicians and other health-care professionals, at the forefront of the treatment of complex medical conditions and conduct most of the research to develop and implement new medical procedures and treatments.

Since *Roe* v. *Wade*, few of the 1.5 million abortions performed annually occurred in teaching hospitals; therefore, many residents in obstetrics and gynecology graduated without systematic exposure to the techniques of uterine evacuation or the newly developing methods of contraception. Reproductive health was not considered an essential aspect of medical education and training. The absence of professional integration played an important role in perpetuating the stigma associated with abortion (see Chapter 8), which persisted in the public's and professional community's perceptions.

Nearly two decades after legalization of abortion, in 1990, the professional organization representing ob-gyns, the American College of Obstetricians and Gynecologists (ACOG) with its 58,000 members, the National Abortion Federation (NAF), the American Board of Medical Specialties (ABMS), the American

Council of Graduate Medical Education (ACGME), along with several other organizations, held a meeting to address what had become an alarming trend: the "graying" of abortion providers [17]. (See Chapter 4.) Most physicians in clinics were self-taught, and no system of educating the next generations existed.

3.3 The ACGME Abortion Mandate, Medical Education Standards and Enforcement

In the USA, the ACGME sets and approves standards for post-graduate (resident and subspecialist) medical education with its specialist-focused Residency Review Committees (RRCs) responsible for updating and enforcing their standards within each teaching hospital. The accreditation of a teaching hospital's residency is dependent on the RRC's periodic reviews. (See Chapter 1.) In addition, The Council on Resident Education in Obstetrics and Gynecology (CREOG), a unit of the American College of Obstetricians and Gynecologists (ACOG), defines resident educational objectives and designs and administers exams for each of the four post-graduate years of training. The American Board of Obstetrics and Gynecology (ABOG) is responsible for administering the final written and oral exams that certify the graduated resident as qualified to practice in the specialty.

The CREOG leadership initiated the establishment of educational objectives for abortion. Dr. Douglas Laube, chair of the CREOG education committee and future president of ACOG, together with Dr. Harry Visscher, vice president of education for ACOG, wrote the first patient-centered draft version of the CREOG Objectives in 1989 and 1990. As the Exam Committee chair, he appointed a family planning expert, Dr. Philip Darney, to write questions about contraception and abortion. After input from residency program directors, a full edition of focused questions was developed over the subsequent two years in consultation with ABOG, whose Executive Director was Dr. Norman Gant, and Joel Polin, the RRC chair. Their effort led to revised RRC guidelines in 1995 along with explicit language about abortion training in the new CREOG objectives. ACOG and its leadership were concerned about political ramifications among its diverse physician membership, but the united voices of ACOG, CREOG, ABOG and the RRC [ACGME] accomplished this essential step for the institutional integration of abortion training.

The leaders of these groups recognized that their professional organizations representing ob-gyns who are focused on reproduction and the reproductive organs had to take the political risk to create a training mandate for teaching future practitioners how to evacuate the uterus, for all indications, including medical emergencies and the woman's desire not to carry the pregnancy to term. The ACGME Board passed an abortion training mandate in 1995, twenty-two years after abortions became legal across the USA:

> . . . access to experience with induced abortion must be part of residency education. This education can be provided outside the institution. Experience with management of complications of abortion must be provided to all residents. If a residency program has a religious, moral, or legal restriction that prohibits the residents from performing abortions within the institution, the program must ensure that the residents receive satisfactory education and experience in managing the complications of abortion. [18]

The Family Medicine Board of the ACGME has not passed a similar requirement for abortion training for family medicine residents [19]. The American Academy of Family Physicians (AAFP), forty-six years after legalization of abortion, passed a statement in support of family medicine practitioners doing medication and first-trimester abortions, provided they were trained to be competent [20]. (See Chapter 15.)

ACGME's ob-gyn professional mandate generated further controversy from Catholic organizations and teaching hospitals. They objected to the mandate, which they considered in conflict with their religious teaching. Teaching hospitals must comply with ACGME mandates in order to be accredited by the Joint Commission on Accreditation of Healthcare Organizations and be eligible for federal funding for post-graduate training. By not complying with the mandate, religiously affiliated hospitals, particular Catholic hospitals could be in danger of losing this essential funding as teaching hospitals.

A year later, in 1996, following congressional hearings to consider "institutional opt-out" provisions brought by Catholic hospitals, the Coats Amendment was passed [21], ensuring that institutions – teaching hospitals – would not be at risk of jeopardizing their accreditation if they chose not to offer the training. Here is an excerpt of Senator Ted Kennedy's objection:

> I reject the belief that the Senate should determine medical residency training criteria as it pertains to issues regarding women. This is the first real attempt to superimpose Congress' view on obstetric and gynecological medical training. . . . Congress should leave the practice of medicine to the doctors. In this case, a highly respected board is attempting to insure [sic] that we have the best-trained physicians in the world. We have already acceded to a conscience clause that protects religious and moral beliefs of institutions and residents. . . . But to go beyond that by passing a law that substitutes congressional and political opinion for medical decision making is wrong. Congress should not interfere with current ACGME policy. It is an inappropriate use of our authority. It is bad policy and it is bad medicine. [22]

The few teaching institutions that maintained an abortion teaching service even before the mandate produced a first generation of family planning experts, clinicians and researchers, including Drs. Philip Stubblefield (Brigham and Women's Hospital, Harvard University), Philip Ferro (SUNY Upstate Medical University), Ronald Burkman (Johns Hopkins University), David

Grimes (University of North Carolina, Chapel Hill) and others who dedicated their professional careers to family planning.

3.4 The Fellowship in Family Planning

In 1991, Dr. Philip Darney, the director of the Women's Options Center at UCSF and contraceptive researcher, started the first Fellowship in Family Planning (FFP) at UCSF. The Fellowship was conceived as an apprentice clinical training model to produce family planning experts and leaders in research, teaching and clinical care – the classic triad of academic medicine [23]. For the FFP, though, a fourth leg of the three-legged stool was essential: advocacy as diagrammed in Figure 3.2. Advocacy training became an added focus early in the history of the Fellowship, and has grown in relevance as institutional barriers to service and state restrictions interfere with service and training. (See Chapter 4.)

Although a formal "Guide to Learning" had not been established, fellows were expected to learn the fundamentals of research by producing a family planning–focused research project. The original vision included an opportunity to learn about family planning and abortion and their impact on women's health abroad through a global health rotation. By 1999, there were five

Fellowships in place but without a unifying structure. The Fellowship needed learning objectives, communication among sites, opportunities for exchange among fellows and directors and systematic outreach and visibility in the professional community. Up to this time, the only gatherings consisted of a yearly meeting with the funder and directors to consider potential new sites. The fellows did not know one other or have opportunities to share clinical or research experiences.

The launch of the Ryan Residency Training Program in 1999 led to the establishment of an administrative National Office (NO). The National Director and founder of the Ryan Program, Dr. Landy, took on the administration of the Fellowships as well as residency training. The FFP soon evolved into a workforce pipeline producing graduates who started Ryan Programs and in turn, Ryan Programs inspired applicants for the Fellowship as shown in Figure 3.3.

3.4.1 The Fellowship in Family Planning: Outreach and Visibility

The first steps toward a unifying structure included designing a brochure for both programs and exhibiting at professional meetings attended by ob-gyn physicians and academics responsible for medical student and physician training. These were the annual meetings of the American College of Obstetricians and Gynecologists (ACOG), Council of University Chairs of Obstetrics and Gynecology (CUCOG), American Gynecological and Obstetrical Society (AGOS) and the Association of Professors of Gynecology and Obstetrics/Council on Resident Education in Obstetrics and Gynecology (APGO CREOG). We later added other organizations such as the

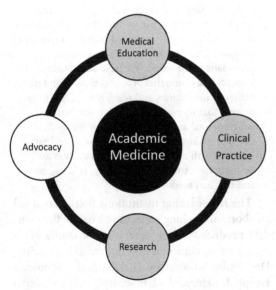

Figure 3.2 Academic medicine's responsibilities

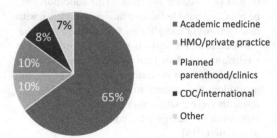

Figure 3.3 Post-Fellowship careers, 2008–2018 [24]

National Abortion Federation (NAF), Medical Students for Choice (MSFC), Abortion Care Network (ACN) and the Society for Maternal-Fetal Medicine (SMFM). Professional visibility became a major programmatic focus.

3.4.2 Setting and Enforcing Standards

Setting standards and a structure to enforce them was paramount. Dr. Dan Mishell and Dr. Mort Stenchever, both founding members of the first two ob-gyn subspecialties – Reproductive Endocrinology and Infertility (REI) and Maternal-fetal Medicine (MFM), drafted the *Guide to Learning* (GTL) and *General Requirements* (GR), defining learning and institutional FFP requirements [24]. The drafts were reviewed by all directors, and the first FFP versions published in 2003.

Applying sites were visited by consultant experts from REI who were current or former department chairs with leadership positions in the other subspecialties and the ABOG together with the National Director or NO staff. A formal evaluation report and recommendations were submitted to the National Director. Sites were approved for one to five years. Once specific protocols were established, site visits were conducted periodically by fellowship directors, a member of the NO staff and, on occasion, department chairs from other FFP sites. Approval status now ranges from one to five years and may include probation. This system of peer review enriched the sites and broadened the fellowship directors' perspectives on mentorship approaches, research and clinical services. By 2005 FFP sites were requested to submit annual reports to the NO to assess compliance with the GTL and GR.

3.4.3 The Pursuit of Subspecialty

It was clear from the outset that this new post-residency training program would be modeled after the other, ABOG approved, subspecialties: Reproductive Endocrinology and Infertility, Maternal-fetal Medicine and Gynecologic Oncology. These were established in the early 1970s by ABOG, which was granted the authority by ACGME to oversee the gynecologic subspecialties. With the formation of the fourth subspecialty in Female Pelvic Medicine and Reconstructive

Surgery in 2011, ACGME reassumed accreditation responsibilities from ABOG. Subspecialties are incorporated into resident training through formal rotations in the clinical area of each, in addition to the rotations in general obstetrics and gynecology.

In 2005, ABOG voted unanimously to approve that family planning become the next subspecialty in obgyn and established a liaison committee to facilitate the process. A meeting of leaders representing ABOG (Drs. Gerson Weiss and William Droegmuller) and the FFP (Drs. Carolyn Westhoff, Philip Darney and Uta Landy) reviewed the requirements for a formal subspecialty: the FFP needed to continue to expand the number of sites (ABOG required a minimum number of twenty-five to thirty) and establish its own subspecialty society. The number of new Fellowship sites increased over the next several years as a result of persistent outreach to the professional communities, particularly department chairs, and the increasing number of Fellowship graduates who started Ryan Programs and Family Planning Fellowships in academic departments around the country as shown in Figure 3.4 [25].

In 2005, Dr. Uta Landy, the national director of the FFP, published an editorial in *Contraception* describing the need for a family planning subspecialty [26]. Over a period of more than twenty years, the FFP established itself as the leader in contraceptive clinical and abortion research. (See Chapters 6 and 7.)

Formation in 2004 of a new subspecialty society (the Society of Family Planning, SFP) was a landmark for the FFP and family planning research. Encouraged by Drs. Leon Speroff and Dan Mishell, leading REI subspecialists whose research emphasized family planning, a group of Fellowship directors organized the SFP, which was initially housed in the NO of the FFP at UCSF, the academic home of SFP's first President, Philip Darney.

From its outset, the SFP reviewed proposals, competitively funded research and organized annual meetings for research protocol discussions and presentations of results into which FFP research was integrated. SFP grew rapidly into a multidisciplinary organization of nearly a thousand members representing the new family planning subspecialty.

In addition to the FFP's contributions to the SFP, NAF and other organizations in the field, FFP graduates participate as investigators of the Contraceptive Clinical Trials Network (CCTN), the US National Institutes of Health's Contraceptive Clinical Trials Network, which now includes a dozen FFP sites and makes substantial contributions to contraceptive development.

3.4.4 Global Health and the FFP

Graduated fellows make substantive contributions in the global health arena with World Health Organization (WHO) and international nongovernmental organizations (NGOs) as staff physicians, medical directors or consultants, often focused on long-acting reversible contraception (LARC) methods and later gestation dilation and evacuation (D&E) uterine evacuation techniques

[27]. Fellows and graduates present at international professional meetings, conduct collaborative research projects with partners from the Global South and play pivotal roles in defining guidelines and standards of abortion and contraception care for the USA through CDC's Medical Eligibility Criteria and globally with the WHO contraception and abortion guidelines.

By 2019, with support of the other subspecialties in obgyn, academic leadership and other professional organizations, the Fellowship was granted subspecialty status by ABMS and ACGME as a Fellowship in Complex Family Planning (see Figure 3.5) [24].

Graduates of the Fellowship serve as consultants, educators and clinicians for patients who present with complex medical conditions for contraception and uterine evacuation with expertise in counseling, ultrasound, uterine evacuation techniques, analgesia and anesthesia

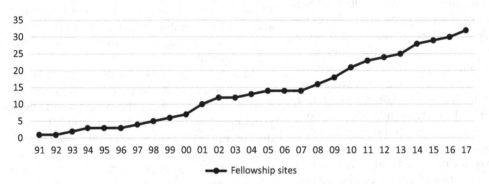

Figure 3.4 Number of Fellowship sites, 1991–2017 [24]

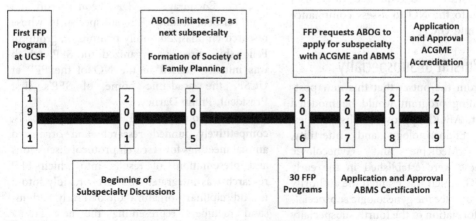

Figure 3.5 Complex Family Planning subspeciality timeline, 1919–2019

management, medically appropriate and patient-centered contraception and management of complications.

3.4.5 Providing Support: Family Planning Fellowship Workshops

The FFP's focus on contraception and abortion means that trainees and graduates must be prepared to contend with political and social controversy, stigma – both personal and professional – and even violence. (See Chapters 24 and 7.) Political interference with medical practice prevents some FFP experts from treating their patients based on the evidence and professional ethics. Bearing witness to the social injustices suffered by their patients places further emotional burdens. In response, the FFP began annual Psychosocial Workshops, addressing such topics as interacting with family and friends; contending with those who object to contraception or abortion; dealing with hostile colleagues, nurses and administrators; understanding the role of religion and professional ethics in providing contraception and abortion; and contending with fears of violence. These workshops, led by diverse senior faculty, Fellowship directors and graduates, became a valued and unique aspect of Fellowship support.

Additional workshops focus on global and domestic rotations, leadership training, communications and, for second-year fellows, career development, which has become an essential guide for fellows searching for academic or other post-Fellowship positions. Research training, provided for fellows by each of their academic departments, and for ten years for graduated fellows by ABOG's Excellence Foundation, is now augmented for first-year fellows by a National Office course to prepare fellows at the beginning of the first year for their required research project. This initial research course presents the *Lancet Handbook of Essential Concepts of Clinical Research* taught by its authors, Drs. David Grimes and Kenneth Schultz, as well as quantitative and qualitative research methodologies, implications of research for health policy, working with Institutional Research Boards (IRBs), publishing and other considerations to support and guide fellows toward the required research project [28].

3.4.6 Creating Community

The need for creating a network and community for the growing number of fellows was apparent from the founding of the Fellowship. Annual meetings brought together the community of current and graduated fellows, their directors and department chairs and NO staff. First- and second-year fellows present their research; next years' incoming fellows are welcomed; clinical, research and policy questions are addressed by national leaders in the field; and a topic of current scholarly or political interest is addressed in depth by nationally recognized experts.

Incoming classes, where many new fellows had become acquainted during the application and interview process, used their first annual meeting to build their own cohort and develop career-long relationships. For fellows and graduates working in hostile political environments and those without other family planning experts in their institutions or cities, these meetings became an important source of reunion and support.

Another important communications tool is the *Fellowship Listserv*, a platform for all current and graduated fellows, directors and research mentors to exchange information and professional updates and present complex clinical cases in search for published evidence or clinical perspectives. (See Chapter 5.)

As the Fellowship has matured with 400 graduates and 28 current sites (Figure 3.6), so has its management and statement of purpose, vision and mission:

The Vision:
To ensure just and equitable abortion and contraception informed by science.

This vision statement is the same as that of the FFP subspecialty Society of Family Planning (SFP).

The Mission:
To develop obstetrician gynecologist leaders in abortion and contraception through training in clinical care, research and education.

Management of the Fellowship in Family Planning and its meetings and communications has moved from UCSF's Bixby Center for Global Reproductive Health, where it was founded in the

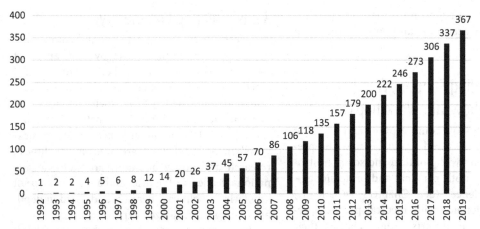

Figure 3.6 Cumulative number of Fellowship in Family Planning graduates:1992–2019 [24]

UCSF Department of Obstetrics, Gynecology and Reproductive Sciences, to its new organizational home, the Society of Family Planning, founded to support the Fellowship's new subspecialty status.

3.5 The Kenneth J. Ryan Program in Abortion and Family Planning: Focus, Growth Documentation

The Ryan Program was founded by Dr. Uta Landy, who had worked as a counselor in one of New York City's first legal outpatient abortion clinics and later became one of the National Abortion Federation's (NAF) founding directors. NAF is the national professional organization of freestanding, outpatient abortion clinics. The Ryan Program's vision was to create dedicated rotations for ob-gyn residents focused on abortion and contraception. Dr. Kenneth J. Ryan, whose outpatient abortion clinic in Boston's leading obstetrical hospital served as a model for resident training, agreed to lend his name to the program. The program was founded at UCSF's Bixby Center for Global Reproductive Health in Obstetrics, Gynecology and Reproductive Sciences so that it could relate from one academic institution to others. Dr. Ryan's prestige as a reproductive scientist who discovered the process of aromatization, as an ethicist who chaired the commission that authored the Belmont Report on the ethics of human research, and as an academic leader as chair of the obgyn department at Harvard's principal teaching hospital (1973–1993), combined with the recognition of

UCSF as a leading center for innovative care and research in women's health, gave the Ryan Program initiative and prestige, which were critical in its early years [29].

3.5.1 Defining the Ryan Residency Training Program

Outcomes of the Ryan Program were based on two premises:

1. Training would be formally integrated into four-year obgyn residency training programs, and
2. An obgyn department would start or enhance an outpatient abortion service to serve as the clinical training site, or, alternatively, develop a collaborative relationship with a clinic to grow and enhance family planning services in the teaching hospital.

When programs are approved, the National Office facilitates funding and offers workshops, mentorship and connection to an ever-growing community of family planning experts. Sites are expected to submit a description of their current level of services and training, and a detailed proposal describing the goals for initiating the program, usually during a two-year period.

3.5.2 Program Outreach

Success in the implementation of a new educational initiative, particularly in an area fraught with controversy and stigma, demanded strategic focus. The program should make itself known not only in the professional world of medical educators and learners but also in the broader field of obgyn. Exhibits at ACOG, CREOG, the organizations representing residency program directors and clerkship directors, the Council of Resident Education in Obstetrics and Gynecology and APGO, the Association of Professors in Gynecology and Obstetrics, along with formal presentations and educational materials were essential in outreach and establishing new training programs. Obgyn department chairs play a pivotal role and must be motivated and inspired to hire a new expert faculty member or identify someone already on faculty in that role, and persuade their deans and hospital administrators to provide initial support.

The Ryan Program gradually gained visibility and respect by attending and eventually presenting its programmatic objectives and results of its program evaluation at professional obgyn meetings, including the Council of University Chairs in Obstetrics and Gynecology (CUCOG). The joint management of Ryan and Fellowship programs made it possible to connect department chairs with graduating Family Planning fellows who were looking for opportunities to apply their expertise and implement resident training. Together, the two programs combined to create and perpetuate the workforce of academics and practitioners in family planning.

Medical students were a critical group of future physicians to reach and inspire. Regardless of their future choice of specialty, students will eventually become practicing physicians who support abortion and contraception as essential components of women's health. Training programs with enthusiastic faculty and residents can inspire students to enter obgyn and later pursue Fellowship training. (See Chapter 20.) Reports from resident interviews at Ryan Program and Fellowship site visits repeatedly demonstrate that medical students, concerned about the limited access to abortion for women in their teaching hospitals, were motivated to select ob-gyn residency and aspire to further training through the Fellowship in Family Planning.

3.5.3 Programmatic Support

The Ryan Program offers support to obgyn departments with guidance for faculty seeking to establish a new training program in writing a proposal as well as several workshops:

1. *Starting a Ryan Program*
2. *Additional workshops* focus on clinical service aspects including sustainability of an outpatient service in the hospital, didactics and various aspects of training and teaching.
3. *Papaya workshops* [30]
4. *Values Clarification and Professionalism workshops*
5. *Career workshops for residents*

Periodic webinars are sponsored by the program with faculty experts on, for example, ultrasound, anaesthesia, publications and writing, contraceptive drug development, implants and removal, sex hormones and contraception, transgender health and various topics on legal, health policy and advocacy aspects of contraception.

This training is provided not just for family planning faculty, fellows and residents but for the entire team of nurses, counselors, administrators and support staff who all play crucial roles in building a successful abortion service in a teaching hospital. (See Chapters 10 and 17.)

3.5.4 Site Visits

National Office staff and an expert physician conduct site visits for new and current programs and those that have completed their Ryan Program support (graduated programs). Site visits serve to ensure compliance with Ryan Program service and training expectations. They also offer opportunities for further mentorship and guidance. For those faculty who need more intensive and specific support, the Ryan Program created the Ryan Initiative in Sustainability and Engagement (RISE) Program, conducted by two graduates of the FFP who successfully started Ryan Programs in their own departments. Each brings expertise in navigating different institutional settings: one in the Northeast at a public hospital serving indigent patients and depending on state funding, the other in the conservative South with numerous institutional and political obstacles. Their guidelines for establishing successful service delivery and training along with periodic personal mentoring have become an important source of support to Ryan Programs facing institutional obstacles. (See Chapter 17.)

3.5.5 Evaluation and Research

Within a few years after its launch, the Ryan Program established evaluation reporting that included the following parameters:

1. Resident self-reported clinical competence in first- and second-trimester abortions, methods of contraception and related skills, for example, contraceptive implant removal, removal of embedded IUDs.
2. Intention to provide abortions before and after the family planning rotation
3. Post-residency practice of abortion
4. Assessment of skills and attitudes of residents who opt out or partially participate
5. Training in Ryan and non-Ryan residency programs
6. Residency program directors', department chairs' and Ryan Program directors' perceptions about the family planning rotation

Systematic collection of these data led to presentations at national professional meetings and to publications describing the Ryan Program. At national meetings, sessions addressed particular aspects of family planning education for students, residents, residency program directors, Ryan Program directors and department chairs. The evaluation efforts and resulting publications enhanced the program's visibility and credibility as a respected new field – Complex Family Planning.

Obgyn residents in the USA are expected to do a research project in order to complete their training. Integrated family planning programs, led by dedicated experts who are teachers and mentors, inspire family planning research interests by residents. Their projects may lead to further research activities or pursuit of a Complex Family Planning Fellowship, and help build the academic standing of family planning in the department and the larger field.

3.5.6 Successes and Challenges

During a period of 20 years, the Ryan Program supported the initiation of 100 resident training programs, including new or expanded clinical services for abortion and contraception and accounting for approximately 40% of obgyn residency training programs in the USA. Since the start of the Ryan Program, ACGME training sites have ranged from 266 to the current total of 284 US programs [31]. The number increased recently, as osteopathy training has become eligible for obgyn residency accreditation.

The majority of the Ryan Programs are based in the 126 teaching hospitals connected to a medical school. We identified these university-affiliated programs as priority sites, as they generally have more residents in training, reach a greater diversity of learners and offer clerkship and elective rotations for medical students from their own and other institutions. These academic medical centers may be part of the state's university system or be located in private medical schools. This distinction can be of far-reaching consequences, as there has been a trend over the past ten years to restrict the clinical activities of employees of state-affiliated teaching hospitals as well as the abortion services they are permitted to provide. This direct interference of state legislators with medical practice and training cannot be levied on private institutions, although dependence on state grants and the level of conservatism of their home states leads to restricted policies in these private institutions as well [32]. (See Chapter 7.) In addition, laws and policies restricting the practice of abortion affect all institutions and individuals who do abortions, whether in private clinics, Planned Parenthood clinics or public or private hospitals.

Geographically, the programs, with a few exceptions in Southern states, have reached virtually every US state with an obgyn residency, and have trained 7,000 residents, despite formidable obstacles of legislative restrictions and interference with evidence-based practice in the hospital and partner clinic setting.

An essential element for success was identifying expert faculty committed to service delivery, teaching and mentorship. While advocacy is understood as a public and legislative educational effort, establishing a program also requires advocacy at many institutional levels to: offer abortions in outpatient settings, expand the availability of abortions within the hospital and create institutional visibility for abortion referrals and contraceptive services, particularly for patients with complex medical conditions. (See Chapter 4.) Opposition by nurses, colleagues within the obgyn department and anaesthesia and the operating room staff are not uncommon obstacles [32].

Even among supportive deans, department chairs and administrators, fear of controversy about abortion can create what may seem insurmountable hurdles for the young physician who joins the faculty as a Complex Family Planning Fellowship graduate eager to pursue structured resident training and expansion of services through a Ryan Program.

3.5.7 Ryan Programs as a Model for Institutionalization of Family Planning Training

The Reproductive Health Education in Family Medicine (RHEDI) Program was formed in 2004 by Dr. Marji Gold, the same time she headed a Family Medicine Fellowship in conjunction with the obgyn Fellowship. The RHEDI Program approach was modeled on the Ryan Program to integrate family planning training into residency, but relied in most of its programs on community rather that academic hospital partnerships.

Some of the obgyn departments offering abortion and contraception training also teach residents from family medicine. Some programs were preceded by family medicine or launched together, others expanded to include family medicine after the training of the obgyn residents was firmly established [33].

Although there was no mandate to include abortion training into the family medicine resident training curriculum, many family practice physicians did abortions and were eager to institutionalize training for residents. Several groups emerged to train in miscarriage management and primarily first-trimester abortions.

3.5.8 The Health and Hospitals Corporation Initiative

In 2002, the Ryan Program was asked by the New York City Health and Hospitals Corporation (HHC) to provide guidance in developing abortion training in the largest public hospital system in the USA: ten public hospitals in the boroughs of New York City. HHC received from newly elected Mayor Bloomberg a mandate to incorporate abortion training in the HHC teaching hospitals [34]. A delegation of administrators, department chairs, chiefs of service and faculty were hosted by the Ryan Program at the UCSF

Women's Options Center (WOC) at San Francisco General Hospital (SFGH), the public hospital of San Francisco, for a three-day review of abortion service and training. The WOC served as a model for staffing, space layout, service delivery and teaching. As a result of that visit, several HHC programs carry the name of Women's Options Center for their abortion services. According to a follow-up study conducted by Guihai et al., the visit inspired HHC leadership to focus their efforts on improving HHC's abortion facilities in order to provide appropriate settings for training young physicians. [35].

3.5.9 The Pathfinder/Vietnam Curriculum Reform Partnership

Similarly, the Ryan Program was asked by Pathfinder International to lead a national reproductive health curriculum reform initiative for the Vietnamese Ministry of Health (MoH). The request resulted in a series of two-week courses in Vietnamese at UCSF for representatives of the MoH, deans and obgyn leadership and faculty from all of the eight public medical schools in Vietnam. The courses were based on principles of curriculum reform, teaching, mentorship and service delivery, taught by UCSF leadership including the vice chancellor and provost, the vice dean for Graduate Medical Education, ethics faculty and residency and medical student curriculum directors. The principles of educational reform used examples from teaching abortion and contraception including simulation training with the hand-held syringe in a "Papaya Workshop." These courses for Vietnamese medical school officials were followed by several courses in Vietnam, including team teaching of medical students by UCSF and local faculty in Vietnamese medical schools to demonstrate curriculum reform through small group sessions and clinical simulation exercises.

In 2008, a delegation including the head of Mexico City's Department of Public Health and other leadership from public hospitals and clinics visited the SFGH WOC to learn about service delivery and training. As a result, several clinics were built in Mexico City's public hospitals to emulate the architectural model and counseling approaches at UCSF for enhancing abortion patient and staff emotional well-being. The visit was followed up with a number of in-service trainings in Mexico City after the new clinics were built. These focused on the emotional aspects of providing abortion care, based on the Psychosocial Workshop of the FFP and second-trimester (D&E) procedures.

In 2015, an international initiative, the Center for International Reproductive Health Training (CIRHT), was launched at the University of Michigan by Dr. Senait Fisseha (see Chapter 29) to integrate abortion and family planning training abroad, beginning with Ethiopia. Dr. Fisseha spent two days with the Ryan Program leadership to learn about the philosophical and practical approaches of institutionalizing resident training, again using the UCSF Women's Options Center as a clinical services and training model. Once CIRHT was launched, the Ryan Program created a two-day intensive workshop for the leaders of CIRHT to describe all aspects of the Ryan Program approach and implementation.

3.5.10 Connecting the FFP and Ryan Program Initiatives to Enhance Success of Both: Creating Workforce Pipelines for Generalists and Subspecialists

Although the connections between the Ryan and Fellowship programs were not apparent initially, the importance of their relationship soon became apparent. The requirements for the Fellowship to meet institutional prerequisites (General Requirements) were assured if a Ryan Program had been started before a Fellowship was applied for [36]. The Fellowship eventually moved to making the establishment of dedicated resident training and the necessary institutional clinical services, and/or community partner collaborations, a prerequisite for Fellowship site approval. There was concern initially that the clinical training of the fellows might interfere with that of the residents. In fact, the presence of fellows enhanced the resident training experience, improved the didactic exercises for both and facilitated clinical and research mentorship. The contributions of the Fellowship to resident training are demonstrated by the frequency with which graduating residents honor their Family Planning Fellowship mentors as outstanding teachers.

The majority of FFP applicants have come from residencies with Ryan Programs [24]. Once fellows graduate, the majority pursue academic careers and start new Ryan Programs or join the faculty of an existing Ryan or Fellowship program. The Fellowship Career Development Workshop evolved to inform second-year fellows about career options, but its main focus is in guiding fellows to learn about and successfully pursue academic positions. The two programs combine to create an efficient and unique workforce pipeline. While most fellows choose academic positions, the Career Workshop also presents opportunities for leadership positions at Planned Parenthood, community clinics and health systems or global health NGOs.

The positive effects of combined Ryan Resident and Fellowship training are described in Fellowship annual reports and site visit reports: FFP graduates become recognized teaching and research mentors, acknowledged with teaching awards given by the residents and by the number of resident research projects in family planning conducted by residents in departments with Ryan and Fellowship programs. (See Chapter 7.)

3.6 Professional Collaborations

Review of the history of family planning training requires description of interactions with relevant professional organizations. The development of these relationships helped to legitimize family planning. For example, shortly after its founding, the FFP decided to hold its annual meeting with ACOG and to invite the president of ACOG to give a meeting keynote address to introduce the community of fellows and Fellowship graduates to ACOG. ACOG presidents have never missed the opportunity to describe ACOG as defining and promoting evidence-based practice of care and advocating on behalf of the specialty with both state and national policy makers. These activities are critical to access to contraception and safe abortion for US women. Since the fellows are trained to be future researchers and advocates, ACOG is able to employ the fellows in advocacy efforts and use their expertise to educate their membership through participation in committees, roundtable discussions and presentations at their annual clinical meeting and meetings of the nine ACOG districts. Collaboration between the FFP and ACOG led to the ACOG LARC initiative, for example.

A growing number of fellows and Fellowship graduates participate in ACOG's advocacy programs (see Chapters 4 and 7), including a one-month ACOG elective rotation for current fellows and, finally, a dedicated one-year post-Fellowship rotation for a graduated fellow – the Darney-Landy ACOG Family Planning Fellowship. Graduated fellows have moved into national committee memberships and ACOG district leadership positions poised to pursue national leadership.

Another national organization, NAF, has welcomed the participation of fellows both on their board and staff with medical director positions, leading evidence-based workshops and scientific presentations. Fellows have become advocates for evidence with a community of practitioners whose pioneering work was steeped in clinical experience.

3.7 The Future of Family Planning and Abortion Education: The Impact of Subspecialty Certification and Accreditation

The Fellowship and Ryan programs are initiatives to make family planning an integral part of services and teaching in US teaching hospitals. The recognition as a subspecialty in Complex Family Planning affirms and further promotes institutional integration, acknowledging that abortion and contraception are essential aspects of obgyn learning objectives for residents and postgraduate training. Subspecialty connotes professional acceptance of a field that faces continuing legislative interference of its clinical and even teaching practice. Subspecialty recognition deepens institutional commitment. It affirms that the work of both programs and its graduates has advanced women's health through clinical care and research, and that, as a subspecialty, it will be better able to improve reproductive health.

Among the practical consequences of subspecialization, the American Board of Obstetrics and Gynecology (ABOG) will have a new division of family planning composed of experts from the field, with its chair becoming a member of the ABOG board; the ACGME will take on the role of setting and enforcing the standards of the new Fellowship in Complex Family Planning, again with the participation of family planning experts. The Residency Review Committee will seek the perspective of a family planning expert to further

ensure that family planning training is an integral part of the formal residency review of US obgyn departments; Complex Family Planning Fellowships will be formally integrated in each institution's office of Graduate Medical Education, an enormous step toward institutional normalization. Subspecialty accreditation institutionalizes clinical training standards based on specific systems applied to other subspecialties. ABOG, in order to develop written and oral exams for the subspecialty, begins with carefully laid out, transparent procedures involving a comprehensive process of practice analysis to define the clinical parameters of the Fellowship. These rigorous examinations ensure that graduates share clearly defined learning objectives that reflect their clinical competence, familiarity with the research in the field and their knowledge of public and health policy. Subspecialty recognition also allows for representation of the subspecialty on the executive board of the ACOG and potential representation within the AMA in setting the procedural billing parameters for services paid by Medicaid.

3.8 Conclusion

While not all of the 7,000 trained or future residents participating in the Ryan Program will make family planning and abortion part of their clinical practices, they have learned the most important lesson of such training: terminating a pregnancy, for any reason, and urgent evacuation of the uterus require training and skills that are based on scientific developments and research. Even if they chose to opt out of some aspects of this training, they understand and accept that ending a pregnancy with abortion is not only a legal right, but a medical and social imperative that should simply be a medical procedure like all others.

Finally, after almost half a century of legalization of contraception and abortion, these residents, together with the more than 400 Fellowship subspecialist graduates, will comprise new generations of health-care providers, educators, researchers and policy advocates, the future medical workforce. For them, the prohibition of abortion or contraception, the interference with their professional clinical practice and their dedication to the continuing advancement of reproductive health is a professional, ethical affront.

The history of abortion and family planning training for ob-gyns in the USA shows that abortion legalization led to women's access to safe abortion. The major professional organizations, while supportive of the change of law, did not recognize the need for integrated training initially. An official training mandate was not passed until more than twenty years later when ACOG, ABOG and the ACGME, despite continuing controversy, concluded that abortion is a professional responsibility and must be part of residency training. The Ryan Residency Training Program and Fellowship in Family Planning were based on the championship of some of the early academic leaders. The programs have built institutionally integrated and sustainable programs that produce a competent and committed professional workforce. A range of incentives and support mechanisms created momentum, fostered institutional support, promoted research and policy leadership and led to the professional recognition for a new subspecialty in Complex Family Planning. Despite unrelenting political interference with medical practice, both initiatives produce new generations of physicians who consider abortion and contraception an essential and normal part of health care.

References

1. Roe v. Wade, 410 U.S. 113 (1973).

2. Greenhouse L, Siegel R. *Before Roe v. Wade: Voices That Shaped the Abortion Debate before the Supreme Court's Ruling.* Rochester, NY: Social Science Research Network; 2012. doi:10.2139/ssrn.2131505

3. Gold RB. Lessons from before Roe: will past be prologue? *Issues Brief (Alan Guttmacher Inst).* 2003;(5):1–4.

4. Tietze C, Lewit S. Joint Program for the Study of Abortion (JPSA): early medical complications of legal abortion. *Stud Fam Plann.* 1972;3 (6):97–122. doi:10.2307/1965375

5. A statement on abortion by one hundred professors of obstetrics. *Am J Obstet Gynecol.* 1972;**112**(7):992–998. doi:10.1016/0002-9378(72) 90826-5

6. Lewit S. *Abortion Techniques and Services.* Amsterdam: Excerpta medica; 1972. http://lib.ugent.be/catalog/rug01:000382479

7. Hodgson JE, ed. *Abortion and Sterilization.* London: Academic Press; 1981. www.elsevier.com/books/abortion-and-sterilization/hodgson/978-0-12-792030-6. Accessed March 31, 2020.

8. Schoen J. Living through some giant change: the establishment of abortion services. *Am J Public Health.* 2013;**103** (3):416–425. doi:10.2105/AJPH.2012.301173

9. Landy U, Lewit S. Administrative, counseling and medical practices in National Abortion Federation facilities. *Fam Plann Perspect.* 1982;**14** (5):257–262.

10. Burkman RT, King TM, Burnett LS, Atienza MF. University abortion programs: one year later. *Am J Obstet Gynecol.* 1974;**119**(1):131–136. doi:10.1016/0002-9378(74) 90327-5

11. Donovan MK. *In Real Life: Federal Restrictions on Abortion Coverage and the Women They Impact.* Washington, DC: Guttmacher Institute; 2017:7. www.guttmacher.org/sites/default/files/article_files/gpr2000116.pdf

12. Freedman L, Langton C, Landy U, Ly E, Rocca C. Abortion care policies and enforcement in U.S. obstetrics–gynecology teaching hospitals: a national survey. *Contraception.* 2017;**96** (4):265. doi:10.1016/j.contraception.2017.07.017

13. Jones RK, Jerman J. Abortion incidence and service availability in the United States, 2014. *Perspect Sex Reprod Health.* 2017;**49**(1):17–27. doi:10.1363/psrh.12015

14. Zekman P. The abortion profiteers. *Chicago Sun-Times*; November 12, 1978. http://dlib.nyu.edu/undercover/abortion-profiteers-pamela-zekman-pamela-warrick-chicago-sun-times. Accessed March 31, 2020.

15. Clendinen D. Abortion clinic bombings have caused disruption for many. *New York Times*; February 6, 1985:14.

16. Grimes DA, Forrest JD, Kirkman AL, Radford B. An epidemic of antiabortion violence in the United States. *Am J Obstet Gynecol.* 1991;**165** (5 Pt 1):1263–1268. doi:10.1016/0002-9378(91) 90346-s

17. Grimes DA. Clinicians who provide abortions: the thinning ranks. *Obstet Gynecol.* 1992;**80** (4):719–723.

18. Committee on Health Care for Underserved Women. ACOG Committee Opinion No. 612: abortion training and education. *Obstet Gynecol.* 2014;**124**(5):1055–1059. doi:10.1097/01.AOG.0000456327.96480.18

19. Herbitter C, Bennett A, Schubert FD, Bennett IM, Gold M. Management of early pregnancy failure and induced abortion by family medicine

educators. *J Am Board Fam Med*. 2013;**26**(6):751–758. doi:10.3122/jabfm.2013.06.120248

20. AAFP Home | American Academy of Family Physicians. www.aafp.org/home.html. Accessed April 3, 2020.

21. www.govinfo.gov › CREC-1996-03-19-pt1-PgS2268

22. www.govinfo.gov/content/pkg/CREC-1996-03-19/html/CREC-1996-03-19-pt1-PgS2268.htm

23. Wessell NY. The triad of medicine. *N Engl J Med*. 1957;**257**(13):603–605. doi:10.1056/NEJM195709262571305

24. Fellowship in Family Planning National Office, 2019 Program Data.

25. Kenneth J. Ryan Residency Training Program in Family Planning and Abortion National Office, 2019 Program Data.

26. Landy U. Is family planning a subspecialty of obstetrics and gynecology? *Contraception*. 2005;**72**(6):399–401.

27. Lathrop E, Landy U. The Fellowship in Family Planning. *Int J Gynaecol Obstet*. 2013;**121**(1):10–13. doi:10.1016/j.ijgo.2012.12.005

28. Schulz KF, Grimes DA. *The Lancet Handbook of Essential Concepts in Clinical Research*. Philadelphia: Elsevier; 2006.

29. *The Belmont Report: Ethical Principles and Guidelines for the Protection of Human Subjects of Research*; 1979. www.hhs.gov/ohrp/regulations-and-policy/belmont-report/read-the-belmont-report/index.html#.

30. Papaya Workshop. About Papaya Workshop. http://papayaworkshop.org/. Accessed April 3, 2020.

31. ACGME. Accreditation Data System (ADS). https://apps.acgme.org/ads/Public/Reports/Report/3. Accessed April 3, 2020.

32. Zeldovich VB, Rocca CH, Langton C, Landy U, Ly E, Freedman L. Abortion policies in United States teaching hospitals: formal and informal parameters beyond the law. *Obstet Gynecol*. 2020;**135**(6):1296–1305. doi:10.1097/AOG.0000000000003876

33. Steinauer J, Dehlendorf C, Grumbach K, Landy U, Darney P. Multi-specialty family planning training: collaborating to meet the needs of women. *Contraception*. 2012;**86**(3):188–190. doi:10.1016/j.contraception.2011.12.001

34. Guiahi M, Westover C, Lim S, Westhoff CL. The New York City mayoral abortion training initiative at public hospitals. *Contraception*. 2012;**86**(5):577–582. doi:10.1016/j.contraception.2012.02.010

35. Guiahi M, Lim S, Westover C, Gold M, Westhoff CL. Enablers of and barriers to abortion training. *J Grad Med Educ*. 2013;**5**(2):238–243. doi:10.4300/JGME-D-12-00067.1

36. Fellowship in Complex Family Planning. General Requirements for a Post-Graduate Program in the Subspecialty Area of Complex Family Planning. 2019.

Chapter

4

The Medical Community, Abortion and the Crucial Role of Physician Advocacy

Philip D. Darney and Carole Joffe

4.1 Introduction

Recognition of abortion as a legitimate component of health care has been dependent on physicians' attitudes and activism. In the nineteenth century, physicians were the dominant voice calling for criminalization of abortion. In the twentieth century, physicians were among the leading voices promoting abortion's legalization and integration into medical practice through patient care and training. In the twenty-first century, as legal abortion is again threatened in the USA, the medical community continues its advocacy efforts in a variety of important ways, as described in this chapter

4.2 The Nineteenth-Century Campaign for Criminalization of Abortion

Until the early 1800s, abortion was a common and accepted practice in many countries. In the USA, abortion was largely unregulated and was acceptable until a pregnant woman felt "quickening" – a standard that was seldom enforced. Abortion was provided by a variety of practitioners including midwives, healers, homeopaths and an assortment of medically untrained individuals, as well as university-trained physicians [1].

In the USA, the movement for the criminalization of abortion came with the founding of the American Medical Association (AMA) in 1847. The new organization made outlawing abortion one of its first and highest priorities. The proponents of criminalization argued abortion was both an immoral and medically dangerous practice because of the incompetence of many abortionists as well as the risks undertaken by women attempting self-abortion. This AMA campaign should be primarily understood as a key component of a larger battle then underway: the attempt

of "regular" or "elite" physicians who had undergone "official" training to attain dominance over the wide range of "irregular" practitioners, some offering abortions [2,3].

During the same period, medical schools, which had previously been private, for-profit, unregulated enterprises, began to affiliate with universities. In 1910, the Flexner Report urged reform of US medical education through stronger standards, including state regulation, and rigorous examinations for licenses to practice. Physicians who had formal academic training, rather than the traditional apprenticeships, sought to improve the standing of their profession and exclude the informally trained by insisting on formal medical school education [1].

Growing societal anxiety in the mid- and late nineteenth century about the flood of immigrants with their large families to the USA from southern and eastern European countries was another element that helped the AMA's campaign find receptive ears in state legislatures. In the industrialized countries, the demographic transition of the mid-1800s led to smaller families among the more affluent. Where immigration was an important component of population growth, this trend toward smaller family size contrasted with the high fertility of recent immigrants. No effective contraception existed at that time. White, married, Protestant middle- and upper-class women used abortion to space and limit births. This practice was contrary to the perceived role of women as mothers and raised concern that poor immigrants would soon outnumber the "better classes" of society [1,3]. Accordingly, control over reproduction, as well as professionalization, became a justification of the medical crusade against abortion. Around this time, Catholic and many Protestant doctrines were reinterpreted to judge abortion, though widely practiced, as immoral [4].

4.3 The Century of Criminalization and Subsequent Push for Re-legalization

By the 1870s, the AMA's campaign had successfully won over politicians in state legislatures, and abortion was illegal in every US state. The new laws stipulated that the only legally permitted abortions were those that were approved by hospital-based physicians in extremely limited circumstances. The newly professionalized physicians soon organized themselves into academic specialties to achieve further distinction from lesser-trained physicians who were not university educated. The first examples from obstetrics and gynecology were the American Gynecological Club (AGC), organized in 1911, and its British counterpart, the Gynaecologic Visiting Society, with the purpose of scholarly communication among leading obgyn departments of the USA and Britain. These organizations and those that came later, like the American Gynecological and Obstetrical Society and the American and Royal Colleges of Obstetricians and Gynecologists, joined in condemnation of abortion as medically dangerous until, decades later, they could no longer ignore the toll illegal abortion took on women's lives.

During this era of criminalization, abortion was not eliminated in the USA; rather, illegality inevitably led to clandestine, incompetent abortions that burdened the hospitals, caused thousands of maternal deaths yearly and left a legacy of contempt for abortionists that persisted after legalization. However, not all those who provided illegal abortions were incompetent; there were also "doctors of conscience," well-trained physicians who performed abortions not for profit but because of compassion for women and revulsion at the deaths and injuries they experienced in the hospital emergency rooms of that period [5].

By the 1960s, much of the medical community as well as the public became frustrated with the inability of American women to obtain a legal, safe abortion, even when a pregnancy was threatened with severe fetal deformities from exposure to drugs like thalidomide or infections like rubella. Wealthy women traveled to countries where abortion was either legal or unpunished, Holland, Sweden and Japan, for example [6]. A few US physicians did illegal abortions in their offices or in hospitals under the guise of other procedures and by inventing indications other than pregnancy, risking their reputations, positions and imprisonment [7]. Most physicians of that era, particularly obstetrician-gynecologists (ob-gyns) who worked in "safety net" hospitals, witnessed in their daily practices the disastrous results of illegal abortion: estimates of the number of women who died each year ranged from 1,000 to 10,000 [8]. Countless others suffered serious medical complications, often leading to hysterectomy and infertility [9].

A major demonstration of physician advocacy and support of legalization occurred at an international meeting convened by John D. Rockefeller III in Hot Springs, Virginia, in 1967. Leaders in gynecology from the UK and USA gathered with legal experts to explore potential strategies toward legalization, safety and access [10].

Doctors who did the few hospital-approved abortions found themselves operating in a gray area, not sure whether such abortions were truly legal. This ambiguity is vividly illustrated by the "San Francisco Nine" of 1966 – an early example of the critical role of physician advocacy for abortion that is the topic of this chapter. These nine gynecologists, faculty at the University of California, San Francisco (UCSF), School of Medicine, did abortions for patients who had contracted rubella during their pregnancies. Rubella, or "German measles," a normally mild disease of children, had not long before been recognized as a cause of severe fetal deformities when contracted by women in the first trimester of pregnancy. The abortions done by these doctors came to the attention of a strongly anti-abortion member of the California Board of Medical Examiners, and the nine doctors were threatened with the loss of their licenses [1,11].

But the threat backfired spectacularly as leaders in academic medicine in California and around the USA mobilized to support their accused nine San Francisco colleagues – an unprecedented show of support for legal abortion within the medical community. More than 200 medical leaders signed an amicus brief, backed up by a legal defense fund, stating: "The Board's action is an unconstitutional interference with the freedom of the licensed physician to prescribe and administer sound and scientific medical treatment, and with the right of the patient to benefit from the best medical care that modern science can provide" [11].

The leader of the accuseds' defense, a professor of obstetrics and gynecology at UCSF, Dr. Edmund Overstreet, stated to the *New York Times*: "We do not believe that violation of an archaic statute is unprofessional conduct, nor that it is unprofessional for a physician to conduct himself in accord with the ethics of the community, the wishes of patients, and the best medical judgment of doctors" [quoted in 11].

The charges against the nine San Francisco doctors were withdrawn, but the incident helped to precipitate the California legislature's reformation of the state's abortion law to conform with a model suggested by the American Bar Association. It required that hospital "therapeutic abortion committees" review and approve women's applications for abortion in light of their physical and mental health [12]. The new law, signed by the future Republican US president Ronald Reagan, reflected the influence of physician leaders, particularly academic ob-gyns, on abortion legality as a key issue in reproductive health. Shortly after the change in the law, Philip Goldstein, chief obstetrician at San Francisco General Hospital, and Gary Stewart, a resident, organized research to demonstrate its effect on women's health [13,14]. Subsequent research worldwide has continued to support legal abortion as a critical element in reducing maternal mortality [15]. (See Chapter 2.)

Physician mobilization for abortion reform continued at a national level. About the same time as the San Francisco Nine incident, doctors in New York, including the eminent gynecologist Professor Alan Guttmacher, chair at Mt. Sinai, formed one of the first prochoice medical organizations, the Association for the Study of Abortion, which supported legalization and published advice on the most effective approaches to advocate for it [16]. (See the Appendix to this chapter for a current guide.)

As additional states legalized abortion, physicians practicing where it was still outlawed began to refer their patients to newly established abortion services in the "abortion reform" states – New York and Washington, DC, in the East and Colorado and California in the West. Voluntary organizations like the Clergy Consultation Service, a New York–based group, guided women from states where abortion remained illegal to legal abortion services in the "liberal states." Obstetricians in states like Georgia, where one author (PD) practiced prior to *Roe*, relied on the Clergy Consultation Service to refer patients from women's clinics known throughout the Southeast as access points to this "underground gateway" to safe, legal abortion, usually in New York.

Because physician training, even of obstetricians, had seldom included abortion, most US doctors had no skills in this previously illegal care. Those familiar with abortion were often immigrant physicians, usually from Eastern Europe, where abortion had been legalized in response to stringent German National Socialist (Nazi) prohibitions of it during their domination of Europe. These physicians worked in US hospitals where they could train some residents in the newly legal surgery, but they also opened freestanding clinics to accommodate the growing referrals to "legal states" from all over the nation. Other physicians were self-taught, developing their skills from the long-standing gynecologic practice of dilating the cervix and emptying the uterus with a sharp curette (D&C) and supplementing that common procedure with suction evacuation at earlier gestations and with forceps at later gestations. Some of these academic obstetricians described their techniques in scholarly publications. [4,17,18].

After a few states and the District of Columbia legalized abortion, medical professional organizations, first the American College of Obstetricians and Gynecologists (ACOG) in 1968, then the AMA in 1970, called for the legalization of abortion nationwide. Leading academic obstetrician-gynecologists prepared their colleagues for legalization with "A Statement on Abortion by One Hundred Professors of Obstetrics," published in April 1972 in the *American Journal of Obstetrics and Gynecology* [19]. Its authors included nearly all the chairs of academic departments of obstetrics and gynecology at the nation's medical schools, including those in states like Alabama, Kansas, Mississippi, Oklahoma and Texas that decades later would restrict access and training in safe abortion.

The 100 Professors statement estimated the numbers of legal abortions needed and described the responsibilities and capacities of their colleagues to provide them, writing "It is our hope that ... physicians prepare for the demand that will be placed upon them ... by the rapidly lessening governmental control of abortion practices." Familiar with the emergency care of women with complications from illegal abortions, they rightly observed that legalization would free up hospital space used to treat complications of illegal abortions to provide safe, legal ones outside of operating rooms with suction under local anesthesia. Their estimations of about one million legal abortions yearly and rapid decreases in maternal mortality (see Chapter 2) were presciently accurate, but their hopes for the role of hospitals, where they led the US obstetrics and gynecology training programs, were not.

4.4 Physician Advocacy after *Roe* v. *Wade*

As the 100 Professors expected, the Supreme Court, in its 1973 *Roe* v. *Wade* decision, legalized abortion. Though they and the prochoice medical community, particularly the previously mentioned "doctors of conscience" [5] who had provided illegal abortions at considerable personal risk, were elated by this decision, things did not go as the 100 Professors had optimistically predicted. Most abortions occurred in freestanding clinics where training and medical research were unlikely to occur. Despite the effective advocacy of academic obstetricians to make abortion legal, a generation of their students and resident physicians had limited access to abortion training – a situation that would persist in many programs for a generation until in 1995 training was required by the Accreditation Council for Graduate Medical Education (ACGME) for all ob-gyn residents and the Ryan Residency Training Program gradually brought abortion services and training to more and more of them. (See Chapters 1, 3 and 5.)

As one of us (PD) has earlier written, "Academic departments of obstetrics and gynecology [did not] welcome skilled abortionists to their ranks. Even though abortion was now legal, a stigma remained on those who had earlier performed illegal abortions" [20]. There was almost immediate response to the *Roe* v. *Wade* decision from Congress with the passage of the Coats Amendment in 1973 (which stipulated no penalties for hospitals or individuals refusing to provide abortions) and the Hyde Amendment in 1976 (which prohibited the use of federal funds for abortion except under very strict circumstances). These actions made clear to a conflict-averse profession that the abortion issue was bound to be contentious, and the obvious controversy dampened enthusiasm for establishing teaching hospital abortion services. Some prochoice doctors were put in the position of having to sue their own hospitals in order for legal abortions to take place [5].

To be sure, several leaders did establish abortion services to serve women and train residents. Notable among them was Prof. Kenneth J. Ryan, chief obstetrician at Boston Hospital for Women of Harvard Medical School (later Brigham and Women's Hospital) at the time *Roe* v. *Wade* was decided [21]. He had earlier persuaded hospital leaders in Cleveland and San Diego to allow abortions under some circumstances in response to the outcome of rubella infections and thalidomide use in the 1960s. Promptly after the *Roe* decision, Prof. Ryan instituted an abortion service at the Boston Lying-in Hospital and required training of all his residents. He later chaired the advisory committee of the resident training program to ensure national availability of ACGME-required abortion training – the program that bears his name. (See Chapter 3.) Other obgyn department chairs also organized abortion services at leading teaching hospitals, including Parkland in Dallas, Johns Hopkins in Baltimore, Grady in Atlanta, Washington Hospital in DC and others, but many of these programs did not survive the backlash against abortion legalization of the Coats and Hyde amendments. Academic obstetricians remained advocates but provided abortions in their teaching hospitals only under special circumstances and, therefore, accomplished little abortion training.

4.5 Physicians' Organizational Advocacy for Abortion

In the decades after *Roe*, academic medical programs persisted in refraining from providing abortions. As of 2017, only 5% of abortions took place in hospitals or private doctors' offices. The freestanding clinics that provide the overwhelming majority of abortions have achieved an excellent safety record and are cost-effective; however, this separation of abortion care from mainstream medicine contributed to the marginalization of abortion services and limited for a generation training opportunities until the founding in 1999 of the Kenneth J. Ryan Residency Training Program. (See Chapters 3 and 9.)

In response to this marginalization, leading academic obstetricians embarked on a new series of abortion advocacy activities. One of the first of these was the founding by Prof. Seymour Romney, chair at Einstein College of Medicine in New York, of the Society of Physicians for Reproductive Choice and Health (now Physicians for Reproductive Health, PRH) in 1992. This organization gave physicians a platform to present evidence of the importance of legal abortion to women's health and to lobby state and national politicians on the need for safe abortion with a major focus of promoting physicians' voices in public debates about abortion. Through its Leadership Training Academy, PRH has taught hundreds of physicians to write op-eds and letters to the editor, appear in the media and offer expert testimony to state legislatures and others considering abortion-related measures. In its first decade, the majority of its trainees were Family Planning fellows (see Chapter 5) who considered the course and its resulting advocacy activities a highlight of their training. These physicians have embraced their roles as advocates for their patients and for evidence-based abortion practice as a central professional obligation. PRH is now led by a Fellowship program graduate, Dr. Jamila Perritt.

The standards for training for the newly certified and accredited Fellowship in Family Planning (FFP) subspecialty, renamed as the Fellowship in Complex Family Planning, acknowledge the importance of professional advocacy for these future leaders in family planning. (See Chapter 5.)

4.6 Institutional Advocacy in Clinical Departments, Hospitals and Medical Schools

While the public advocacy forum is essential for legislative and legal action, advocacy also must occur in the hospitals where physicians provide abortion care. Fellowship training must include this "institutional advocacy" to contend with the practical problems of providing abortion care and training at teaching hospitals, particularly in states with restrictive policies toward abortion [22,23]. This form of advocacy ranges from convincing reluctant hospital administrators to permit abortion care up to the state's gestational limit; to negotiating with department chairs in restrictive states to begin a "Ryan Abortion Training" program; to assuring that there will be cooperating nurses and anesthesiologists in the operating room for medically complicated abortions and those later in pregnancy.

One of the most delicate – and desperate – of such local advocacy efforts occurs in those situations where abortions are permitted only because of a threat to a woman's life – and the attending physician has to convince others that the patient's death is likely imminent [24]. To give a sense of the complexity of the "institutional advocacy" required from providers in hospital settings, a national study by a team of UCSF researchers found that in order to offer abortion in the second trimester or later, the patient's physician typically had to secure permission from some combination of the maternal-fetal medicine specialists in the hospital, the chair of obstetrics, the hospital ethics committee, a special abortion committee and hospital lawyers. This involved process, even if successful, delays treatment of the threatened woman until approval for abortion is secured from all of these officials [25].

4.6.1 Influencing Hospital Policy

When abortion policy is developed by hospital leadership, family planning experts can contribute to evidence-based decisions. Their knowledge of research as well as of clinical and patient access implications is critical, but also important are respect for formal and informal institutional policies and familiarity with statements by professional organizations. For example, a reminder of the ACGME's training and educational mandates [26] for family planning along with the ACOG's statement that abortion services are an important component of women's health care [27,28] affirms the importance of abortion in gynecologic training and practice:

Facts are very important, especially when discussing the health of women and the American public. The fact is, abortion is an essential component of women's health care.

The American College of Obstetricians and Gynecologists (ACOG), with over 57,000 members, maintains the highest standards of clinical practice and continuing education for the nation's women's health physicians. Abortion care is included in medical training, clinical practice, and continuing medical education.

4.7 Institutional Advocacy in Response to Legislative Interference

In the past ten years, the US federal and state legislatures have enacted more than 400 laws that intervene in the health care of women and the physician–patient relationship. They typically require physicians to provide to patients information that is not scientifically supported, mandate uncomfortable and useless diagnostic tests and medications and require inappropriate office visits and waiting periods.

Residency program directors and chairs play key roles in institutional response to legislative initiatives that threaten education and practice. These department leaders can advocate with a broader audience to which other physicians may not have access. They can consult with national colleagues who may have had experience at their own medical schools and university hospitals in contending with restrictions and political interference.

State academic medical centers rely on public funds for education and research programs and for support of the care of patients who are uninsured. When institutional leaders are able to draw on policies written by prestigious organizations such as the Association of American Medical Colleges (AAMC) [28], ACOG [29,27], ACGME [26] and the National Academy of Medicine (NAM) [30], they will likely feel prepared and more comfortable educating trustees and members of the legislature.

Other opportunities for advocacy are meetings with legislative liaisons to describe the clinical services provided by the reproductive health program, the prestige it brings to medical education and physician training and the competitive gains that accrue to the institution; a crucial role of the abortion leadership from Ryan and Fellowship programs in the academic medical center is to arm institutional leaders with information and language for even broader advocacy.

4.8 Confronting Stigma

Another advocacy-related task facing Fellowship in Family Planning graduates – in the hospital setting, at professional meetings, with individual patients, and in conversation with the general public – is countering the pervasive abortion stigma in American society [31]. Dr. Lisa Harris, who leads the Fellowship in Family Planning at the University of Michigan, has been one of the most creative leaders in this effort. (See Chapter 24.) She has developed workshops for fellows and others to share feelings about their work, including the stigma they face [32]. She also led a team exploring the most effective messages for abortion providers to reach various audiences, including their own institutional leaders. This chapter's Appendix presents the team's suggestions for physician communications on abortion.

4.9 The Society of Family Planning's Role in Advocacy

In order to pursue subspecialty status for the Fellowship in Family Planning (FFP), a professional society, similar to those of other obgyn subspecialties, was required. Accordingly, the Society of Family Planning (SFP) was established in 2004 to give graduated fellows a scholarly forum for presentation of their research and to provide funding for research in areas like abortion, where government support is restricted. Sixteen years after its founding, the membership was 60% physicians, most from the FFP community, but also including some non-FFP clinicians and many social scientists from a broad range of disciplines. SFP grew over two decades into the leading organization for those who investigate clinical and social aspects of abortion and contraception.

Though the advocacy activities of SFP are less directly political than those of some other organizations, its support for and promotion of research that provides the evidence base for political and judicial advocacy is critical. Its annual meeting has become the primary US forum on the clinical, policy and social science aspects of family planning. Research and publications as a result of its grants and in the SFP's journal, *Contraception*, have lent weight and legitimacy to all aspects of clinical and social research in family planning and are often cited in policy and legal decisions. (See Chapters 6 and 7.)

4.10 Creating the Evidence Base for Advocacy

An example of the importance of the evidence produced by the Fellowship is the National Academy of Medicine's 2017 report, *The Safety and Quality of Abortion Care in the United States*, where nearly one third of 500 international citations of studies of abortion were published by members and graduates of the Fellowship in Family Planning and its associated medical school academic departments [30]. The editors of *Obstetrics and Gynecology*, the leading obgyn specialty journal, in an analysis of the importance of the various subspecialties' contributions to the science it had published, found family planning literature to have the highest "impact factor" [33].

4.11 The Fellowship in Family Planning's Inter-professional Collaborations

In 2012, in response to the alarming increase in legislative interference with medical practice, specifically family planning services and training as described above, the Fellowship in Family Planning convened the first Academic Leadership meeting (ALM), a gathering of scholarly organizations including ACOG, the Council on Resident Education in Obstetrics and Gynecology (CREOG), the American Gynecological and Obstetrical Society (AGOS), the Association of Professors of Gynecology and Obstetrics (APGO) and department chairs representing states which suffered some of the most severe legislative attacks. Since then, the ALM has met annually and has grown to include all of the subspecialty societies in obstetrics and gynecology, for example, Maternal-fetal Medicine (MFM) and Reproductive Endocrinology and Infertility (REI), and relevant pediatric and nursing groups. The deliberations of this group of eleven academic professional societies affirmed the importance of comprehensive women's health care, including abortion [34].

Since 1982, ACOG has held an annual Congressional Leadership Conference (CLC) where a growing number of Fellowship in Family Planning physicians learn about the legislative process, meet with legislative representatives and develop skills in opinion and editorial writing and social media as advocacy tools.

4.12 Continued Advocacy by Academic Obstetrician-Gynecologists

In further response to increasing restriction of abortion access and training, leading academic obstetrician-gynecologists published a reassessment of the "100 Professors" statement in the same *American Journal of Obstetrics and Gynecology*

where the first 100 had commented 40 years earlier [35]. It, too, was authored by "100 Professors," but missing this time were those from medical schools in several states that had in the 40-year interim restricted abortion access and training. Professors from these states said they were reluctant to sign on because of fears of reprisals from their legislatures such as reductions in funding for indigent women's obstetrical care through the Affordable Care Act, for family planning clinics through Title X and for their own medical schools. The new statement examined the original one "in light of medical advances and legal changes" and suggested a "further course of action for obstetricians and gynecologists . . . in consideration of current legislative threats to the autonomy of our patient relationships, to evidence-based medical practice, to the training of our students and residents, and ultimately to the health of our patients" [35]. They affirmed their academic responsibilities to:

(1) teach future practitioners about all methods of contraception and about uterine evacuation throughout pregnancy, which ranges from miscarriage management to emergent evacuations and the treatment of complications in accordance with our professional mandate from the Accreditation Council for Graduate Medical Education;

(2) provide evidence-based information to all patients who seek family planning or pregnancy termination;

(3) provide evidenced-based information to legislators who propose laws requiring inaccurate information or unindicated procedures for women seeking to terminate a pregnancy;

(4) insist that the hospitals where we care for women and teach students and residents admit patients who require hospital-based pregnancy terminations, and

(5) ensure the availability of all methods of contraception, particularly long-acting reversible contraception (LARC) methods, to reduce the need for abortion.

4.13 The American College of Obstetricians and Gynecologists (ACOG)

ACOG is considered the most powerful legislative presence in advocating for women's health, and was the first physician organization to advocate for women's access to contraception and abortion. ACOG has trained Family Planning Fellows in advocacy efforts and also used the fellows' specialized expertise to educate their membership through committee publications, roundtable discussions and presentations at ACOG's Annual Clinical Meeting. Graduated fellows serve on national committee positions and in ACOG district leadership positions poised to pursue national leadership. To gain more skills in political advocacy, forty-eight fellows have spent a month at ACOG in Washington, DC. Over the years, collaborations with the FFP led to the ACOG LARC initiative, participation of growing numbers of fellows and Fellowship graduates in ACOG's advocacy programs and a dedicated one-year post-Fellowship advocacy rotation for a graduated fellow – the Darney-Landy ACOG Fellowship, named after the Fellowship in Family Planning's founders.

To demonstrate its commitment to family planning access in women's health, the president of ACOG has spoken to the annual meeting of the FFP every year since the Fellowship was founded. This address serves to introduce the community of fellows and Fellowship graduates to the professional organization, which defines and promotes evidence-based practice of care and advocates on behalf of the specialty with both state and national policy makers. ACOG has taken stands on other abortion-related issues in past years: for example, ACOG has spoken out forcefully against state bans on the most common second-trimester abortion procedure (dilation and evacuation), against legislative interference in open and truthful informed consent regarding abortion and against other restrictions on abortion practice that endanger women [36]. In the wake of the rise of self-managed abortions in recent years, ACOG has called for women making such attempts to not be criminally prosecuted [36].

4.14 Medical Student Advocacy of Abortion Care and Training

The leading student family planning advocacy effort in the USA is Medical Students for Choice (MSFC), organized in 1993 by a group of medical students led by Jody Steinauer at UCSF. The first murder of an abortion doctor that spring and outrage at a vulgar antiabortion pamphlet sent to many medical students by an extremist group were primary motivations for MSFC's founding. (See Chapters 20 and 21.) MSFC began by requesting more teaching about abortion and contraception in medical education. These topics had often been ignored in medical school curriculae. Since 1993, MSFC has spread to hundreds of medical school campuses in the USA and, more recently, globally, and has expanded its activities to include internships at academic medical centers that are Ryan Program or Fellowship in Family Planning sites, where they often participate in abortion and contraception research. MSFC also provides students opportunities to learn the fundamentals of family planning care at its regional and national conferences, where they learn about the clinical and social aspects of abortion as well as the role of advocacy. These experiences have inspired MSFC members from all over the USA to pursue residencies in obstetrics and gynecology at institutions having Ryan abortion training. Many Fellowship in Family Planning applicants started as MSFC chapter founders, participants or leaders.

4.15 National Abortion Federation

The National Abortion Federation (NAF), founded in 1977, is an abortion advocacy organization representing freestanding clinics. NAF advocates for both abortion patients and providers and educates the public about abortion. Although not involved in formal medical education that is the topic of this book, NAF, in its early days under the direction of Dr. Uta Landy, brought together academic experts in public health (eg, from the Centers for Disease Control and Prevention) and clinical aspects of abortion and physicians from freestanding clinics to establish evidence-based standards for abortion care at periodic seminars. NAF has welcomed the participation of fellows both on its board and staff with medical director positions, as well as in leading evidence-based workshops. Fellows have become advocates for research with a community of practitioners whose pioneering work was steeped in clinical experience.

One of NAF's most significant advocacy events took place in 1990, when the organization, in collaboration with ACOG and with funding from the Ford and George Gund foundations, held a symposium on the predicted shortage of abortion providers available to work in member clinics as the early practitioners aged. The symposium brought together, for the first time, leaders from academic medicine and the professional organizations including NAF, Planned Parenthood, ACOG, the Council on Resident Education in Obstetrics and Gynecology (CREOG) and the Accreditation Council for Graduate Medical Education (ACGME) to consider workforce and training issues regarding abortion. Symposium participants emphasized the need for abortion training in obgyn residency programs and the need for systematic inclusion of abortion in CREOG standards and evaluations, encouraging the eventual ACGME mandate (1996) for abortion training in obgyn residency programs. Thirty years after the meeting, the Ryan and Fellowship in Family Planning programs have achieved most of the goals set for training. For example, ACGME set standards for the Fellowship in Family Planning in the newly accredited obgyn subspecialty of Complex Family Planning specifically for training in the science and practice of abortion and contraception. (See Chapters 3 and 5.)

4.16 Abortion Advocacy in Family Medicine

Obstetrician-gynecologists and their organizations have taken primary responsibility for physician family planning advocacy efforts. The two family medicine professional groups did not promote abortion care or advocacy but individual practitioners have. For example, the Reproductive Health Access Project (RHAP), which was founded in 2005, grew out of family medicine physicians' efforts to enhance abortion training and provision in primary care using the model of the Ryan Program for obgyn residents. Similarly, the Reproductive Health Education in Family Medicine (RHEDI) program, founded around the same time, established abortion training in some family medicine residencies. These training activities by RHAP and RHEDI are supplemented by lectures and advocacy of abortion-related issues at meetings of the American Academy of Family Medicine and the Society of Teachers of Family Medicine. (See Chapter 15.)

4.17 Advocacy in Courts of Law

Though, as this chapter argues, there has always been a need for physician advocacy, this need dramatically increased beginning in 2010 with the passage of hundreds of new state restrictions on abortion care. These legislative measures, which addressed, among other things, hospital abortion policy and training, created opportunities for physicians from SFP and the Fellowship in Family Planning to testify before state legislatures to oppose restrictive legislation. After the enactment of restrictions, pro-choice physicians similarly testified before state and federal courts, including the US Supreme Court, to argue that the new laws are threats to women's health and autonomy and ought to be invalidated. Research from the Fellowship is often cited as evidence against restrictive legislation.

In 2016, as the Supreme Court was preparing to hear the landmark *Whole Woman's Health* case, which addressed admitting privileges and ambulatory surgery center requirements in Texas, collaborative research between physicians and social scientists at the University of Texas and other universities, and the participation of a UCSF family planning professor, Daniel Grossman, as an expert witness, were repeatedly cited by the Court as reason to rule these restrictions unconstitutional. The *Whole Woman's Health* v. *Hellerstedt* case provides a recent and compelling example of the power of evidence in court determinations. This case was appealed to the US Supreme Court by the State of Texas. At trial, research and testimony from SFP scientists was conclusive in setting aside a Texas law that would have reduced the number of abortion clinics in this large and populous state by two thirds, with devastating effects on the women of Texas.

Other examples of expert testimony by SFP members and Fellowship in Family Planning graduates include the federal Partial-Birth Abortion Ban Act, which was enacted, but has had little effect on abortion practice, and legislation, enacted in twenty-three states, requiring that women under age eighteen obtain parental consent to terminate a pregnancy. Evidence-based testimony about parental consent has succeeded in blocking harmful legislation in a number of states, including California.

This Supreme Court research and testimony from the Fellowship in Family Planning continued in the US Supreme Court Louisiana case, *June Medical Services L. L. C. et al* v. *Russo* which, like Texas, required admitting privileges and was refuted. Moreover, many former Fellowship in Family Planning fellows serve as expert witnesses in court cases and offer testimony before state legislatures. Specific examples include former fellows' evidence-based testimony in favor of medication abortion via telemedicine and against the progestogen "abortion reversal" messages required in some state-mandated abortion consent. Research specific to these legislative questions provides the base for advocacy. For example, data developed by researchers at the UCSF supported the successful campaign that saw the passage in California of a bill mandating that the state's public universities and four-year colleges offer medication abortion at their health centers.

4.18 Physician Advocacy Efforts in Other Countries

The USA provides more examples of the role of physician advocacy than any other country. But family planning doctors all over the world have been instrumental in changing restrictive abortion laws and arguing to judges, politicians and societies that access to safe abortion is critical to women's health. (See Chapter 2.) Other chapters in this book demonstrate that physicians in Colombia, Uruguay, Mexico, Nepal, Ethiopia and Ghana, among many others, have provided expertise and passion to convince their public and politicians of the need for safe abortion. Global advocacy by physicians is demonstrated by their authorship of many influential books presenting the public health and ethical aspects of abortion, several of which are previously cited in this chapter [6,4,17,20].

Appendix 4.1 Countering Abortion Stigma
Lisa Harris, MD

Questions to Consider in Developing Your Advocacy Message

1. How can I talk about the shared values, related to health, family and helping others, that drive my work and shape who I am? (ie, being with people in life's important moments, called to help others in times of need)

2. How am I establishing my credibility/experience as a doctor who provides abortion care? (ie, type of practice, years of experience, providing a range of reproductive care or other medical care in addition to abortion care)

3. What can I share about myself and my life experience that fosters shared humanity and disrupts flawed beliefs about doctors who provide abortion care? (eg, person of faith, parent)

4. How can I describe my journey or motivations for including abortion care in the health-care work I do? (ie, life moments/experiences/values/learning that led you to provide abortion care as part of your practice)

5. How will I paint a picture of the process when women seek abortion care? What details can I include to contextualize abortion care as part of health care and women's health care broadly? What lived experiences can I share to disrupt flawed beliefs about people who seek abortion care and doctors who provide it? (ie, seeing women from all walks of life, involving women and their loved ones in care decisions, providing women with options/information/counseling/support, giving a woman time to decide or change her mind)

6. How can I normalize conflicted feelings? Am I modeling compassion and empathy for people who are conflicted about abortion, even if that's not how I feel? (ie, many people have complex and conflicting views on abortion, abortion can sometimes feel complicated and also be important and necessary in women's lives, life is complicated, no two situations are the same)

7. What leads me to feel called as a doctor to share my experience and speak out about this topic now? (e., duty as a doctor, commitment to patients, protecting patients from harm, ensuring laws are based on sound science and good medical practice)

(For further information, contact doctorstories@goodwinsimon.com.)

REFERENCES

1. Reagan LJ. *When Abortion Was a Crime: Women, Medicine, and Law in the United States, 1867–1973*. Berkeley: University of California Press; 1997.

2. Mohr JC. *Abortion in America: The Origins and Evolution of National Policy*. Oxford University Press; 1978.

3. Luker K. *Abortion and the Politics of Motherhood*. Berkeley: University of California Press; 1984.

4. Potts M, Diggory P, Peel J. *Abortion*. New York: Cambridge University Press; 1977.

5. Joffe C. *Doctors of Conscience*. Boston: Beacon Press; 1996.

6. Grimes D. *Every Third Woman in America: How Legal Abortion Transformed Our Nation*. Carolina Beach, NC: Daymark; 2014.

7. Joffe C. Physician provision of abortion before *Roe v. Wade*. *Res Sociol Health Care*. 1991;9:21–32.

8. Cates W, Rochat RW, Grimes DA, Tyler CW. Legalized abortion: effect on national trends of maternal and abortion-related mortality (1940 through 1976). *Am J Obstet Gynecol*. 1978;**132**(2):211–214. doi:10.1016/0002-9378(78)90926-2

9. Fathalla MF, Sinding SW, Rosenfield A, Fathalla MMF. Sexual and reproductive health for all: a call for action. *Lancet*. 2006;**368**(9552):2095–2100. doi:10.1016/S0140-6736(06)69483-X

10. Garrow DJ. *Liberty and Sexuality: The Right to Privacy and the Making of Roe v. Wade.* Berkeley: University of California Press; 1998.

11. Dynak H, Weitz T, Joffe C, Stewart F, Arons A. *Honoring San Francisco's Abortion Pinoeers.* San Francisco: UCSF Center for Reproductive Health Reseach & Policy; The Regents of the University of California; 2003.

12. Leavy Z, Kummer JM. Criminal abortion: human hardship and unyielding laws. *South Calif Law Rev.* 1962;**35**(123):24.

13. Stewart GK, Goldstein PJ. Therapeutic abortion in California. Effects of septic abortion and maternal mortality. *Obstet Gynecol.* 1971;**37**(4):510–514.

14. Goldstein P, Stewart G. Trends in therapeutic abortion in San Francisco. *Am J Public Health.* 1972;**62**(5):695–699. doi:10.2105/AJPH.62.5.695

15. Arulkumaran S, Hediger V, Manzoor A, May J. *Saving Mothers' Lives: Transforming Strategy into Action.* Global Health Policy Summit, Report of the Maternal Health Working Group. London: Imperial College; 2012.

16. Guttmacher AF. Abortion: odyssey of an attitude. *Fam Plann Perspect.* 1973;**4**:10–14.

17. Zatuchni GI, Sciarra JJ, Speidel JJ, eds. *Pregnancy Termination: Procedures, Safety, and New Developments.* Hagerstown, MD: Harper & Row; 1979.

18. Margolis AJ, Overstreet EW. Legal abortion without hospitalization. *Obstet Gynecol.* 1970;**36**(3):479–481.

19. A statement on abortion by one hundred professors of obstetrics. *Am J Obstet Gynecol.* 1972;**112**(7):992–998. doi:10.1016/0002-9378(72)90826-5

20. Darney PD, Training physicians in elective abortion technique in the United States. In U Landy, SS Ratnam (Eds.), *Prevention and Treatment of Contraceptive Failure: In Honor of Christopher Tietze.* New York: Plenum Press; 1986: 133–147.

21. Ryan KJ. Abortion or motherhood, suicide and madness. *Am J Obstet Gynecol.* 1992;**166**(4):1029–1036. doi:10.1016/s0002-9378(11)90587-0

22. Freedman L. *Willing and Unable: Doctors' Constraints in Abortion Care.* Nashville: Vanderbilt University Press; 2010.

23. Freedman L, Landy U, Darney P, Steinauer J. Obstacles to the integration of abortion into obstetrics and gynecology practice. *Perspect Sex Reprod Health.* 2010;**42**(3):146–151. doi:10.1363/4214610

24. Blackwell S, Louis JM, Norton ME, et al. Reproductive services for women at high risk for maternal mortality: a report of the workshop of the Society for Maternal-Fetal Medicine, the American College of Obstetricians and Gynecologists, the Fellowship in Family Planning, and the Society of Family Planning. *Am J Obstet Gynecol.* 2020;**222**(4): B2–B18. doi:10.1016/j.ajog.2019.12.008

25. Zeldovich VB, Rocca CH, Langton C, Landy U, Ly E, Freedman L. Abortion policies in United States teaching hospitals: formal and informal parameters beyond the law. *Obstet Gynecol.* 2020;**135**(5):1296–1305. doi:10.1097/AOG.0000000000003876

26. Clarification on Requirements Regarding Family Planning and Contraception Review Committee for Obstetrics and Gynecology. www.acgme.org/portals/0/pfassets/programresources/220_obgyn_abortion_training_clarification.pdf. Accessed June 2, 2019.

27. American College of Obstetricians and Gynecologists. College Statement of Policy. Abortion Policy. November 2014. www.acog.org/clinical-information/policy-and-position-statements/statements-of-policy/2017/abortion-policy

28. Association of American Medical Colleges. Accredited Medical Education Programs in the U.S. February 26, 2020. www.printfriendly.com/p/g/gK5Aec. Accessed April 8, 2020.

29. American College of Obstetricians and Gynecologists. Facts Are Important. Abortion Is Health Care. www.acog.org/-/media/Departments/Government-Relations-and-Outreach/FactsAreImportantABisHC.pdf?dmc=1&ts=20190803T1459203762. Accessed August 3, 2019.

30. National Academies of Sciences, Engineering, and Medicine, Health and Medicine Division, Board on Health Care Services, Board on Population Health and Public Health Practice, Committee on Reproductive Health Services: Assessing the Safety and Quality of Abortion Care in the U.S. *The Safety and Quality of Abortion Care in the United States.* Washington, DC: National Academies Press; 2018. www.ncbi.nlm.nih.gov/books/NBK507236/. Accessed March 30, 2020.

31. Norris A, Bessett D, Steinberg JR, Kavanaugh ML, De Zordo S, Becker D. Abortion stigma: a reconceptualization of constituents, causes, and consequences. *Womens Health Issues.* 2011;**21**(3 Suppl):S49–S54. doi:10.1016/j.whi.2011.02.010

32. Debbink MLP, Hassinger JA, Martin LA, Maniere E, Youatt E, Harris LH. Experiences with the Providers Share Workshop method: abortion worker support and research in tandem. *Qual Health Res.* 2016;**26**(13):1823–1837. doi:10.1177/1049732316661166

33. Parikh LI, Benner RS, Riggs TW, Hazen N, Chescheir NC. Subspecialty influence on scientific peer review for an obstetrics and gynecology journal with a high impact factor. *Obstet Gynecol.* 2017;**129**(2):243–248. doi:10.1097/AOG.0000000000001852

34. Espey E, Dennis A, Landy U. The importance of access to comprehensive reproductive health care, including abortion: a statement from women's health professional organizations. *Am J Obstet Gynecol.* 2019;**220**(1):67–70. doi:10.1016/j.ajog.2018.09.008

35. One Hundred Professors of Obstetrics and Gynecology. A statement on abortion by 100 professors of obstetrics: 40 years later. *Am J Obstet Gynecol.* 2013;**209**(3):193–199. doi:10.1016/j.ajog.2013.03.007

36. Cohen DS, Joffe C. *Obstacle Course.* Berkeley: University of California Press; 2020.

5

The US Fellowship in Family Planning as a Community of Practice

Uta Landy and Jody Steinauer

5.1 Background

Community is an essential concept of human interaction and productivity. It can be built around religion, political orientation, artistic interests and other shared beliefs and activities. Community creates a sense of belonging, connection and support, and allows groups to accomplish specific tasks.

In the USA, medical organization was initially propelled by the need to create standards of competence. (See Chapter 4.) The Flexner Report, addressing medical education and the responsibilities of the medical community regarding the education of its practitioners, led to major changes ensuring that medical education is based on scientific advancements in university-based medical schools and to produce a medical workforce prepared to lead reforms and changes in health care. Medical organizations were formed to accept and promote these responsibilities.

In the USA, these medical organizations gradually formed societies to represent specialties and subspecialties, to set learning objectives and standards of care and address questions of health-care policy. A major breakthrough occurred in the field of gynecology with scientific discoveries involving human reproduction and reproductive control, that is, the role of hormones to prevent pregnancy and the development of scientific techniques to terminate a pregnancy.

These advances in contraception and abortion, the development of new social norms regarding sexuality and the role of women and the tragic deaths of young women who did not want to be or remain pregnant led to advocacy efforts among established societies (eg, American College of Obstetricians and Gynecologists and the American Medical Association) and the formation of new medical societies and organizations to promote the legalization of contraception and abortion, and, once legalized, define standards of care. One such new organization, the National Abortion Federation, was launched to represent the emerging practitioners of abortion in outpatient settings, define practice standards within its community and create a community. (See Chapter 3.) Another organization to address training and access was the Fellowship in Family Planning.

5.2 The Fellowship in Family Planning

The Fellowship in Family Planning (FFP) began in 1991 with the founding of a first Fellowship site to establish advanced training in contraception and abortion, create medical leadership in the field and begin to create an academic professional community (Figures 5.1 and 5.2). Community and the support it provides become urgent and meaningful to practitioners when their clinical focus is controversial and stigmatized. Contraception and abortion are unique to medical practice in that they moved from illegal to legal status over the course of a century and continue to be embroiled in controversy decades after legalization, as is the case in the USA.

The FFP community can be considered a "community of practice," as described by a social learning theory about learning and identity formation within communities. The theory of communities of practice, originally articulated by Lave and Wenger [1], posits that learning is a social activity, takes place within communities and is influenced by culture. A community of practice is a "persistent, sustaining social network of individuals who share and develop an overlapping knowledge base, set of beliefs, values, history and experiences, focused on a common practice and/or mutual enterprise" [2]. In order to qualify as a community of practice, Wenger writes, the group must have mutual engagement by members, be

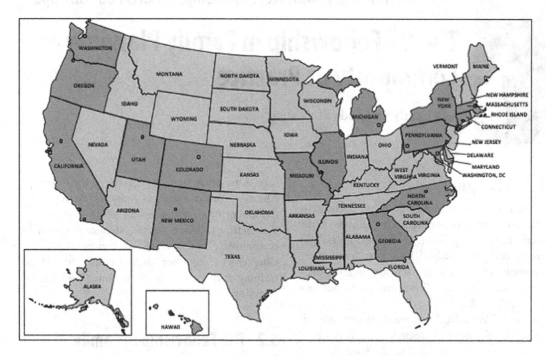

28 Ob-Gyn Fellowship sites in 17 states and Canada
2 Family Medicine Fellowship Sites

11/2019

Figure 5.1 Map of US Fellowship in Family Planning sites

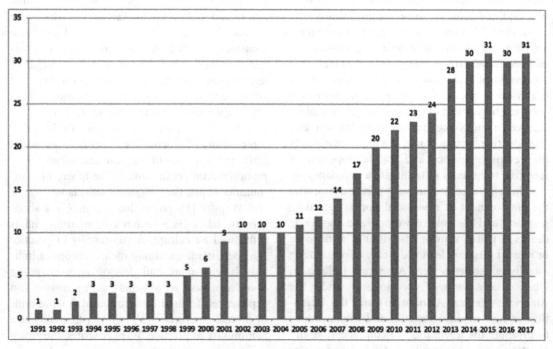

Figure 5.2 Growth of the US and Canadian Fellowship in Family Planning

focused on a joint enterprise that is negotiated by the community and have a shared repertoire – for example, shared language and ways of doing things – that the community has produced and has incorporated into its practice [3].

An individual joins the community and moves from being a peripheral, novice participant to being acknowledged as a full member.

Educational activities created by the group support new participants to adopt the knowledge, skills and identity shared by the group so they can become full members of the community. These educational activities additionally serve to further define the community's enterprise or goals.

Soon after the FFP formed an organizational structure by hiring a national director and staff, creating a National Office and Fellowship directors serving as an advisory board, creating structures and systems to promote a community of practice became an early priority. New fellows, having finished either obstetrics and gynecology residency or family medicine residency training, join the community after an application and selection process, based on a residency match system, with each fellow joining the Fellowship at an individual academic program. The fellow begins clinical and research training within the matched program and department like other US graduate medical education fellowships. Under the supervision of the local faculty mentor team, fellows take classes on research skills, design a research study and acquire clinical skills. The local institution and mentors support the fellow to meet the Fellowship learning objectives and goals.

In the early days of the FFP, when it lacked professional recognition and stature, directors and fellows could feel alone and surrounded by controversy within their teaching hospital or from other faculty. Support by the department chair, other faculty and administration could vary greatly. Over the years, and with the growth and recognition of the Fellowship, the family planning faculty and fellows have come to be respected and valued in their departments and institutions, demonstrated by the awards that fellows and Fellowship faculty receive from residents and others.

When the establishment of a Ryan Residency Training Program and its concomitant integration of family planning into the department became a requirement for the approval of new ob-gyn Fellowship sites, the groundwork to ensure institutional support and acceptance had been laid. In addition to the family planning community of each Fellowship site, the fellows' development into family planning experts and leaders is supported by the larger, national Fellowship community. The FFP intentionally developed programs and activities to ensure the community's ongoing learning and development. (See Table 5.1 and Chapter 3.)

5.3 Activities to Support the Family Planning Community of Practice

From the beginning of the FFP's operation, the community was brought together for learning, networking and providing support for graduated fellows, directors and novice members, which include both incoming and current fellows. The support encompasses the members' many roles as researchers, clinicians, academic educators, advocates and leaders in a newly developing subspecialty, recognizing that their work is innovative and groundbreaking, but sometimes controversial and stigmatized.

Table 5.1 summarizes the in-person and virtual meetings we describe in this chapter, with each meeting and session coded by its focus: Research (R), Clinical (C), Advocacy (A), Education (E), Leadership (L), Psychosocial support (P) and Global placement (G). Figure 5.3 shows the timeline of the in-person meetings.

5.3.1 The First and Most Effective Community-Building Event of the FFP: The Fellowship Annual Meeting

The FFP Annual Meeting has been one of the most valued and effective community-building Fellowship gatherings. Until recently, it was held in conjunction with the Annual Clinical Meeting of the American College of Obstetricians and Gynecologists (ACOG) (see Chapter 3). The Annual Meeting addresses all Fellowship objectives and topics: research, clinical innovation, policy, leadership, legal and legislative aspects of abortion and contraception and global health.

By adding the "Fellows' Spotlight," highlighting the work of a particular graduated fellow and presenting special Fellowship awards, everyone learns about one another's work, successes and challenges. A special lecture on the state of the

Table 5.1 Meetings and sessions of the US-based Fellowship in Family Planning community

Meeting	Description, each session marked as a focus on Research (R), Clinical (C), Advocacy (A), Education (E), Leadership (L), Psychosocial support (P) and Global placement (G)
Fellowship Community In-person Meetings	
Annual Fellowship meetings 2000–present	Opportunity to learn about and support fellows' research projects, learn about the highlights of the National Office and Fellowship and individual fellows' accomplishments and celebrate the community with an annual dinner and keynote presentations from the leadership of the American College of Obstetricians and Gynecologists and other leaders in the field (all)
One-day symposia associated with Fellowship meetings 2004–present	<ul><li>2019 - "Diversity, Equity and Inclusion" (L, A, E, P)</li><li>2018 - "The Future of Complex Family Planning Training and Service Delivery" (L)</li><li>2017 – "Post-Election Battles: Putting on our Fatigues" (A)</li><li>2016 – "2nd-Trimester Abortion – Clinical and Policy Updates" (C)</li><li>2015 – "Science, Policy and Politics" (A)</li><li>2014 – "Second Trimester Abortion" (C)</li><li>2013 – "Simulation Training in Family Planning" (E)</li><li>2012 – "Abortion, Contraception, and Medical Education under Assault" (A)</li><li>2011 - "Politics, Policy, and Evidence," "Working with the Media" (A)</li><li>2010 - "Family Planning Experts as Health Policy Makers" (L)</li><li>2009 - "Second Trimester Abortion Care" (C)</li><li>2008 - "LARC Workshop" (C, E)</li></ul>
Fellowship directors' business meetings 2001–present	Annual (until 2011) or biannual business meetings of directors to discuss the management aspects of the Fellowship program, including the pursuit of subspecialty status. Management transitioned to an Advisory Committee and then Advisory Board in 2014
Fellows' meetings 2000–present	Annual networking time for fellows. Sample topics include the following plus time for class and cohort discussions:<ul><li>2019 - "Legislative Testimony: Strategies for Using Your Physician Voice" (A)</li><li>2018 - "What Can SFP Do for You?" (All)</li><li>2017 - "Diversity and Inclusion: Becoming an Intercultural Ally" (L)</li><li>2016 - "Media and Advocacy 101" (A)</li><li>2015 - "Best Practices in Grants Management" (L)</li><li>2014 - "Journal Reviewer Training" (R)</li><li>2013 - "Research Proposal Development" (R)</li><li>2013 - "Ryan Program 101 – for Second Year Fellows" (L)</li><li>2012 - "Designing and Funding a Research Project" (R)</li><li>2012 - "Building Community" (L)</li><li>2011 - "Advocacy and Its Challenges: A Facilitated Discussion" (A)</li><li>2010 - "Professional Development and Mentorship" (L)</li><li>2009 - "Creating and Negotiating a Package for a Career in Academics" (L)</li><li>2009 - "Protocol Updates" (C)</li><li>2008 - "Job Placement Post-Fellowship" (L)</li><li>2008 - "Psychosocial Needs" (P)</li><li>2007 - "Lessons for Graduating Fellows" (L)</li><li>2007 - "Post Fellowship Research" (R)</li><li>2007 - "Involvement in ACOG" (L)</li><li>2006 - "Post-Fellowship Job Opportunities" (L)</li><li>2005 - "Balancing Work and Family Life" (P)</li><li>2005 - "International Placements" (G)</li></ul>

Table 5.1 (*cont.*)

Meeting	Description, each session marked as a focus on Research (R), Clinical (C), Advocacy (A), Education (E), Leadership (L), Psychosocial support (P) and Global placement (G)
	• 2005 - "Fellowship Research" (R) • 2004 - "Academics – How to Succeed" (L) • 2003 - "Generalist vs. Subspecialist" (L) • 2003 - "Planning the Next PALM Course" (A) • 2002 - "Advocacy and Media Training for Fellows (A) • 2002 - "Life after the Fellowship" (L) • 2002 - "Collaborations among Fellows" (L)
Building a Ryan Program Workshop academic family planning training program workshop 2002–present	Annual, two-day workshop to create and sustain a family planning residency training program and family planning and abortion services in a teaching hospital. The workshop is typically attended by recently graduated fellows and family planning–focused faculty and program managers. The workshop was initiated by a group of early Fellowship graduates and includes such details as negotiating with leadership for support and billing. (See Chapter 17.) (C, A, E, L)
Global placement workshop 2004–present	A half-day to day-long meeting to help fellows plan for their low-resource-setting placements. Formerly focused on global work, low-resource domestic settings were added as alternative options. (G) Faculty are composed of fellows who describe the successes and challenges of their placement experience and Fellowship leaders who work in global settings.
Career workshop 2011–present	A two-day workshop for fellows entering their second year of Fellowship to guide fellows' search for academic or other post-Fellowship positions. (L)
Research workshop 2018–present	A four-day workshop in research methods and Fellowship research project development. Fellows attend at the beginning of their first year of Fellowship. (R)
Psychosocial workshop 2007–present	Annual, two-day workshop to provide psychosocial support for fellows and directors. Topics include stigma, discussing work with friends and family, religion and spirituality, conscientious provision, finding meaning in our work and policy restrictions. (P)
Social science perspectives on abortion 2009–present	Annual, online course run by sociologist Dr. Carole Joffe about the history and sociology of abortion in the USA. (A)
Fellowship in Family Planning and Ryan Project Communities' Online Workshops	
Online, webinar educational training seminars 2010–present	We host approximately six webinar training sessions per year to enhance the curriculum of residents and fellows. Sample topics include the following: 2019: • "Introduction to Mixed Methods in Family Planning Research and Scholarship" (R) • "Provision of Affirming Healthcare at the Intersection of Transgender Health, Family Planning, and Reproductive Justice" (C) • "Role of Research in the Current and Future Landscape of Abortion Policy Law" (R, A) • "Informing Legal and Policy Work with Research: How Clinical Researchers Can Engage in the Process" (R, A) • "Fertility Awareness Methods for Contraception" (C) • "The Open Access Debate: A 360-Degree View" (R) • "Non-Palpable Implant Removal" (C) • "Drug Development and Regulatory Oversight" (R)

Table 5.1 (cont.)

Meeting	Description, each session marked as a focus on Research (R), Clinical (C), Advocacy (A), Education (E), Leadership (L), Psychosocial support (P) and Global placement (G)
	2018: • "Reactions to Provider Voices" (A) • "Combined Hormonal Contraception 101: Back to Basics" (C) • "Collaboration between University Researchers and Industry" (R) • "Self-Managed Abortion in the US" (C) • "FFP Milestones: Information and Implementation" (E) • "Closing the Floodgates: Hemorrhage in Second Trimester Abortion" (C) 2017: • "Partial Participation and Abortion Training in Residency" (E) • "Patient-Centered Support for Contraceptive Decision Making" (C) • "The Role of Family Planning in the Zika Response" (C) • "The Fellowship in Family Planning and Subspecialty Status" (L) • "Contraception and Chronic Medical Conditions" (C) • "Adolescent Sexual and Reproductive Health: What Do I Need to Know Now?" (C) 2016: • "State of the States: A Look at 2015's Legislative and Hospital Abortion Restrictions and How to Work within Them" (A) • "Billing and Coding" (L) • "Endocrinology and Family Planning" (C) • "New Tools and Resources from Innovating Education" (E) • "What's in the Pipeline? The Future of Contraception" (C) 2015: • "Incorporating Simulation into Family Planning Training" (E) • "Incoming Fellows Research Webinar" (R) • "Developing Research Infrastructure" (R) • "Contraception and HIV" (C) • "Demography Research" (R)
Mid-career workshop 2014 and 2017	One-day workshop for associate professors in the Fellowship and Ryan Program communities to learn leadership skills and strategies for professional advancement. (L)
Ryan Community In-Person Meetings	
Ryan meetings 2002–present	Biannual business and educational meetings for Ryan Program directors, managers and faculty. Topics vary and include: • 2019 - "Billing and Coding 101" (L) • 2019 - "20 Years of Integrating Abortion and Contraception into Resident Training" (E) • 2018 - "Clinical Protocol Showcase" (C) • 2018 - "Research, Advocacy and Practice in Resident Training" (R, A) • 2017 - "Using Data for Sustainability" (L) • 2017 - "Psychosocial Workshop" (P) • 2016 - "Revamp Your Style – Tools for Medical Education" (E) • 2015 - "Sustainability Meeting: The Good, the Bad, the Ugly – The Operating Room" (L) • 2015 - "Building and Sustaining a Ryan Program: Difficult Dilemmas" (L) • 2014 - "Sustainability Meeting: Shifting Culture through Patient-Centered Services" (C)

Table 5.1 (cont.)

Meeting	Description, each session marked as a focus on Research (R), Clinical (C), Advocacy (A), Education (E), Leadership (L), Psychosocial support (P) and Global placement (G)
	• 2014 - "Advancing Contraception: Techniques and Technology" (C)
	• 2013 - "Sustainability Workshop: Business, Finances and Marketing" (L)
	• 2012 - "Long-Term Sustainability: Outlining Support and Moving Forward" (L)
	• 2012 - "Increasing Access to Second Trimester Abortion" (C)
	• 2011 - "Reaching Out to Novel Patient Populations to Strengthen Your Service" (C)
	• 2011 - "Engaging Trainees and Staff" (E)
	• 2010 - "Amplifying your Sustainability: Expanding Services, Developing Support, Maximizing Returns" (L)
	• 2010 - "Long-Acting Reversible Contraception: Training and Clinical Use" (C)
	• 2009 - "Amplify Your Assets: Coding, Collecting and Staff" (L)
	• 2009 - "Setting-Specific Challenges to Second Trimester Training and Services" (C, E)
	• 2008 - "Ensuring Sustainable Clinical Services" (L)
	• 2008 - "Best Practices for Documentation, Coding and Billing" (L)
	• 2008 - "Developing a Financial Sustainability Plan" (L)
	• 2008 - "Transforming Training Expectations" (E)
	• 2008 - "Teaching Values Clarification" (E)
	• 2008 - "Setting Rotation Expectations: Refining Your Opt Out Policy" (E)
	• 2007 - "Ryan Program Evaluation: Billing/Financial Management" (L)
	• 2006 - "Didactic Curriculum in Family Planning" (E)
	• 2006 - "Opportunities for Educational Research" (R)
	• 2006 - "Resident Training in Second Trimester Procedures" (E)
	• 2005 - "Financial Planning for a Sustainable Service" (L)
	• 2005 - "Building Enthusiasm for Training among Residents" (E)
	• 2004 - "Hospital-Based and Collaborative Model (C)
	• 2004 - "Resources, Evaluation and Family Practice Training" (E)

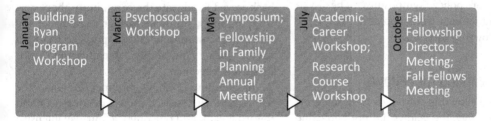

Figure 5.3 Timeline of in-person meetings of the Fellowship in Family Planning community

art of new and future research, practice and policy issues in contraception and abortion provides a review of the field's advances in national and international research and policy. Academic leaders, for example, department chairs, are invited to present their perspectives on the impact of a family planning program, the role of the Fellowship in enhancing research and training and advancing policy initiatives within their institution and nationally. (See Chapter 6.)

See the following excerpt from the 2003 FFP newsletter for a sample description:

> Annual Meetings of Fellows and Directors at ACM of ACOG

We held our fourth Annual Meeting of Fellows and Directors at the Annual Clinical Meeting of ACOG in New Orleans. What began four years ago as a half day meeting for seven directors and an informal networking luncheon for ten former and current fellows . . . the meeting has grown into a one and a half day meeting of 50 fellowship directors, co directors, fellows and former fellows. Our customary meeting room set up – a U shaped table with the screen at one end had to be so long that it was difficult to read the slides from the far end of the table. . . . Dr. Beverly Winikoff, president of Gynuity Health Projects, our guest speaker during lunch, presented about Gynuity's innovate work on medical abortion. (Fellowship newsletter)

A few years after holding regular meetings, the annual meetings expanded to include fellows' research project presentations and clinically relevant discussions presented by Fellowship directors. From 2001 to 2004, these were relatively small meetings. By 2005, an additional annual symposium on clinical and policy topics, highlighting research by the Fellowship community and other experts in the field, was added in conjunction with the FFP Annual Meeting. Topics have included updates about medication abortion, dilation and evacuation, contraception and policy.

Over the course of 20 years, the annual meetings became a four-day gathering to accommodate the growing number of fellows' research presentations, a separate session for fellows' networking and community building, a business meeting for the Fellowship directors and a one-day clinical or policy symposium. The Ryan Program held its own workshop either before or after the Fellowship meeting.

5.3.2 Networking for Fellows

Although the Fellowship started in 1991 and grew to six sites by 1999, the fellows did not know one another. While the Annual Meetings, once formalized, were primarily focused on the work of the sites and directors, fellows were invited in the following years to meet, network, discuss their sites and post-Fellowship positions. The following is the minutes from a 2004 fellows' meeting:

After introductions among the group were complete, one representative from each fellowship program described the structure of their program

and their clinical and academic training. Many participants openly discussed the parts of their programs that were outstanding and the parts that needed improvement. Subsequently, former fellows described the types of jobs they currently have and those they've had in the recent past. Fellows about to graduate spoke about the jobs they planned to take. . . . Dr. Landy then presented the experiences of several recent fellowship graduates who have established or are trying to establish Ryan residency training programs at new sites and described potential job opportunities for current fellows.

These early fellow networking meetings eventually grew into formal meetings for current and graduated fellows and orientations for incoming fellows. The Global Health Workshop, renamed the Low Resource Placement Workshop, offered another opportunity for networking and support for the required Global and more recently added Low Resource Placement, which included the USA.

5.3.3 Community of Researchers

Within a few years of Fellowship directors' meetings, fellows were invited to formally present their research projects. Over time, a schedule was established where first-year fellows reported ideas for their research projects in brief presentations, fielded questions and received feedback to improve study design and research focus. Then, as soon-to-graduate second-year fellows, they reported their study findings to the community. These formal presentations and community feedback served to educate the community about new study findings, stimulate further research for the Fellowship community and support the fellow to move into community membership with increasing expertise.

In addition to these meetings to guide the fellows in their research project development and toward meaningful outcomes, a four-day intensive research course (see Chapter 3) was added for first-year fellows in 2017. The research course is the first structured occasion for fellows to connect both professionally and personally, after meeting informally during their interviews at various sites. During the Research Course, the new fellow cohort not only develops and exchanges early ideas and concepts for projects but also begins the process of building community. For example, the new fellows initiated their own listserv after the last course.

A unique rigorous research review process further enhances membership of the community. Mentored by their site directors, attending institutional research courses and pursuing their Master of Public Health or Science degree studies, fellows submit their research proposals through a multistep, peer-reviewed process, managed by the National Office (NO), to maximize the quality of their projects. Publication of research continues to be important for the academic advancement of fellows pursuing academic careers and to impact clinical and policy aspects and status of the family planning field. By 2006, an external evaluation of the FFP reported that more than 75% of former fellows reported publishing research in peer-reviewed journals during the prior two years.

The community of researchers has grown to encompass many roles and contexts, each reinforcing community. Fellowship in Family Planning directors and graduates are investigators in the National Institutes of Health's Contraceptive Clinical Trials Network (CCTN); journal editors and editorial board members; Centers for Disease Control and Prevention (CDC) abortion surveillance and World Health Organization (WHO) committee members and program staff; contributors to contraception, abortion and HIV guidelines worldwide; advisors to and committee and board members of the Society of Family Planning (SFP) and committee members and leaders within ACOG, Council on Resident Education in Obstetrics and Gynecology (CREOG) and Association of Professors of Gynecology and Obstetrics (APGO); grant recipients and reviewers; and experts in other research roles. (See Chapter 7.)

5.3.4 Community of Clinicians: The Fellowship Listserv and Other Platforms of Communication

To further enhance the network and collegiality among current and former fellows and directors, the FFP Listserv was launched in 2003 with fifty-eight former and current fellows. Initially, the purpose of the Listserv was to obtain feedback about research, job opportunities (especially from the growing list of departments of obstetrics and gynecology looking to establish Ryan Programs by hiring FFP fellows), listings of international opportunities, upcoming conferences, abstract submission deadlines, public affairs training, courses on establishing a Ryan Program, working internationally and other Fellowship-related topics.

Since its inception, the listserv has grown into a frequently, sometimes daily, used forum to support the memberships' roles as clinicians and advocates. Participation on the listserv has expanded beyond fellows and directors to include research mentors. Members pose clinical questions about complex patient scenarios to the community, which responds with suggestions for possible interventions and strategies, based on research evidence and clinical experience. Recipients typically summarize the advice, send it back to the community and describe the clinical care and outcomes.

The listserv serves an important role not only in harnessing the expertise of the Fellowship community, enabling its members to use the most effective and evidence-based treatments and have feedback in urgent patient scenarios, but also in identifying the many areas of clinical care that need further evidence. A sample of Listserv topics from the past year included questions about medication abortion care for patients with rare medical conditions, patient questions about contraceptives not available in the USA (eg, one-month contraceptive pill and two-rod implant), discussion of vaginal administration of combined oral contraceptives to decrease nausea, strategies for implant localization and difficult IUD removals and advice about clinical systems, for example, for obtaining mifepristone for management of early pregnancy loss. An unexpected benefit of the listserv and its national network is finding access to care for patients who need specialized care in another part of the country.

By 2005, the FFP launched its first newsletter, which highlighted fellows' activities. These included a fellow's work at Orientame, a clinic in Bogota, Colombia; a fellow's establishment of a contraceptive service in a local jail, which grew into an educational opportunity for residents and medical students; and fellows' personal announcements about the arrival of new babies. Now, the Fellowship, with more than 400 graduated and current fellows, has grown too large to maintain this national personal touch, but each year's cohort continues to bond, connect and uphold the traditions of community and fellowship.

5.3.5 Community of Educators

The FFP has also focused on developing the community members' skills as educators. Symposia, webinars and fellow meetings address topics pertaining to fellow, resident and medical student education, and ensure expertise in clinical teaching. Graduated fellows have developed innovative family planning curricula (see Chapters 18 and 22), become experts in educational research and presented at national and international meetings about family planning training. (See Chapter 6.) Their curricular innovations include the Papaya Workshop, Values Clarification and Professionalism workshops, Team-Based Learning, clinical clerkships and in-service trainings and presentations about equity and diversity which they share with educators around the country [4,5,6,7].

A growing number of Fellowship directors and graduates have taken on the roles of residency program and clerkship directors within their departments, ensuring that family planning is an integral part of resident and student education. They attend the national meetings of those educators (CREOG and APGO), and form community within those organizations. They have moved into positions of department chairs and vice chairs for research and education, and into dean roles such as vice/associate dean for curricula and for diversity, equity and inclusion. (See Chapter 7.)

5.3.6 Community of Leaders

The fellows are prepared to become leaders and change agents in the field of family planning and experts in the field as clinicians, educators, researchers and advocates. All educational programs of the FFP are designed to prepare for and inspire leadership roles. Some Fellowship workshops address the subject of leadership directly.

The Leadership Workshop, held by academic leaders and family planning experts, described leadership roles outside and within the institution. Fellows learned to understand their own personal psychological dynamics and how to persuade institutional leaders and policy makers and become effective change makers. The course also presented a lecture on the principles of implementation science and closed with ACOG advocacy staff summarizing leadership opportunities within its national and district structures.

The Career Workshop, held annually, focuses on the search for professional opportunities, covers academic advancement, negotiation, organizational change, and diversity, equity and inclusion, as well as other roles for leadership in health care settings outside of academia. Graduated fellows, fellowship directors and department chairs serve as faculty and inspirational mentors.

For graduated fellows, specific leadership workshops have been designed to define and explore leadership in their current and future roles, academic advancement and the dynamics of effective negotiation. For example, Communications Workshops for graduated fellows have focused on communication styles, approaches for effective presentations, communication strategies with different audiences and conflict management to achieve the desired outcomes.

5.3.7 Community of Advocates

Abortion, while a common experience for women and an essential aspect of reproductive health care throughout the world, is often considered controversial and stigmatized even after it becomes legal. In the USA, abortion stigma and controversy have led to significant legal, hospital and clinical restrictions on abortion, driven by a complex combination of antiabortion attitudes, religious beliefs, politically perpetuated controversy and ignorance about the crucial role of safe abortion and contraception for women's health. (See Chapter 24.) The controversy has led to decreased access to care, targeting of clinics and physicians through protests and sometimes violent action and intentional interference with physicians' ability to provide scientifically informed and ethical care for their patients.

The constant controversy and flow of misinformation about abortion led the FFP to include the unique requirement of advocacy skills in the FFP's *Guide to Learning* (GTL). (See Chapters 3 and 4.)

The GTL and *General Requirements* (GR) state that fellows "demonstrate knowledge and expertise of the influences of public policy and means of influencing government agencies, policy makers, and the media with respect to contraception and abortion."

While fellows are eager to embrace all aspects of Fellowship learning, advocacy plays a unique role. Many come to the Fellowship inspired by a prior experience that made them aware of the tragic situations, driven by state laws, institutional restrictions or personal and economic circumstances, which prevent women from ending their pregnancy. They may have founded or participated in Medical Students for Choice chapters at their medical schools. (See Chapter 21.)

The Fellowship, in close collaboration with ACOG, has developed several advocacy training opportunities – for example, fellows are welcome to participate in ACOG's national and state advocacy efforts. (See Chapter 3 and 4.) The Fellowship hosts an annual, online course under the direction of sociologist Dr. Carole Joffe about the history and sociology of abortion in the USA. This course ensures that the fellows are educated about the complex political history of abortion.

The Fellowship annual symposia are frequently focused on advocacy. Since 2005, the president of ACOG has been invited to give a keynote address at the annual meeting of the fellowship. As ACOG plays a critical role in advocating for women's health in the USA, inviting the president to speak gives the community insight into ACOG's advocacy efforts and priorities and, ideally, motivation to participate in those efforts. Joining the FFP community in turn reminds ACOG leadership about the strength, commitment and resources offered by the fellows, and helps to reinforce ACOG's attention to abortion in its overall women's health mission.

Fellows distinguish themselves from other advocates in that their advocacy is informed by their work as clinicians, researchers and educators. For example, one learning objective in the GTL is for fellows to "gather and communicate medical evidence, including in regard to health consequences, in order to counter myths and stigma." The political commitments and passions they bring to the Fellowship are powerful sources of connection and community building. Attending the FFP annual meeting, ACOG's advocacy programs and Physicians for Reproductive Health's Leadership Training Academy strengthens their advocacy skills and bonds. They become inspired and trained to advocate for access to care, responding to specific legislation and within the teaching hospitals where they work. (See Chapters 4 and 10.) In addition to direct advocacy efforts, their range of activities, from clinical care to research to institutional and public education, can and does influence institutional and public policy [8]. (See Chapter 3 and 4.)

5.3.8 Psychosocial Support for Fellows

The continuing political controversy and stigma and the resulting tension can be a burden for the Fellowship community and its individual members. Stigma adds an additional emotional layer to the work done as family planning experts.

As first-year fellows join the movement to establish a new field of practice, they are met with opportunities and challenges in learning how to handle the political and social controversies over abortion. As a result, in the early years of fellowship and their career, fellows can feel isolated or overwhelmed and may not feel supported within their family and friend communities. Oftentimes, their mentors and colleagues are dealing with similar conflicts and emotions. By introducing fellows to a broader community of practice, they are able to find support and learn how to manage the emotional challenges this field brings.

In recognition of the emotional aspect of abortion, the FFP launched the first Psychosocial Workshop in 2007, which has become a yearly opportunity for fellows to come together and connect. (See Chapter 3.) Here, fellows speak about their feelings and interactions with patients and others and the controversy and social stigma associated with their work. A combination of individual and panel presentations, interspersed with small group discussions, promote reflection about the meaning of abortion work, strategies to manage personal and professional conflict and hostile encounters. Other topics include stigma, finding support in our communities, discussing work with friends and family, religion and spirituality, conscientious provision and policy restrictions. The faculty includes graduated fellows and national experts.

5.4 The Ryan Program

The Kenneth J. Ryan Residency Training Program in Abortion and Family Planning (the Ryan Program) supports obstetrics and gynecology residency programs to integrate abortion and family planning training (see Chapter 3 and Figures 5.4 and 5.5). During its growth, it has developed a community of practice, in which faculty learn from and support one another to provide care and train learners. The Ryan

2019: 99 RYAN PROGRAMS

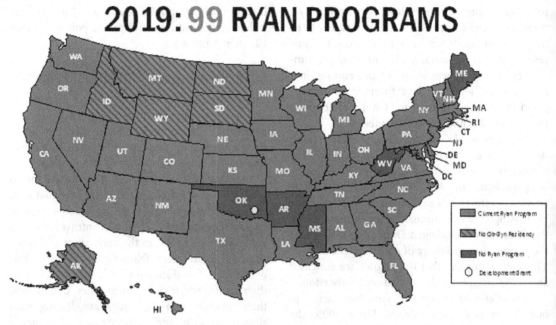

Figure 5.4 Map of the sites of the US Kenneth J. Ryan Residency Training Program in Abortion and Family Planning, 2019

Number of Ryan Programs per Year

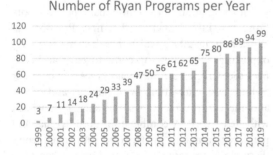

Figure 5.5 Growth of the Kenneth J. Ryan Residency Training Program in Abortion and Family Planning, 1999–2019

Program parallels the Fellowship, with many interrelationships of shared programs, all with the intention of promoting community and enhance both programs' effectiveness. The Fellowship and Ryan Program are closely connected: fellows become Ryan Program directors, providing the workforce for the Ryan Program, and the Ryan Program produces the majority of Fellowship applicants. Ryan and Fellowship graduates start or join established Ryan or Fellowship programs to increase faculty depth or join partner-training clinics.

The first workshop for the Ryan Program – How to Start a Ryan Program – was launched by graduated fellows who started Ryan Programs and wanted to share their expertise with others. This

annual workshop helps build further community around the strategies and challenges of integrating formal resident training, expanding hospital services and changing hospital culture. Both fellowship-trained and generalist family planning specialists connect, mentor and inspire one another, and continue their interactions when they have clinical or administrative questions using the listserv and other meetings and workshops.

In addition to the Starting the Ryan Program Workshop, the Ryan Program has added additional workshops held in conjunction with the Fellowship's annual meeting and the annual meeting of the Society of Family Planning, formerly known as the FORUM meeting. Here, topics of common interest include the rollout of the CDC's updated Medical Eligibility Criteria and Selected Practice Recommendations [9] for contraception, billing and coding, sustainability of the programs and services and engaging learners (see Table 5.1). Another important workshop sponsored by the Ryan Program is the Resident Career Workshop, similar to the Fellowship's Career Workshop, but designed for residents. Topics include potential career paths in family planning, including pursuing fellowship in family planning and opportunities to work with clinics where they can apply their clinical skills and commitment to reproductive health. In addition, a midlevel and senior faculty career development workshop is offered to Fellowship and other expert faculty to encourage and explore professional growth and leadership roles in academic settings. To supplement in-person education meetings, the Ryan Program hosts online discussions and education sessions covering a variety of topics for the community.

Often faculty at individual Fellowship and Ryan programs face challenges such as knowledge gaps within their departments or institutions, which require outreach to the other departments. These faculty can utilize a grand rounds program in which they invite speakers to present grand rounds and often additional teaching sessions for faculty, residents or staff. Not only does this reinforce evidence-based, high-quality care principles at these Ryan and Fellowship institutions but bringing a prestigious speaker supports the faculty in their efforts. Finally, similar to the Fellowship, the Ryan Program hosts a listserv for Ryan faculty, learners and staff, which offers another opportunity for support and exchange. As many fellowship graduates are Ryan Program directors, the exchanges of the FFP and Ryan Program listservs frequently overlap, and again, reinforce a community of practice.

5.5 Conclusion

The Fellowship and Ryan Program education initiatives are focused on reproduction and its control, surrounded by continuing controversy. In order to succeed in ensuring clinical practice, scientific advancement and access to care, the members of this unique community needed to form professional and emotional bonds and connections. In fact, the community from the start called itself a family. Despite their successful growth, both programs continue to uphold, over more than two decades, the principles of community of practice as defined by Wenger [3]. To succeed, it requires mutual engagement and trust by its members. The trust and respect are apparent even in the manner in which the listserv postings seeking advice are addressed: *Dear braintrust / communal brain / community*. The annual meeting, workshops and communications offer support through in-person and virtual gatherings, allow members to share knowledge and teach one another and provide mentorship to its new members, fellows, Fellowship graduates and Ryan directors, all joined through their passionate commitment to women's health.

References

1. Lave J, Wenger E. *Situated Learning: Legitimate Peripheral Participation*. Cambridge: Cambridge University Press; 1991.

2. Barab SA, Barnett M, Squire K. Developing an empirical account of a community of practice: characterizing the essential tensions. *J Learn Sci.* 2002;**11**(4):489–542.

3. Wenger E. *Communities of Practice: Learning, Meaning, and Identity*. Cambridge: Cambridge University Press; 1998.

4. Mody SK, Kiley J, Gawron L, Garcia P, Hammond C. Team-based learning: a novel approach to medical student education in family planning. *Contraception.* 2013; **88**(2):239–242.

5. Steinauer J, Preskil F, Devaskar S, Landy U, Darney P. The Papaya Workshop: using the papaya to teach intrauterine gynecologic procedures. *MedEdPORTAL.* 2013.

6. Steinauer J, Hawkins M, Preskill F, Koenemann K, Dehlendorf C. Caring for Challenging Patients Workshop. *MedEdPORTAL.* 2014.

7. Espey E, Ogburn T, Chavez A, Qualls C, Leyba M. Abortion education in medical schools: a national survey. *Am J Obstet Gynecol.* 2005;**192**(2):640–643.

8. Advocacy Essentials: Reproductive Rights, Health, and Justice. 2018.

9. Curtis KM, Jatlaoui TC, Tepper NK, et al. U.S. selected practice recommendations for contraceptive use, 2016. *MMWR Recomm Rep.* 2016; **65**(4):1–66.

Building Evidence through Research

The Benefits of Integrating Research Training into Fellowship in Family Planning Programs

Maria I. Rodriguez and Alisa B. Goldberg

Family planning research is fundamental to optimizing individual and population-level health, informing policy and eliminating reproductive health disparities. A structured research program, focusing on contraception and abortion, facilitates the translation of bench research into improved clinical and population health [1]. The Fellowship in Family Planning (FFP) provides an abundance of examples of how training in research methodology and implementation paired with integration of formal research programs with clinical training can lead to meaningful improvements to scientific knowledge, clinical outcomes, education and health-care delivery.

Improving health-care systems requires the concurrent pursuit of three aims: improving the individual quality of care, improving the health of populations and reducing health-care costs [2]. Evidence-based medicine is a core strategy for improving health. Evidence-based medicine seeks to apply the best information available in making decisions about the care of individual patients [3,4]. Evidence-based practice integrates clinical experience, patient values and the best available data [5]. Research is the cornerstone of evidence-based practice. An evolving, robust body of biomedical, clinical and public health research is needed to ensure that up-to-date knowledge is available to inform health care.

Evidence is particularly important in guiding sensitive and controversial topics in health care, where bias may be more likely to enter. In the USA and globally, stigma has permeated attitudes toward both recipients and providers of reproductive health care [6]. *Stigma* is commonly described as a negative social, cultural or psychological attitude [6,7]. The health consequences of the stigmatization of sexual and reproductive health services, in particular abortion, has far-reaching

consequences. Stigmatization may cause individuals to avoid testing for sexually transmitted infections and the use of modern, effective contraception and to seek out unsafe abortion [6,8,9]. Research can contribute to the reduction of stigma by counteracting myths and misperceptions with science.

During the past twenty-seven years, the FFP has greatly expanded research in all aspects of contraception and abortion. Since 1997, the FFP has produced nearly 2,000 articles in peer-reviewed publications on abortion, contraception and complex family planning topics. These works have helped create the evidence base to support medical practice guidelines, health policy decisions and the development of professional standards for training students and residents.[10–18]. This evidence base spans biomedical, clinical and health systems research.

For example, members of the Fellowship community have designed and conducted bench research identifying new, potential contraceptive targets. This work has contributed to the development of novel types of contraception including new, non-surgical methods for female permanent contraception [19–27]. Basic science research supported by the FFP has also demonstrated the increased risk obese women may have for contraceptive failure and examined how genetic variations may influence etonogestrel levels among implant users [28–32]. Fellows have led a diverse array of clinical research studies, contributing to knowledge of how to best manage pain control during abortions, dispelling misconceptions regarding the safety of intrauterine devices and developing best practices in postpartum sterilization [33–43]. The Fellowship community has conducted a breadth of policy and health systems research demonstrating the importance of safe and accessible family planning services on improving health outcomes and reducing public costs [44–51]. The FFP has produced a broad array of evidence to further science, guide health care and improve public health.

To demonstrate the impact that a structured research program for early stage investigators that encompasses training in methodology, funding for studies and mentorship can have, we present two case examples. First, we focus on the role research from the FFP has played in the dramatic increase in use of long-acting reversible contraception (LARC) in the USA. We then review how scientists from the community have contributed to the availability and safety of second-trimester surgical abortion.

LARC methods, consisting of the intrauterine device (IUD) and implant, are the most effective forms of reversible contraception available [52]. Women relying on LARC for contraception have a significantly reduced risk of unintended pregnancy, and many forms of LARC have additional health benefits such as reduction in heavy menstrual bleeding [52,53]. However, despite the addition of a new progestin-containing IUD to the US market in 2000, many barriers to LARC use existed at the patient, provider and system levels [54,55]. Examples of these barriers included the following: the myth that the IUD could cause infertility; the misperception that nulliparous women could not use an IUD; and insurance restrictions on reimbursement for LARC placed in the immediate postpartum period [56]. In 2002, two years after the new progestin-containing IUD came to the US market, 2% of reproductive-age women used an IUD. In 2014 in the USA, 14% of all contraceptive users relied on a LARC method, a historic increase [57].

While the increase in LARC use is attributed to many factors, the role of research from the FFP community has been significant in promoting access to and acceptability of LARC. The most notable example is the Contraceptive CHOICE project, which was a prospective cohort study of 9,256 women led by Dr. Jeffrey Peipert at Washington University [58]. The Contraceptive CHOICE project's primary objective was to remove several of the greatest barriers to LARC use: lack of patient education, limited access to preferred methods and cost. Subsequent studies included the impact on LARC acceptance, utilization and associated health outcomes. The team of investigators expanded knowledge and improved acceptance of LARC by utilizing standardized contraceptive counseling describing the effectiveness, advantages and disadvantages of reversible contraceptives, in order of contraceptive effectiveness [59]. They further expanded access by implementing protocols that enabled same-day initiation of LARC methods. The study removed financial barriers to LARC by providing participants with the contraceptive method of their choice at no cost. The results from the CHOICE study have been transformative in how women and clinicians view LARC. When access barriers to LARC were removed, three quarters of study participants selected a LARC method for use [59,60]. Not only was initial uptake of LARC high, but satisfaction and continuation of LARC persisted throughout the study period. At 24 months, 77% of LARC users were continuing their method, as compared with 41% of non-LARC users [60]. The impressive findings from the Contraceptive CHOICE project have been widely disseminated in more than 65 peer-reviewed publications contributing to a sea change in LARC use in the USA [54]. The CHOICE project also contributed to the education and career development of a large number of individuals. The vast majority of publications from the CHOICE project involved trainees in various stages of their education, including medical students, residents, family planning fellows as well as recent FFP graduates establishing their academic careers.

Members of the FFP have collaborated with the American College of Obstetricians and Gynecologists (ACOG) and state legislatures to remove policy barriers to postpartum contraception, in particular immediate postpartum (IPP) LARC [61]. Research conducted by Fellowship members has demonstrated the need for postpartum contraception and the role that IPP LARC can play in promoting maternal health and reducing Medicaid costs [46,62–65].

IPP LARC, or provision of LARC prior to hospital discharge after childbirth, is a safe and effective strategy to promote maternal health and reduce rapid, repeat pregnancy. A third of all second- or higher-order births in the USA occur less than 18 months from the previous birth, resulting in worse health outcomes for the woman and child [66,67]. Despite the proven efficacy of LARC to prevent rapid, repeat pregnancy, only 6% of US women are using a LARC method by

3 months postpartum [68]. Fellowship researchers have contributed to the growing availability in the USA of IPP LARC through clinical research to determine optimal placement technique and how to reduce expulsion of IUDs, as well as how to best train providers on insertion [40,69–74].

Research from the Fellowship in Family Planning has both evaluated the impact of policy restrictions on access to IPP LARC and supported progressive policy change [46,64,65,75]. Important disparities in rapid, repeat pregnancy exist [76]. Minority and low-income women are more likely to have rapid, repeat pregnancy as a result of unintended pregnancies than white women [66]. A unique population at particular risk for unintended pregnancy is low income, immigrant women.

Unauthorized and authorized immigrants, within the first five years of residence in the USA, are excluded from participation in full Medicaid [77]. Immigrants who meet the financial criteria to enroll in Medicaid are restricted to coverage for emergency services only. For pregnancy-related care, this includes a hospital admission for childbirth, but no prenatal or postpartum care. A portfolio of research from Oregon demonstrated the impact of expanding access to prenatal care for immigrant women and children [78,79]. Investigators leveraged the staggered county-by-county rollout of a policy change, which expanded coverage during pregnancy to include prenatal care and delivery for low-income immigrant women. Prior to this policy change, the state, consistent with federal law, covered the delivery only. The study used rigorous, quasi-experimental methods to demonstrate that expanding prenatal care coverage to include new immigrants enrolled in Emergency Medicaid significantly reduced infant mortality, and improved receipt of infant well-child care through the first year of life [78].

Cost-benefit analyses from Oregon, relying on hospital and Medicaid claims data, demonstrated that expansion of Emergency Medicaid to include postpartum care, in particular contraception, was a cost-saving strategy for both state Medicaid programs and society at large. They demonstrated that covering IPP LARC for the Emergency Medicaid population would save state Medicaid programs $2.94 for every dollar spent. This body of evidence was shared with state public health leadership and the legislature, and together with

academic publications led to the successful passage of Oregon's Reproductive Health Equity Act, which expanded coverage, regardless of citizenship, to all low-income individuals capable of becoming pregnant. Oregon's Reproductive Health Equity Act provided access to 60 days of postpartum coverage and full-scope contraception, including IPP LARC, as well as no-cost abortion.

Evidence from the FFP has also contributed greatly to the body of research strengthening access, safety and the quality of abortion care. As an example of how rapidly the portfolio of abortion research has grown, consider the case of the World Health Organization (WHO)'s Safe Abortion guidelines, the international standard for technical guidance. In 2003, the first edition of the guidance was published, representing an important contribution to ensuring high-quality abortion care globally. A standard guideline process using rigorous and transparent methods to systematically review and assess the quality of research informing the clinical guidelines was utilized. The development of the guidelines was led by a former FFP fellow. The impact of the Fellowship is most clearly seen, however, when examining the difference in the quantity and quality of the evidence available in the first edition of the guidelines (2003) to the second edition, published in 2012 [80]. Similarly, research from the FFP was instrumental in the development of the US National Academy of Medicine's 2018 report on the safety and quality of abortion care in the USA [81]. This report summarizes the state of the science that guides current provision of medical and surgical abortion and emphasizes the overall safety of abortion care in the USA. It heavily cites research from the FFP community that led to current standards of care and delineates the need for timely access to care that meets these standards, especially in light of "state regulations that have created barriers to optimizing each dimension of quality care" (p.9).

While the majority of abortions occur in the first trimester, improving access to safe abortion in the second trimester was identified as a key research priority by international experts in 2003. Over the next decade, research from the Fellowship was designed, conducted and implemented to address that knowledge gap [82–85]. A key clinical consideration was optimal cervical preparation for second-trimester surgical abortion, which ensures surgical abortion is both feasible and safe. Multiple studies conducted by current and former FFP fellows compared pharmacologic cervical preparation (misoprostol) to osmotic dilators [86]; the role of osmotic dilators plus adjunctive medications (misoprostol, mifepristone, digoxin) [87–89]; and the optimal length of time needed for various methods [90,91].

In an effort to evaluate cervical preparation for later surgical abortions with a large sample size and in various practice settings, in 2012 the Society of Family Planning sponsored a multicenter study of cervical preparation before dilation and evacuation (D&E). This multicenter, blinded, randomized trial compared osmotic dilators alone to osmotic dilators plus either adjunctive mifepristone or misoprostol and found comparable operative times in all three groups, but subjectively easier procedures in the later gestational cohort with adjunctive mifepristone. Additionally, mifepristone was well tolerated, while misoprostol was associated with more side effects. All of the clinical trial sites included graduated FFP fellows. These results, supported by additional research conducted by graduated fellows that similarly showed benefit to the use of mifepristone for cervical preparation before D&E, have led many abortion providers to incorporate adjunctive mifepristone into their D&E practice [88,91,92].

The Fellowship in Family Planning demonstrates how a structured research program can shape the development of evidence and guide practice to improve contraceptive utilization and the safety and quality of abortion care. Fellows have made a substantial contribution to the enormous increase in LARC use over the past decade in the USA to advancing the quality of abortion services and to evaluating and promoting clinical interventions that simplify care and help expand access to abortion.

Integrating a family planning research program with a strong clinical services and education program can strengthen both missions. Researchers can complement clinical care by evaluating new interventions and clinical practices, as well as evaluating and monitoring programs. Trainees benefit from engagement in research by building expertise in research design and analysis and becoming more informed consumers of medical literature.

The Fellowship in Family Planning has facilitated the development and support of research programs housed both within academic settings and in Planned Parenthood affiliates nationally. Creating and sustaining a family planning research program requires attention to three key areas: funding for studies, stability of infrastructure and mentorship.

It is widely recognized that today's early career investigators face greater obstacles in securing independent research funding than in years past. An increasing number of scientists are competing for a decreasing amount of funding, and the success rate for National Institutes of Health grants is below 20%. This means that investigators must spend an increasing amount of time applying for grants. New investigators, by virtue of having less experience than senior scientists, face greater challenges in securing funding. Furthermore, the nature of grant-funded research is cyclic – financial support for studies will ebb and flow. Additionally, in the USA, federal funding cannot be used to support abortion-related research, further restricting funding options for family planning investigators interested in abortion research.

Maintaining a research center that can withstand the vagaries of funding requires strong institutional support, including the availability of bridge funding and early career support for researchers. The FFP provides fellows with seed funding for a research project. Fellows design and write a study protocol that undergoes rigorous peer review. This funding allows fellows to complete a project that can support the establishment of an academic niche and facilitate acquisition of subsequent grant funding. This Fellowship-project seed funding, provided to the Fellowship institution year after year, can help establish and then sustain a stable research staff. For example, at some institutions the Fellowship research seed funding has enabled the institution to hire and sustain support for a research assistant. Fellowship programmatic funding has also been used to support statisticians and others who help implement projects to enable the creation of a solid foundation for a research program. Upon graduation, fellows often stay at their home institution and go on to conduct post-Fellowship research funded by private, industry and government grants. These grants then grow and further support research infrastructure at the home institution.

Emphasizing the importance of mentorship in building successful researchers, effective teams and a successful research program is essential. Mentoring is critical, not only to foster the direct knowledge of skills and methods but also to help inform career trajectories and development. Mentors are responsible for sharing their knowledge and expertise, supervising the trainee's work, helping the trainee connect within the research community and providing career guidance. Mentees play a proactive role in their learning and contribute by providing enthusiasm, work hours and a novel perspective.

How to create an excellent mentor-mentee team is rarely taught. Fostering a structured mentored relationship through a mutually negotiated and explicit agreement on responsibilities can help ensure success. Early in the mentoring relationship, the mentor and trainee should create an agreement outlining the goals of the relationship. Is the mentor going to serve primarily in a career-development role or as the primary mentor on the mentee's research project? If both, time should be allotted for each. At the outset of a project-specific mentorship, the expected time frame for the study, key deliverable due dates and ownership of data should be discussed and authorship should be negotiated.

Research helps ensure innovation and excellence in clinical care and promotes population health. Integrating a structured research program within a clinical training program in family planning can help strengthen both the educational and clinical services of an institution. Developing an effective research program requires funding for studies and attention to maintaining core infrastructure while facilitating mentorship. Mentorship in turn can help develop a new generation of leaders in family planning who can provide clinical services, educate future generations of care providers and researchers and continue to advance the evidence base that moves our field forward.

References

1. Fort DG, Herr TM, Shaw PL, Gutzman KE, Starren JB. Mapping the evolving definitions of translational research. *J Clin Transl Sci.* 2017;**1**(1):60–66.

2. Berwick DM, Nolan TW, Whittington J. The triple aim: care, health, and cost. *Health Aff (Millwood).* 2008;**27**(3):759–769.

3. Sackett DL, Rosenberg WM, Gray JA, Haynes RB, Richardson WS. Evidence based medicine: what it is and what it isn't. *Clin Orthop Relat Res.* 2007;**455**:3–5.

4. Sackett DL, Rosenberg WM. The need for evidence-based medicine. *J R Soc Med.* 1995;**88**(11):620–624.

5. Straus SE, Glasziou P, Richardson S, Haynes RB. *Evidence-Based Medicine: How to Practice and Teach EBM.* 5th ed. London: Churchill Livingstone; 2018.

6. Cook RJ, Dickens BM. Reducing stigma in reproductive health. *Int J Gynaecol Obstet.* 2014;**125**(1):89–92.

7. Cook RJ, Cusack S, Dickens BM. Unethical female stereotyping in reproductive health. *Int J Gynaecol Obstet.* 2010;**109**(3):255–258.

8. Norris A, Bessett D, Steinberg JR, Kavanaugh ML, De Zordo S, Becker D. Abortion stigma: a reconceptualization of constituents, causes, and consequences. *Womens Health Issues.* 2011;**21**(3 Suppl):S49–S54.

9. Geibel S, Hossain SM, Pulerwitz J, et al. Stigma reduction training improves healthcare provider attitudes toward, and experiences of, young marginalized people in Bangladesh. *J Adolesc Health.* 2017;**60**(2S2):S35–S44.

10. Guiahi M, Davis A. First-trimester abortion in women with medical conditions: release date October 2012 SFP Guideline #20122. *Contraception.* 2012;**86**(6):622–630.

11. Diedrich J, Drey E. Induction of fetal demise before abortion. *Contraception.* 2010;**81**(6):462–473.

12. Roe AH, Bartz D. Society of Family Planning clinical recommendations: contraception after surgical abortion. *Contraception.* 2019;**99**(1):2–9.

13. American College of Obstetricians and Gynecologists. Practice Bulletin No. 143: medical management of first-trimester abortion. *Obstet Gynecol.* 2014;**123**(3):676–692.

14. Kerns J, Steinauer J. Management of postabortion hemorrhage: release date November 2012 SFP Guideline #20131. *Contraception.* 2013;**87**(3):331–342.

15. Newmann S, Dalve-Endres A, Drey EA. Clinical guidelines. Cervical preparation for surgical abortion from 20 to 24 weeks' gestation. *Contraception.* 2008;**77**(4):308–314.

16. Lohr PA, Lyus R, Prager S. Use of intrauterine devices in nulliparous women. *Contraception.* 2017;**95**(6):529–537.

17. Levy BS, Ness DL, Weinberger SE. Consensus guidelines for facilities performing outpatient procedures: evidence over ideology. *Obstet Gynecol.* 2019;**133**(2):255–260.

18. Allen RH, Singh R. Society of Family Planning clinical guidelines pain control in surgical abortion part 1 – local anesthesia and minimal sedation. *Contraception.* 2018;**97**(6):471–477.

19. Han L, Padua E, Hart KD, Edelman A, Jensen JT. Comparing cervical mucus changes in response to an oral progestin or oestrogen withdrawal in ovarian-suppressed women: a clinical pilot. *Eur J Contracept Reprod Health Care.* 2019;**24**(3): 209–215.

20. Han L, Padua E, Edelman A, Jensen JT. Appraising cervical mucus: a new approach to evaluating contraceptives. *Eur J Contracept Reprod Health Care.* 2018;**23**(1): 78–83.

21. Han L, Taub R, Jensen JT. Cervical mucus and contraception: what we know and what we don't. *Contraception.* 2017;**96**(5): 310–321.

22. Patil E, Thurmond A, Edelman A, et al. Pressure dynamics in the non-gravid uterus: intrauterine pressure cannot confirm tubal occlusion after non-surgical permanent contraception. *Contraception.* 2017;**96**(5):330–35.

23. Jensen JT, Hanna C, Yao S, Thompson E, Bauer C, Slayden OD. Transcervical administration of polidocanol foam prevents pregnancy in female baboons. *Contraception.* 2016;**94**(5):527–533.

24. Slayden OD, Lee DO, Yao S, Jensen JT. Polidocanol induced tubal occlusion in nonhuman primates: immunohistochemical detection of collagen I-V. *Contraception.* 2016;**94**(5): 521–526.

25. Jensen JT, Hanna C, Yao S, Bauer C, Morgan TK, Slayden OD. Characterization of tubal occlusion after transcervical polidocanol foam (PF) infusion in baboons. *Contraception.* 2015;**92**(2):96–102.

26. Jensen JT, Hanna C, Yao S, et al. Blockade of tubal patency following transcervical administration of polidocanol foam: initial studies in rhesus macaques. *Contraception.* 2014;**89**(6):540–549.

27. Jensen JT, Rodriguez MI, Liechtenstein-Zabrak J, Zalanyi S. Transcervical polidocanol as a nonsurgical method of female sterilization: a pilot study. *Contraception.* 2004;**70**(2): 111–115.

28. Luo D, Westhoff CL, Edelman AB, Natavio M, Stanczyk FZ, Jusko WJ. Altered pharmacokinetics of combined oral contraceptives in obesity – multistudy assessment. *Contraception.* 2019;**99**(4): 256–263.

29. Edelman A, Trussell J, Aiken ARA, Portman DJ, Chiodo JA, 3rd, Garner EIO. The emerging role of obesity in short-acting hormonal contraceptive effectiveness. *Contraception.* 2018;**97**(5):371–377.

30. Edelman AB, Cherala G, Blue SW, Erikson DW, Jensen JT. Impact of obesity on the pharmacokinetics of levonorgestrel-based emergency contraception: single and double dosing. *Contraception.* 2016;**94**(1): 52–57.

31. Edelman AB, Cherala G, Munar MY, McInnis M, Stanczyk FZ, Jensen JT. Correcting oral contraceptive pharmacokinetic alterations due to obesity: a randomized controlled trial. *Contraception.* 2014;**90**(5):550–556.

32. Lazorwitz A, Aquilante CL, Oreschak K, Sheeder J, Guiahi M, Teal S. Influence of genetic variants on steady-state etonogestrel concentrations among contraceptive implant users. *Obstet Gynecol.* 2019; **133**(4):783–794.

33. Renner RM, Edelman AB, Nichols MD, Jensen JT, Lim JY, Bednarek PH. Refining paracervical block techniques for pain control in first trimester surgical abortion: a randomized controlled noninferiority trial. *Contraception.* 2016;**94**(5): 461–466.

34. Allen RH, Fortin J, Bartz D, Goldberg AB, Clark MA. Women's preferences for pain control during first-trimester surgical abortion: a qualitative study. *Contraception.* 2012; **85**(4):413–418.

35. Romero I, Turok D, Gilliam M. A randomized trial of tramadol versus ibuprofen as an adjunct to pain control during vacuum aspiration abortion. *Contraception.* 2008;**77**(1): 56–59.

36. Dragoman MV, Grossman D, Kapp N, et al. Two prophylactic medication approaches in addition to a pain control regimen for early medical abortion < 63 days' gestation with mifepristone and misoprostol: study protocol for a randomized, controlled trial. *Reprod Health.* 2016;**13**(1):132.

37. Conti JA, Lerma K, Shaw KA, Blumenthal PD. Self-administered lidocaine gel for pain control with first-trimester surgical abortion: a randomized controlled trial. *Obstet Gynecol.* 2016;**128**(2): 297–303.

38. Carr S, Espey E. Intrauterine devices and pelvic inflammatory disease among adolescents. *J Adolesc Health.* 2013;**52**(4 Suppl): S22–S28.

39. Bryant AG, Kamanga G, Stuart GS, Haddad LB, Meguid T, Mhango C. Immediate postpartum versus 6-week postpartum intrauterine device insertion: a feasibility study of a randomized controlled trial. *Afr J Reprod Health.* 2013;17(2):72–79.

40. Chen BA, Reeves MF, Creinin MD, Schwarz EB. Postplacental or delayed levonorgestrel intrauterine device insertion and breast-feeding duration. *Contraception.* 2011;84(5): 499–504.

41. Wolfe KK, Wilson MD, Hou MY, Creinin MD. An updated assessment of postpartum sterilization fulfillment after vaginal delivery. *Contraception.* 2017;96(1):41–46.

42. Zite N, Wuellner S, Gilliam M. Failure to obtain desired postpartum sterilization: risk and predictors. *Obstet Gynecol.* 2005;105(4):794–799.

43. Rodriguez MI, Seuc A, Sokal DC. Comparative efficacy of postpartum sterilisation with the titanium clip versus partial salpingectomy: a randomised controlled trial. *BJOG.* 2013;120(1):108–112.

44. Dilley SE, Havrilesky LJ, Bakkum-Gamez J, et al. Cost-effectiveness of opportunistic salpingectomy for ovarian cancer prevention. *Gynecol Oncol.* 2017;146(2): 373–379.

45. Rodriguez MI, Darney BG, Elman E, Linz R, Caughey AB, McConnell KJ. Examining quality of contraceptive services for adolescents in Oregon's family planning program. *Contraception.* 2015;91(4):328–335.

46. Rodriguez MI, Chang R, Thiel de Bocanegra H. The impact of postpartum contraception on reducing preterm birth: findings from California. *Am J Obstet Gynecol.* 2015;213(5): 703 e1–e6.

47. Krashin JW, Edelman AB, Nichols MD, Allen AJ, Caughey AB, Rodriguez MI. Prohibiting consent: what are the costs of denying permanent contraception concurrent with abortion care? *Am J Obstet Gynecol.* 2014;211(1):76e1–e10.

48. Burlone S, Edelman AB, Caughey AB, Trussell J, Dantas S, Rodriguez MI. Extending contraceptive coverage under the Affordable Care Act saves public funds. *Contraception.* 2013;87(2):143–148.

49. Jarlenski M, Borrero S, La Charite T, Zite NB. Episode-based payment for perinatal care in medicaid: implications for practice and policy. *Obstet Gynecol.* 2016;127(6): 1080–1084.

50. Zite N, Wuellner S, Gilliam M. Barriers to obtaining a desired postpartum tubal sterilization. *Contraception.* 2006;73(4):404.

51. Gilliam ML, Neustadt A, Gordon R. A call to incorporate a reproductive justice agenda into reproductive health clinical practice and policy. *Contraception.* 2009;79(4): 243–246.

52. Hatcher RA. *Contraceptive Technology.* 21st ed. New York: Ardent Media; 2018: xxx.

53. Hubacher D, Grimes DA. Noncontraceptive health benefits of intrauterine devices: a systematic review. *Obstet Gynecol Surv.* 2002;57(2): 120–128.

54. Hubacher D, Kavanaugh M. Historical record-setting trends in IUD use in the United States. *Contraception.* 2018;98(6): 467–470.

55. Hubacher D, Finer LB, Espey E. Renewed interest in intrauterine contraception in the United States: evidence and explanation. *Contraception.* 2011;83(4):291–294.

56. MacIsaac L, Espey E. Intrauterine contraception: the pendulum swings back. *Obstet Gynecol Clin North Am.* 2007;34(1):91–111, ix.

57. Kavanaugh ML, Jerman J. Contraceptive method use in the United States: trends and characteristics between 2008, 2012 and 2014. *Contraception.* 2018;97(1):14–21.

58. Secura GM, Allsworth JE, Madden T, Mullersman JL, Peipert JF. The Contraceptive CHOICE Project: reducing barriers to long-acting reversible contraception. *Am J Obstet Gynecol.* 2010;203(2): 115 e1–e7.

59. McNicholas C, Madden T, Secura G, Peipert JF. The Contraceptive CHOICE Project round up: what we did and what we learned. *Clin Obstet Gynecol.* 2014;57(4): 635–643.

60. O'Neil-Callahan M, Peipert JF, Zhao Q, Madden T, Secura G. Twenty-four-month continuation of reversible contraception. *Obstet Gynecol.* 2013;122(5):1083–1091.

61. Rodriguez MI, Evans M, Espey E. Advocating for immediate postpartum LARC: increasing access, improving outcomes, and decreasing cost. *Contraception.* 2014;90(5): 468–471.

62. Teal SB. Postpartum contraception: optimizing interpregnancy intervals. *Contraception.* 2014;89(6): 487–488.

63. Han L, Teal SB, Sheeder J, Tocce K. Preventing repeat pregnancy in adolescents: is immediate postpartum insertion of the contraceptive implant cost effective? *Am J Obstet Gynecol.* 2014;211(1): 24 e1–e7.

64. Rodriguez MI, Jensen JT, Darney PD, Little SE, Caughey AB. The financial effects of expanding postpartum contraception for new immigrants. *Obstet Gynecol.* 2010;115(3):552–558.

65. Rodriguez MI, Caughey AB, Edelman A, Darney PD, Foster DG. Cost-benefit analysis of state- and hospital-funded postpartum intrauterine contraception at a university hospital for recent immigrants to the United States. *Contraception*. 2010;**81**(4): 304–308.

66. Gemmill A, Lindberg LD. Short interpregnancy intervals in the United States. *Obstet Gynecol*. 2013;**122**(1):64–71.

67. Ball SJ, Pereira G, Jacoby P, de Klerk N, Stanley FJ. Re-evaluation of link between interpregnancy interval and adverse birth outcomes: retrospective cohort study matching two intervals per mother. *BMJ*. 2014;**349**: g4333.

68. White K, Teal SB, Potter JE. Contraception after delivery and short interpregnancy intervals among women in the United States. *Obstet Gynecol*. 2015;125(6):1471–1477.

69. Gurney EP, Sonalkar S, McAllister A, Sammel MD, Schreiber CA. Six-month expulsion of postplacental copper intrauterine devices placed after vaginal delivery. *Am J Obstet Gynecol*. 2018;**219**(2):183 e1–e9.

70. Whitaker AK, Endres LK, Mistretta SQ, Gilliam ML. Postplacental insertion of the levonorgestrel intrauterine device after cesarean delivery vs. delayed insertion: a randomized controlled trial. *Contraception*. 2014;**89**(6): 534–539.

71. Jatlaoui TC, Marcus M, Jamieson DJ, Goedken P, Cwiak C. Postplacental intrauterine device insertion at a teaching hospital. *Contraception*. 2014;**89**(6): 528-33.

72. Prager S, Gupta P, Chilambwe J, et al. Feasibility of training Zambian nurse-midwives to perform postplacental and postpartum insertions of intrauterine devices. *Intl J Gynaecol Obstet*. 2012;**117**(3): 243–247.

73. Chen BA, Reeves MF, Hayes JL, Hohmann HL, Perriera LK, Creinin MD. Postplacental or delayed insertion of the levonorgestrel intrauterine device after vaginal delivery: a randomized controlled trial. *Obstet Gynecol*. 2010;**116**(5): 1079–1087.

74. Hayes JL, Cwiak C, Goedken P, Zieman M. A pilot clinical trial of ultrasound-guided postplacental insertion of a levonorgestrel intrauterine device. *Contraception*. 2007;**76** (4):292–296.

75. Rodriguez MI, Edelman A, Wallace N, Jensen JT. Denying postpartum sterilization to women with Emergency Medicaid does not reduce hospital charges. *Contraception*. 2008;**78** (3):232–236.

76. Dehlendorf C, Rodriguez MI, Levy K, Borrero S, Steinauer J. Disparities in family planning. *Am J Obstet Gynecol*. 2010;**202**(3):214–220.

77. DuBard CA, Massing MW. Trends in emergency Medicaid expenditures for recent and undocumented immigrants. *JAMA*. 2007;**297** (10):1085–1092.

78. Swartz JJ, Hainmueller J, Lawrence D, Rodriguez MI. Expanding prenatal care to unauthorized immigrant women reduces infant mortality. *Obstet Gynecol*. 2017;**130**(5):938–945.

79. Swartz JJ, Hainmueller J, Lawrence D, Rodriguez MI. Oregon's expansion of prenatal care improved utilization among immigrant women. *Matern Child Health J*. 2019;**23**(2):173–182.

80. *Safe Abortion: Technical and Policy Guidelines*. Geneva: World Health Organization; 2012.

81. Calonge BN, Gayle HD. The safety and quality of abortion services in the United States: what does the evidence indicate? *Ann Intern Med*. 2018;168(12):878–880.

82. Goldberg AB, Fortin JA, Drey EA, et al. Cervical preparation before dilation and evacuation using adjunctive misoprostol or mifepristone compared with overnight osmotic dilators alone: a randomized controlled trial. *Obstet Gynecol*. 2015;**126**(3):599–609.

83. Shaw KA, Shaw JG, Hugin M, Velasquez G, Hopkins FW, Blumenthal PD. Adjunct mifepristone for cervical preparation prior to dilation and evacuation: a randomized trial. *Contraception*. 2015; **91**(4):313–319.

84. Drey EA, Benson LS, Sokoloff A, Steinauer JE, Roy G, Jackson RA. Buccal misoprostol plus laminaria for cervical preparation before dilation and evacuation at 21–23 weeks of gestation: a randomized controlled trial. *Contraception*. 2014;**89**(4):307–313.

85. Newmann SJ, Dalve-Endres A, Diedrich JT, Steinauer JE, Meckstroth K, Drey EA. Cervical preparation for second trimester dilation and evacuation. Cochrane Database Syst Rev. 2010;(8):CD007310.

86. MacIsaac L, Grossman D, Balistreri E, Darney P. A randomized controlled trial of laminaria, oral misoprostol, and vaginal misoprostol before abortion. *Obstet Gynecol*. 1999;**93**(5 Pt 1):766–770.

87. Goldberg AB, Drey EA, Whitaker AK, Kang MS, Meckstroth KR, Darney PD. Misoprostol compared with laminaria before early second-trimester surgical abortion: a randomized trial. *Obstet Gynecol*. 2005;**106**(2):234–241.

88. Shaw KA, Shaw JG, Hugin M, Velasquez G, Hopkins FW, Blumenthal PD. Adjunct mifepristone for cervical preparation prior to dilation and evacuation: a randomized trial. *Contraception*. 2015;**91**(4): 313–319.

89. Jackson R, Teplin V, Drey E, Thomas L, Darney P. Digoxin to facilitate late second-trimester abortion: a randomized, masked, placebo-controlled trial. *Obstet Gynecol*. 2001;**97**(3):471–476.

90. Edelman AB, Buckmaster JG, Goetsch MF, Nichols MD, Jensen JT. Cervical preparation using laminaria with adjunctive buccal misoprostol before second-trimester dilation and evacuation procedures: a randomized clinical trial. *Am J Obstet Gynecol*. 2006;**194**(2): 425–430.

91. Casey FE, Ye PP, Perritt JD, Moreno-Ruiz NL, Reeves MF. A randomized controlled trial evaluating same-day mifepristone and misoprostol compared to misoprostol alone for cervical preparation prior to second-trimester surgical abortion. *Contraception*. 2016;**94**(2):127–133.

92. Shaw KA, Topp NJ, Shaw JG, Blumenthal PD. Mifepristone-misoprostol dosing interval and effect on induction abortion times: a systematic review. *Obstet Gynecol*. 2013;**121**(6):1335–1347.

Impact of Integrated Family Planning Training
Culture Change and Access to Care

Courtney Schreiber, Philip D. Darney and Uta Landy

7.1 ACGME Requirement

In 1996, the Accreditation Council for Graduate Medical Education (ACGME) Obstetrics and Gynecology Program Requirement IV.A.2.d asserted that although no program or resident with a religious or moral objection shall be required to provide training in or to perform induced abortions, access to experience with induced abortion must be part of residency education [1]. This requires programs to allow residents to opt out of, rather than opt into, abortion training. Military residency programs may have difficulty fulfilling these requirements because they are subject to additional federal restrictions. In Catholic hospitals, religious dogma limits abortion training opportunities for residents. (See Chapter 13.)

Training in abortion includes many skills that are applicable to general obstetrics and gynecology practice, including counseling in topics such as pregnancy options, early gestational ultrasonography, pain management for gynecology-based office procedures, cervical dilation and the use of manual vacuum aspiration for early pregnancy loss. Most residents who partially participate in abortion training affirm the value of a dedicated family planning rotation to obtain these skills. (See Chapter 23.) Residency program directors reported that 82% of residents rank the family planning rotation higher than other outpatient gynecology rotations [2].

In response to the need for organized resident education in abortion care, the Kenneth J. Ryan Residency Training Program was founded in 1999; currently, 100 US and Canadian obstetrics and gynecology residencies include Ryan Programs. A survey of residents and residency directors demonstrated significant improvement in knowledge and skills related to family planning and abortion for residents involved in this program, even for those who opted out of some aspects of training [3].

In 1991, the first fully developed Fellowship in Family Planning (FFP) was launched at the University of California, San Francisco (UCSF), by Dr. Philip Darney. In the two decades since, the Fellowship, led by Dr. Uta Landy, has changed the field and culture of obstetrics and gynecology practice, as well as expanded access to family planning and abortion care in communities where Fellowship graduates practice. The FFP provides post-residency obstetrician-gynecologists (ob-gyns) the opportunity to study research methods and obtain advanced clinical skills in complex family planning and abortion care. The Fellowship is designed broadly to develop leadership and strengthen credibility in a field that has experienced withering funding for research, aging of service providers and diminishing access to services resulting from a complex combination of sociopolitical forces such as harassment and attacks on providers, insurance-related restrictions and a long history of religious and political stigmatization. (See Chapter 4.)

Graduated FFP fellows have created or improved many new education, service, and training programs. They have founded new Ryan Residency Programs, created family planning rotations for medical students, enhanced staff training in family planning, improved clinical care for pregnancy options, provided counseling and lectures on abortion and contraception to other medical and nursing school departments, developed new curricula on family planning, and improved medical education for medical students and residents [4]. They have also made family planning research a foundation for many academic departments and created new service delivery sites, with improved provider counseling and prescribing practices for family planning. Some respondents reported changing or creating institutional policies and promoting changes in the international programs of many countries. (See Chapters 27–35.) At the ten-year fellowship anniversary, 80% of fellows and former fellows indicated that they are engaged in some form of advocacy activity aimed at the goal of increasing access and availability of FP and abortion services [5].

As of 2020, twenty-three obstetrics and gynecology departments of the twenty-eight Fellowship in Family Planning sites across the country have instituted sections or formal divisions in family planning, led by expert family planning faculty. More than eighteen graduated fellows hold leadership positions at Planned Parenthood, and some have started their own independent abortion clinics in underserved areas [4].

7.2 Research and Contribution to Science

Prior to the Fellowship, there was little funding or academic community for family planning research, which had been left behind by the focus of reproductive endocrinologists on new infertility treatments. The Fellowship filled the void in contraceptive research and created new investigators in abortion research, making family planning a true subspecialty of obstetrics and gynecology.

Among the many requirements for recognition of a family planning subspecialty was an organization to serve as an academic home for the research that would be produced by fellows and graduates and provide a source of funding for abortion research that had neither a scholarly society nor governmental support. The Society of Family Planning (SFP), first conceived of by leading reproductive endocrinologists Leon Speroff and Daniel Mishell Jr. as a forum for researchers to share ideas, develop protocols, review work in progress and provide career development for emerging investigators, became this home.

From its founding, the SFP has had a partnership with the Fellowship, funding and presenting a wide range of contraception and abortion research. Through grants, hosting an annual meeting and publication of the journal *Contraception*, the growth of both SFP and the Fellowship has legitimized family planning as a subspecialty through advances in its science.

Fellowship graduates and directors have served on the editorial boards and as reviewers for the major peer-reviewed journals in ob-gyn, including *Contraception*, *Obstetrics and Gynecology*, and the *American Journal of Obstetrics & Gynecology*.

In just under fifteen years, the quality and quantity of family planning–related science has improved so much that along with *Contraception*, family planning–focused articles are frequently published in journals such as the American College of Obstetricians and Gynecologists's (ACOG) *Obstetrics and Gynecology*, the *American Journal of Obstetrics & Gynecology*, *JAMA*, *Lancet*, and *The New England Journal of Medicine*. This growth in the evidence base has led to changes in guidelines and protocols for clinical practice, not just in academic medical settings, but in freestanding abortion care clinics, Title X family planning centers, Planned Parenthood clinics and health-care organizations of all kinds.

An example of research by fellows and graduates that has had a great impact is medication abortion. When approved by the US Food and Drug Administration (FDA) in 2000, the mifepristone and misoprostol regimen included three clinical visits, a costly and high dose of mifepristone and rigid timing for starting misoprostol. Research published by the Fellowship community resulted in alternative protocols for the administration of the two medications that were more efficacious, more flexible, less costly for both patients and providers and more acceptable for patients. The adoption of these off-label, evidence-based regimens by the majority of abortion care providers, including Planned Parenthood–affiliated clinics, led to the eventual relabeling of mifepristone by the FDA in 2016. Fellowship investigators are now working to remove the final major restriction on evidence-based use of mifepristone, the FDA's Risk Evaluation and Mitigation Strategy (REMS) requirements [6,7].

Fellowship-related research on abortion care safety and methods informed the 2018 National Academies of Sciences, Engineering, and Medicine publication *The Safety and Quality of Abortion Care in the United States* [8]. This comprehensive report included the expertise of sixty-eight former fellows during the Academies' gathering of testimony and comprehensive review of evidence. As evidenced by the ninety-eight citations authored by the Fellowship community, the National Academy of Medicine's report focused on areas of abortion care that have been standardized through evidence collected largely through the Fellowship and its graduates in areas such as abortion safety, procedural protocols for cervical dilation, sedation and pain control, medication abortion use and complication management. The report also acknowledged the important role of the Fellowship in training physicians in advanced gestational care.

Contraception practice guidelines have also changed significantly as a result of the science developed by Fellowship-trained clinicians, particularly for patients post-abortion and birth, those with complex medical conditions and for younger patients.

Long-acting reversible contraception (LARC) methods have long been not only the most effective methods of birth control, but also often the most difficult to access for patients due to cost and limited research to demonstrate safety for younger, nulliparous patients, and for patients post-abortion and immediately postpartum. Focused research on the safety of LARC methods by Fellowship-trained physicians has led to a revolution in the use of LARC methods over the course of the past decade, as rates of use of highly effective contraceptives have doubled in the USA between 2008 and 2014 [9].

Fellow-led research has changed the use of intrauterine devices (IUDs), once reserved only for patients who had experienced a vaginal delivery. IUDs have now been shown to be safe and effective for nulliparous patients, as well as adolescents, and for women post-abortion and postpartum. The evidence is so strong in support of adolescent LARC use that a 2014 American Academy of Pediatrics report and a 2018 ACOG Committee Opinion recommended LARCs, including the IUD, to be first line contraceptives for adolescents, citing research accomplished through the Fellowship in Family Planning [10,11].

7.2.1 Impact on LARC Access

The Ryan LARC Program was launched in 2008 as a new component of the Ryan Residency Training program. The program's aims were

twofold: (1) to increase evidence-based training of ob-gyn residents regarding all methods of long-acting reversible contraceptive methods; (2) to increase access for women otherwise not able to receive devices (postpartum, post-abortion, adolescents, women with comorbidities) through the provision of free LARC devices [12]. Over a period of 11 years, nearly 100,000 LARC devices were distributed to 90 Ryan Residency Training Programs in the USA [13].

Overall, evaluation of the program showed that it accomplished its goals. The distribution of no-cost LARC devices increased counseling, training and, subsequently, access to LARC at almost all of the program sites, and had a significant effect on expanding contraceptive options otherwise limited by insurance coverage barriers. Through the Ryan LARC program, residents and other health-care providers incorporated counseling and offered LARC more consistently and became adept at insertion.

The LARC initiative was launched at a time when the use of LARC was not yet widespread. Over time, the LARC program led to a culture change among trainees and future ob-gyn practitioners, creating new generations of skillful LARC providers, and making a significant contribution to acceptance by both patients and physicians and subsequent access to LARC.

7.2.1.1 The Choice Project

Dr Jeffrey Peipert, while Fellowship and Family Planning Director at Washington University in Saint Louis, and his research team led by Dr. Gina Secura, organized the Contraceptive CHOICE project – a prospective cohort study that enrolled 9,256 women in the St. Louis, Missouri, area. The project was designed to address what family planning specialists had long believed: that women who wanted to avoid unintended pregnancy could succeed with increased use of highly effective LARC methods. To provide this opportunity to the women of Saint Louis, the project set out to reduce the most common barriers cited for low use of highly effective contraception: cost, patient knowledge and access. Ultimately, the CHOICE project succeeded in reducing unintended pregnancy on a population level in the St. Louis area [14]. Not only did women choose LARC methods at unprecedented rates, they also had high rates of continuation and satisfaction [9].

7.2.1.2 The Colorado Initiative (2009–2015)

In a public and private partnership, the state of Colorado's Department of Public Health launched in 2009 the Colorado Family Planning Initiative (CFPI) to make LARC methods both accessible and affordable as a family planning method. The Initiative used well-established Title X family planning clinics, which receive federal funding for their services as the CFPI's service provider network. The goal of the initiative was to make family planning services more accessible and allow women to choose a method, including LARC, without consideration of cost.

After 2015 when the program ended, it became sustainable through increased state family planning funding, as it demonstrated effective public health policy. The teen birth rate was cut nearly in half, high-risk pregnancies dropped significantly and key maternal and infant health measures improved. Birth and abortion rates fell by 50%. Eventual cost savings far outweighed initial investments, which convinced the policy makers to increase public funding after the program ended in 2016. Essential to CFPI's success was the extensive training of clinic staff in the technical aspects of LARC, counseling and addressing misconceptions about LARC methods. The FFP experts in Colorado played an essential role in this initiative [15].

7.2.2 Impact on Clinical Care

The work of fellows has also resulted in a critical shift in public health science, resulting in an increased interest in helping women with comorbid conditions to safely plan their pregnancies. This work has contributed to the evidence for safe and effective contraceptive care for vulnerable populations including those at high risk of premature birth [16].

In 2014, fellowship-trained physicians Rebecca Allen and Carrie Cwiak published *Contraception for the Medically Challenging Patient*, the first reference of its kind. Studies had demonstrated that many women with comorbid conditions were not receiving contraception counseling or care due to misconceptions about their own ability to conceive, as well as a lack of clear guidance for providers. Despite Centers for Disease Control and Prevention (CDC) guidelines for contraceptive counseling for patients with complex conditions, there was a significant gap in patients actually receiving appropriate contraceptive management. The publication of this guide was made possible by the work of Fellowship-trained physicians across the country who had focused their efforts on providing care for patients referred by generalist gynecologists or primary care providers unfamiliar with contraceptive care for patients with serious illnesses [17].

Given the rising maternal mortality rate in the USA over the past three decades, addressing the risks associated with rapid repeat pregnancy and delivery through postpartum contraception and pregnancy spacing has been an important strategy in improving maternal health. Most of the research and available evidence on the appropriateness of and best practices for postpartum contraception come through research conducted at Fellowship sites. Fellowship-led clinical trials have resulted in recommendations on postpartum contraceptive implant use, and the immediate postpartum placement of IUDs from professional organizations like the CDC, ACOG, the American Academy of Family Physicians, and the Centers for Medicaid and Medicare Services [18,19,20,16].

7.2.3 Contraceptive Research and Development

Pharmaceutical companies now partner with investigators at Fellowship sites across the country to develop new contraceptive methods, improve and diversify methods and increase the value of existing methods. One example of the success of these collaborations is the recent intrauterine contraceptive Liletta, developed in cooperation with Allergan, a global pharmaceutical company, and Meds360, a global health-care non-profit. The FDA approved Liletta, an IUD with a one-hand inserter and hormone profile similar to Mirena, in 2015. The most significant difference between Liletta and Mirena, however, was not the inserter, but the values-based development of the IUD and commitment of Allergan and Meds360 to address the expense of IUDs for patients and providers. Their commitment to the public health benefits of contraception led them to offer the IUD at extremely reduced rates in order to ensure that the most underserved and marginalized communities would have access to effective, long-acting contraceptive methods [21,22].

The National Institutes of Health (NIH) has recognized the value of fellowship research by enrolling 12 of its sites in the nation's largest contraceptive development program, the Contraceptive Clinical Trials Network (CCTN) [23]. NIH-sponsored contraceptive research at these universities is usually led by their fellowship directors. The CCTN collaborates with non-profit research groups like the Population Council and FHI 360 to use combinations of private foundation and government funding to advance contraceptive development. An exemplary product is the Annovera one-year vaginal contraceptive ring – a product of the Population Council, NIH, pharmaceutical industry and Fellowship site collaborations over several years.

The Fellowship in Family Planning has advanced contraception and abortion research through two unique programs for its graduates. The first is a placement at the World Health Organization's (WHO) Center for Reproductive Health Research in Geneva. A recently graduated fellow is selected by a WHO and Fellowship panel to work alongside WHO career researchers on global contraceptive and abortion evaluations for one to two years. Eleven fellowship graduates have participated in this placement since its inception in 2006.

Unlike WHO scientists, these Fellowship graduates are active clinicians who bring to WHO patient care and health system perspectives. WHO-assigned fellows have been particularly valuable in developing and updating guidelines and manuals used around the world for contraceptive and abortion care. Publications include the *Clinical Practice Handbook for Safe Abortion*, *Eligibility Criteria for Contraceptive Use (MEC)* and *Selective Practice Recommendations (SPR)*. Fellows contributed to recommendations for misoprostol use for obstetric and gynecologic indications. WHO's technical and policy guidance for health systems on safe termination of pregnancy led the development of a new guideline on medication abortion, developed evidence-based recommendations of medical management of missed, incomplete and induced abortions and helped create the Global Abortion Policies Database (GAPD) [8,24–29]. Fellows led capacity-strengthening workshops, multi-center international trials and more than fifteen systematic reviews of topics such as emergency contraception, hormonal contraceptive use and HIV/AIDS

and other medical conditions, providers of safe pregnancy care, contraceptive implants and telemedicine for medication abortion. Several former fellows remained at WHO beyond their initial two-year assignment as staff scientists and mentors to newly assigned fellows or worked with international agencies in leadership and advisory roles. Because of the success of the "WHO Assignments," the Fellowship developed a similar program with the Division of Reproductive Health at the CDC in 2010. As with WHO, CDC and Fellowship representatives select from among applicant fellows one to join the CDC reproductive health research group for the following two years. As at WHO, these recent Fellowship graduates bring a fresh clinical perspective to the work of the Division of Reproductive Health, where they have been particularly useful in adapting WHO contraceptive practice guidelines and standards to the US situation and conducting surveillance of US abortion trends and safety. As with WHO, some of these fellows accept career positions at the CDC. They can then serve as mentors to newly arriving fellows. Since its inception, nine fellowship graduates participated in the CDC assignment. They work closely with WHO, updating and preparing for its own US MEC and US SPR and to add new topics for guidance such as IUD placement postpartum and after pelvic infection [30–35]. Their focus is on the maintenance, dissemination and implementation of the CDC contraception guidelines. This has included working on systematic reviews (in primary and support roles), participating in the WHO reproductive health collaboration and contributing to the CDC's abortion surveillance program. Fellows also assisted with the data management, analysis and manuscript preparation for the 2015 Abortion Surveillance Report.

The FFP fellows who want specialized research training can take advantage of one- or two-month assignments in contraceptive development at the Population Council's Biomedical Research Center at Rockefeller University in New York City [36].

7.2.4 Charlotte Ellertson Social Science Postdoctoral Fellowship in Abortion and Reproductive Health

Social science research on abortion is critically important to inform policy debates and improve services and access, yet few organizations and researchers conduct abortion research. Abortion is politicized and polarizing, leading many researchers to shy away from addressing it, even though it is a central issue at stake in our elections, and in powerful government decisions shaping individuals' opportunities and social views of gender and sexuality. In 2003, Ibis Reproductive Health in partnership with the University of California, San Francisco (UCSF), Bixby Center for Global Reproductive Health, launched the Charlotte Ellertson Social Science Postdoctoral Fellowship in Abortion and Reproductive Health to foster talented researchers committed to reproductive health and rights. The Ellertson Fellowship was inspired by and emulated the model of the clinical ob-gyn Fellowship in Family Planning. As a postdoctoral two-year program with salary and research support, it advanced training for social scientists in research, leadership, advocacy and interdisciplinary policy-relevant work in contraception and abortion. The Fellowship extended to several other sites, including Columbia University Mailman School of Public Health, Johns Hopkins University Bloomberg School of Public Health and the Guttmacher Institute.

This highly competitive fellowship attracted an impressive pool of applicants from across the globe, and graduated fellows have made important contributions, complementing the clinical contributions of family planning fellows. The fellowship set the precedent for collaboration between the clinical and social sciences, which is reflected in the Society of Family Planning's research agenda and support. The Ellertson fellows came from a cross section of social science disciplines, with doctoral degrees in psychology, sociology, anthropology, demography, epidemiology, public health and psychology. The fellows have gone on to take prestigious jobs at universities and at private research institutions, and their work continues to advance reproductive health research. Fellows have produced a body of high-quality research, demonstrating that abortion does not cause mental health problems, including, for example, depression and anxiety. Their research has also scrutinized abortion access for imprisoned women, abortion stigma and the reproductive health experiences of women of color. Globally, their work has investigated abortion restrictions in Poland and other

countries. Rigorous research also demonstrated the positive impact of the legalization of services in Nepal and Mexico City on safety and maternal health [37].

7.3 Clinical Care and the Ryan and Fellowship in Family Planning Programs

Research creates the evidence base to improve clinical practice and population health. This evidence is translated into better health through well-trained practitioners. Other chapters of this book describe the academic and clinical programs that train many types of clinicians to provide family planning care in hospitals and freestanding clinics around the world. In the USA and elsewhere, the growth of the Fellowship in Family Planning has had an enormous positive impact on access to abortion care in hospitals, clinics and traditional office practices.

As the Fellowship has grown over the past 20 years, graduates of the program have gone on to start Ryan Residency Programs across the country. Eighty percent of all Ryan programs have fellowship-trained physicians leading them. As a result, of the more than 280 ob-gyn residency programs in the USA, 100 are homes to Ryan programs that offer abortion care training for all residents. Ongoing evaluations of the impact of these training programs show that nearly all graduates did abortions during residency (median of 31, including all medical and procedural techniques) [13]. A third of those trained reported that they intended to do abortions in their current hospital, clinic or office practice. Another third who said they want to provide abortions do not do them because of state or practice site restrictions on abortion care for their patients [13].

In Massachusetts, a state with wide access to abortion care, only 13% of the reproductive-aged women live in a county without an abortion provider [38]. This wasn't always the case, and abortion access in Massachusetts provides an example of the impact of the Ryan and Fellowship in Family Planning programs. Brigham and Women's Hospital established a residency training program in abortion in 1973 and a Fellowship in Family Planning in 2005. Referrals to the hospital were common, and women came from all over New England to get hospital-based care. Since then, many graduating residents and fellows have stayed in the region and have increased access to second trimester abortion care.

Though access to abortion care is one fundamental way to measure the success of the Fellowship, it is not the only aspect of women's health in which the Fellowship has had a positive impact. At the University of Pennsylvania Hospital in Philadelphia, the development of a Fellowship program led to a new model of care for patients experiencing early pregnancy complications or a pregnancy loss. In 2013, the University of Pennsylvania program noted that, though miscarriage is the most common complication of pregnancy, few patients were treated for miscarriage in their physicians' offices. Because traditional prenatal care generally begins when a patient is already eight to ten weeks pregnant, few women receive care during the early first trimester, the time during which a miscarriage is most likely to occur. During those weeks, most patients with problem pregnancies go to an emergency department for care, despite the fact that miscarriage is rarely a medical emergency [39,40]. Often these patients experience multiple, confusing and expensive visits to a busy emergency department ill equipped to manage either the medical or the complex emotional component of pregnancy complications, and eager to discharge a patient who is not experiencing a true medical emergency [41].

Managing a miscarriage, either with medication or surgery, is identical to providing abortion care, and often very similar in terms of emotional care for the patient. Through qualitative interviews with patients who have experienced miscarriage, along with studies of cost, it became clear that finding a way to integrate miscarriage management into an office-based abortion care setting would benefit patients and health-care systems. This model allowed patients to access care in a specialized practice with clinicians expert in pregnancy loss throughout pregnancy. As a consequence, residents and fellows learned to direct care efficiently, with appropriate emotional support, and using evidence-based practices such as offering mifepristone in conjunction with misoprostol for early miscarriage management, or for cervical preparation during dilation and evacuation procedures for pregnancy losses that happen later in pregnancy [7].

By integrating pregnancy loss into the abortion care practice and developing a health service–wide system for pregnant patients to access care throughout their pregnancies, this program is giving physician learners and advanced-practice clinician learners experience in managing complex pregnancies in an evidence-based, shared decision-making model. Treatment of all aspects of pregnancy loss, from early miscarriage to later fetal demise, and abortion, exposes learners to the complex and inequitable system of pregnancy care, leading some to become researchers and advocates.

7.4 Family Planning Training and Advocacy

A unique requirement of the Fellowship in Family Planning is developing physician advocates. (See Chapter 4.) Integrated into the Fellowship experience, along with clinical and research training and experience, is advocacy skill building and training through programs like Physicians for Reproductive Health's (PRH) Leadership Training Academy and the ACOG Congressional Leadership Conference and Darney-Landy Fellowship [42]. The skills developed through these immersive experiences prepare Fellowship physicians to be leaders in reproductive health advocacy through media training, experience lobbying legislators and public testimony when antiabortion legislation is proposed, as well as advocates in their own departments, medical schools and health systems. This integration of advocacy is important in strengthening physicians' connections to the reproductive health, rights and justice community. As a result, the collaborations between abortion-providing physicians and advocacy organizations have promoted policy changes, successful court challenges and a greater understanding of the importance of family planning and abortion to the public. (See Chapter 4.)

7.5 Political and Legal Effects of Fellowship Advocacy

Fellowship physicians have used their academic experience, evidence-based practices and clinical expertise to help defeat state and local laws, including gestational limit bans, abortion method bans, mandatory ultrasound bills and parental consent laws. In Pennsylvania, the work of

Fellowship graduates was instrumental in preventing a dangerous legal prohibition of the common dilation and evacuation abortion method (D&E), which would have prevented the use of D&E in any circumstance, including miscarriage or fetal demise. In Georgia, Fellowship graduates' testimonies helped to stop a law limiting abortion to no more than 20 weeks' gestation. If the efforts of reproductive health, rights and justice advocates do not prevent the passage of legislation harmful to health, they are often successful in the court battles that follow [43].

Not all of fellowship physicians' advocacy is focused on defeating antiabortion legislation. In some states, they work on proactive policies that expand access to abortion and contraception. All but nine states in the USA have "physician-only" laws, disallowing advanced-practice clinicians (APCs) from providing abortions. (See Chapters 16 and 26.) California was the first state to pass legislation explicitly allowing APCs to provide first-trimester abortions using safety data from research at Fellowship sites. Providers in Maine and Montana are now suing to overturn physician-only laws for abortion provision based on the success of access expansion in California [44].

7.6 Culture Change

Along with effecting policy change, Fellowship-trained physicians are also changing the cultural narratives of abortion. Personal storytelling from people who experience abortion has long been known to have an impact on how the public perceives those who seek abortion. Storytelling by physicians is proving to have a similar impact.

Ryan and Fellowship program graduates with faith-based backgrounds describe their call to abortion practice as a part of their faith practices through writings, speaking engagements and social media to challenge false narratives about abortion [45]. Many open their practices to journalists, the public and the media to demystify and normalize abortion [46,47,48]. Studies of the media show that this openness is working to shift public perceptions of abortion. TV and film audits show a slow but steady shift toward more accurate, positive representations of abortion in shows and movies [49].

Though geographic disparities in access to abortion and complex family planning persist, the Ryan and Fellowship programs have improved quality and access. The National Academies of Science, Engineering, and Medicine's comprehensive 2018 report on abortion care in the USA noted that access to care is very much dependent on the existence of a residency training program or Fellowship in the region. Unfortunately, political action to restrict abortion and contraceptive access creates challenges for improving women's health in the most underserved regions of the country. Fellowship research has shown that those regions provide generally poor health services for women and children having, for example, high maternal mortality rates in comparison to regions that are not restrictive [47]. If Ryan Program and Fellowship graduates can continue to integrate abortion into their practices and advocate for evidence-based care in their regions, measurable improvements in maternal and infant mortality will result.

7.6.1 Crossing the Threshold of Formal Certification and Accreditation

The Fellowship in Family Planning has influenced institutions, services, professional organizations and social change more than its founders anticipated. Former fellows report that they are actively working to change their institutions to ensure greater access and improved quality of family planning and abortion services. In their teaching of medical students and residents, they are directly influencing the attitudes and skills of future providers, and often win "outstanding teacher" awards from their medical schools, where many serve in the influential administrative positions of student clerkship directors, residency program directors and section and division heads, and an increasing few are department chairs and deans. Outside their own departments and schools, graduated fellows hold leadership positions in national professional organizations like the American Board of Obstetrics and Gynecology (ABOG), ACOG, Planned Parenthood, SFP, National Abortion Federation (NAF) and PRH and serve as advisors to the National Institute of Child Health and Human Development (NICHD), WHO pharmaceutical companies, and nongovernmental organizations like IPAS, JHPIEGO, Engender Health and Population Services International (PSI). With certification and accreditation of Complex Family Planning's subspecialty status, representation will grow to include ABOG and ACGME. (See Chapter 1.)

The culmination of the Fellowship's institutional impact was the American Board of Obstetrics and Gynecology's submission of the application for certification of the Complex Family Planning subspecialty to the American Board of Medical Specialties (ABMS) in April 2018. This submission was supported by letters from the SFP, PRH, Catholics for Choice (CFC), CDC, Society for Maternal-Fetal Medicine (SMFM) and the American Society for Reproductive Medicine (ASRM). In October 2018, the ABMS Board of Directors voted to approve ABOG's application, a hard-earned victory for which the organization is indebted to ABOG's dedicated and persistent leadership, specifically Drs. George Wendel, its Executive

Director; Laurel Rice, chair of ABOG's ad hoc Family Planning Committee; and Dr. Debbie Driscoll, ABOG's chair at the time.

Soon after ABOG received the news from ABMS, ABOG submitted a proposal to the Accreditation Council for Graduate Medical Education (ACGME) for accreditation. In 2019, the ACGME's board approved Complex Family Planning for accreditation. Accreditation of sites and certification of subspecialists are currently underway.

The systematic integration of family planning through two national initiatives and the resulting clinical, research, education, advocacy and global leadership have contributed to far-reaching changes to the academic status, policies and access to care related to all aspects of family planning.

References

1. Committee on Health Care for Underserved Women. ACOG Committee Opinion No. 612: abortion training and education. *Obstet Gynecol.* 2014;**124**(5):1055–1059. doi:10.1097/01. AOG.0000456327.96480.18

2. Steinauer JE, Turk JK, Pomerantz T, Simonson K, Learman LA, Landy U. Abortion training in US obstetrics and gynecology residency programs. *Am J Obstet Gynecol.* 2018;**219**(1):86.e1–86.e6. doi:10.1016/j.ajog.2018. 04.011

3. Steinauer JE, Turk JK, Fulton MC, Simonson KH, Landy U. The benefits of family planning training: a 10-year review of the Ryan Residency Training Program. *Contraception.* 2013;**88**(2):275–280. doi:10.1016/j. contraception.2013.02.006

4. Fellowship in Family Planning National Office, 2019 Program Data.

5. Miller RA. *Evaluation of the Family Planning Fellowship.* Oakland: Public Health Institute; 2006:89.

6. Renner R-M, Nichols MD, Jensen JT, Li H, Edelman AB. Paracervical block for pain control in first-trimester surgical abortion: a randomized controlled trial. *Obstet Gynecol.* 2012;**119** (5):1030–1037. doi:10.1097/ AOG.0b013e318250b13e

7. Schreiber CA, Creinin MD, Atrio J, Sonalkar S, Ratcliffe SJ, Barnhart KT. Mifepristone pretreatment for the medical management of early pregnancy loss. *N Engl J Med.* 2018;**378**(23):2161–2170. doi:10.1056/NEJMoa1715726

8. National Academies of Sciences, Engineering, and Medicine, Health and Medicine Division, Board on Health Care Services, Board on Population Health and Public Health Practice, Committee on Reproductive Health Services: Assessing the Safety and Quality of Abortion Care in the U.S. *The Safety and Quality of Abortion Care in the United States.* Washington, DC: National Academies Press 2018. www.ncbi.nlm.nih.gov/books/ NBK507236/. Accessed March 30, 2020.

9. Secura GM, Madden T, McNicholas C, et al. Provision of no-cost, long-acting

contraception and teenage pregnancy. *N Engl J Med.* 2014;**371**(14):1316–1323. doi:10.1056/NEJMoa1400506

10. American Academy of Pediatrics. AAP Updates Recommendations on Teen Pregnancy Prevention. http:// www.aap.org/en-us/about-the- aap/aap-press-room/Pages/ AAP-Updates- Recommendations-on-Teen- Pregnancy-Prevention.aspx. Accessed April 7, 2020.

11. ACOG Committee Opinion No. 735: adolescents and long- acting reversible contraception: implants and intrauterine devices. *Obstet Gynecol.* 2018;**131**(5):e130–e139. doi:10.1097/ AOG.0000000000002632

12. Simonson K, Pomerantz T, Mullersman K, Ly E, Landy U. Improving evidence-based practice for LARC: evaluation of the Ryan LARC program. Oral presentation at the International Federation of Gynaecology and Obstetrics meeting; 2015.

13. Kenneth J. Ryan Residency Training Program in Family Planning and Abortion National Office, 2019 Program Data.

14. Welcome to Family Planning Fellowship | Family Planning Fellowship. www .familyplanningfellowship.org/. Accessed April 6, 2020.

15. Colorado's success with long-acting reversible contraception (LARC). Department of Public Health and Environment; January 6, 2017. www.colorado .gov/pacific/cdphe/cfpi-report. Accessed April 6, 2020.

16. Rodriguez MI, Chang R, Thiel de Bocanegra H. The impact of postpartum contraception on reducing preterm birth: findings from California. *Am J Obstet Gynecol*. 2015;**213** (5):703.e1–6. doi:10.1016/j. ajog.2015.07.033

17. Allen RH, Cwiak C, eds. *Contraception for the Medically Challenging Patient*. New York: Springer-Verlag; 2014.

18. Thiel de Bocanegra H, Chang R, Menz M, Howell M, Darney P. Postpartum contraception in publicly-funded programs and interpregnancy intervals. *Obstet Gynecol*. 2013;**122**(2 Pt 1):296–303. doi:10.1097/ AOG.0b013e3182991db6

19. Thiel de Bocanegra H, Chang R, Howell M, Darney P. Interpregnancy intervals: impact of postpartum contraceptive effectiveness and coverage. *Am J Obstet Gynecol*. 2014;**210**(4):311.e1–311.e8. doi:10.1016/j.ajog.2013.12.020

20. Rodriguez MI, Jensen JT, Darney PD, Little SE, Caughey AB. The financial effects of expanding postpartum contraception for new immigrants. *Obstet Gynecol*. 2010;**115**(3):552–558. doi:10.1097/ AOG.0b013e3181d06f96

21. Darney PD, Stuart GS, Thomas MA, Cwiak C, Olariu A, Creinin MD. Amenorrhea rates and predictors during 1 year of levonorgestrel 52 mg intrauterine system use. *Contraception*. 2018;**97**

(3):210–214. doi:10.1016/j. contraception.2017.10.005

22. Archer DF, Merkatz RB, Bahamondes L, et al. Efficacy of the 1-year (13-cycle) segesterone acetate and ethinylestradiol contraceptive vaginal system: results of two multicentre, open-label, single-arm, phase 3 trials. *Lancet Glob Health*. 2019;7(8):e1054–e1064. doi:10.1016/S2214-109X(19) 30265-7

23. Contraceptive Clinical Trials Network (CCTN). www.nichd .nih.gov/research/supported/ cctn.. Accessed April 6, 2020.

24. *Clinical Practice Handbook for Safe Abortion*. Geneva: World Health Organization; 2014. www.ncbi.nlm.nih.gov/books/ NBK190095/. Accessed April 6, 2020.

25. Centers for Disease Control and Prevention (CDC). U S. Medical Eligibility Criteria for Contraceptive Use, 2010. *MMWR Recomm Rep Morb Mortal Wkly Rep Recomm Rep*. 2010;59(RR-4):1–86.

26. Curtis KM, Jatlaoui TC, Tepper NK, et al. U.S. Selected Practice Recommendations for Contraceptive Use, 2016. *MMWR Recomm Rep*. 2016;65 (4):1–66. doi:10.15585/mmwr. rr6504a1

27. Tang J, Kapp N, Dragoman M, de Souza JP. WHO recommendations for misoprostol use for obstetric and gynecologic indications. *Int J Gynaecol Obstet*. 2013;121 (2):186–189. doi:10.1016/j. ijgo.2012.12.009

28. Lavelanet AF, Schlitt S, Johnson BR, Ganatra B. Global Abortion Policies Database: a descriptive analysis of the legal categories of lawful abortion. *BMC Int Health Hum Rights*. 2018;18(1):44. doi:10.1186/ s12914-018-0183-1

29. *Medical Management of Abortion*. Geneva: World Health Organization; 2018.

www.ncbi.nlm.nih.gov/books/ NBK536779/. Accessed April 6, 2020.

30. Hannaford PC, Ti A, Chipato T, Curtis KM. Copper intrauterine device use and HIV acquisition in women: a systematic review. *BMJ Sex Reprod Health*. 2020;**46** (1):17–5. doi:10.1136/bmjsrh-2019-200512

31. Jatlaoui TC, Eckhaus L, Mandel MG, et al. Abortion surveillance – United States, 2016. *MMWR Surveill Summ*. 2019;**68**(11):1–41. doi:10.15585/mmwr.ss6811a1

32. Lathrop E, Romero L, Hurst S, et al. The Zika Contraception Access Network: a feasibility programme to increase access to contraception in Puerto Rico during the 2016–17 Zika virus outbreak. *Lancet Public Health*. 2018;3(2):e91–e99. doi:10.1016/S2468-2667(18) 30001-X

33. Li R, Simmons KB, Bertolli J, et al. Cost-effectiveness of increasing access to contraception during the Zika virus outbreak, Puerto Rico, 2016. *Emerg Infect Dis*. 2017;**23** (1):74–82. doi:10.3201/ eid2301.161322

34. Curtis KM, Tepper NK, Jatlaoui TC, et al. U.S. medical eligibility criteria for contraceptive use, 2016. *MMWR Recomm Rep*. 2016;**65** (3):1–103. doi:10.15585/mmwr. rr6503a1

35. Gavin L, Moskosky S, Carter M, et al. Providing quality family planning services: recommendations of CDC and the U.S. Office of Population Affairs. *MMWR Recomm Rep*. 2014;**63**(RR-04):1–54.

36. The Center for Biomedical Research | Population Council. www.popcouncil.org/cbr. Accessed April 6, 2020.

37. Charlotte Ellertson Social Science Postdoctoral Fellowship in Abortion and

Reproductive Health. Ibis Reproductive Health; May 1, 2011. www .ibisreproductivehealth.org/ projects/charlotte-ellertson- social-science-postdoctoral- fellowship-abortion-and- reproductive-health. Accessed April 6, 2020.

38. Guttmacher Institute. State Facts about Abortion: Massachusetts; January 26, 2016. www.guttmacher.org/ fact-sheet/state-facts-about- abortion-massachusetts. Accessed April 6, 2020.

39. Lang B, Sammel M, Meisel Z, Schreiber C. Most patients with bleeding and cramping in early pregnancy can be safely triaged to the ambulatory setting. *Contraception.* 2019;**100**:325. doi:0.1016/j. contraception.2019.07.070

40. Shorter JM, Atrio JM, Schreiber CA. Management of early pregnancy loss, with a focus on patient centered care. *Semin Perinatol.* 2019;**43**

(2):84–94. doi:10.1053/j. semperi.2018.12.005

41. Miller CA, Roe AH, McAllister A, Meisel ZF, Koelper N, Schreiber CA. Patient experiences with miscarriage management in the emergency and ambulatory settings. *Obstet Gynecol.* 2019;**134** (6):1285–1292. doi:10.1097/ AOG.0000000000003571

42. ACOG Congressional Leadership Conference (CLC). www.acog.org/en/Education. Accessed April 6, 2020.

43. Lathrop v. Deal, 801 S.E.2d 867 (Ga 2017).

44. Weitz TA, Taylor D, Desai S, et al. Safety of aspiration abortion performed by nurse practitioners, certified nurse midwives, and physician assistants under a California legal waiver. *Am J Public Health.* 2013;**103**(3):454–461. doi:10.2105/AJPH.2012.301159

45. Parker W. *Life's Work: A Moral Argument for Choice.* New York: 37 Ink; 2017.

46. Gordon M, McCammon S. A drug that eases miscarriages is difficult for women to get. NPR; January 10, 2019. www.npr.org/sections/ health-shots/2019/01/10/ 666957368/a-drug-that-eases- miscarriages-is-difficult-for- women-to-get

47. Harris LH. My day as an abortion care provider. *New York Times*; October 24, 2019:23.

48. Hardy-Fairbanks A. Mother and abortion provider – I can be both. *Newsweek*; May 11, 2019. www.newsweek.com/ abortion-provider-mother- opinion-1409871

49. Abortion Onscreen. Abortion Onscreen in 2019. San Francisco: Advancing New Standards in Reproductive Health; 2019:19. www.ansirh .org/sites/default/files/ publications/files/Abortion% 20Onscreen%20Report% 202019.pdf. Accessed April 7, 2020.

Chapter

8

Conscientious Provision and Objection in Medical Training in the Context of the Abortion Controversy

Wendy Chavkin

8.1 Conscientious Objection

In recent years around the globe, many have cited "conscientious objection" to justify their refusal to participate in politically contested changes in medical and social practices. Conscientious objection has been defined as the refusal to participate in an activity that an individual considers incompatible with his/her religious, moral, philosophical or ethical beliefs [1]. This originated as opposition to mandatory military service but has increasingly been raised in a wide variety of controversial settings, such as education (eg, evolution, climate change, sex), capital punishment, driver's license requirements, marriage licenses for same-sex couples and medicine and health care. For example, conscientious objection has been invoked in the USA by those resisting racially discriminatory laws and the Vietnam War; providing sanctuary to Central American refugees denied political asylum; and by those opposed to legal abortions, emergency contraception, end-of-life care, vaccination, blood transfusion, stem cell research, same-sex marriage licenses and wedding cakes [2].

Conscientious objection to sexual and reproductive health care (eg, refusal to perform abortion, assisted reproductive technologies, prenatal diagnosis, contraception, including emergency contraception and sterilization, care for transgender people) has become a widespread global phenomenon and constitutes a barrier to these services for many. Although there are few rigorously obtained data regarding prevalence of this practice, estimates vary widely, according to context [3]. Thus, in Scandinavia, where sexual and reproductive health care is accepted as normative, only a small minority claim conscientious objector status regarding abortion provision, whereas in Ghana two surveys indicate that more than a third of obstetrician-gynecologists (obgyns) object to providing abortion and more than 80% do so in Italy [3,4].

Conscientious objection raises the profound question of when and how to draw the line between support for individual belief and integrity and support for those with other beliefs who are entitled to legally permitted goods, services and protections [5]. Non-theocratic states are obligated to treat all citizens' beliefs equally and fairly and to negotiate the boundaries between rights in tension. Health-care providers have additional specific obligations, known as fiduciary duties, to put the needs of patients first, ahead of their own [2].

The International Covenant on Civil and Political Rights, a central pillar of human rights that gives legal force to the 1948 UN Universal Declaration of Human Rights, states in Article 18(1) that:

> Everyone shall have the right to freedom of thought, conscience and religion. This right shall include freedom to have or to adopt a religion or belief of his choice, and freedom, either individually or in community with others and in public or private, to manifest his religion or belief in worship, observance, practice and teaching. [1]

Article 18(3), however, states that:

> Freedom to manifest one's religion or beliefs may be subject only to such limitations as are prescribed by law and are necessary to protect public safety, order, health or morals or the fundamental rights and freedoms of others. Many other international covenants and national constitutions, including that of the US, protect freedom of belief and speech, but also stipulate that their exercise may not compromise the rights of others. [1]

This concept is key, as otherwise, those who refuse to participate in a contested social requirement extend their objection beyond personal participation, and effectively seek to govern the conduct of others who do not share their religious or moral beliefs [6]. By so doing, they undermine their own position by subverting pluralism, the animating value underlying protection of individual conscience from the dictates of the majority.

American society has many rules and directives that individuals must follow regardless of how their consciences compel them. Business owners, for example, must comply with tax requirements, worker protection and antidiscrimination laws and policies. Government employees and elected officials must fulfill basic obligations of public service, including adherence to all laws and regulations that provide equal opportunity for all Americans regardless of race, color, religion, sex *education*, national origin, age or disability, and in some jurisdictions, regardless of gender identity and sexual orientation [7].

Moreover, the state is responsible for advancing the social good by promoting public health measures and fundamental values such as pluralism and equity and requires citizens and residents to fulfill duties that contribute to these values. Examples include mandatory military service, compulsory education and mandated compliance with measures to halt the spread of infectious diseases. Those objecting must comply with alternative requirements to ensure that they do not undermine these social goods and shared values (eg, alternative service for those refusing combat or California's and New York's exclusion from school for unvaccinated children) [8,9]. However, those invoking conscientious objection today often seek exemption from legal or professional consequences for refusing to perform a duty.

8.2 Conscientious Objection and Medical Practice

In the domain of health care, the situation is further complicated, as those who choose to work in these professions have additional obligations. As licensure conveys monopoly and power over provision of that service, with attendant social benefits, the profession becomes a kind of public utility, with consequent obligations to the public trust. In exchange for being granted such privileges as self-governance by the state, professionals (eg, physicians, lawyers and financial advisors) are expected to fulfill fiduciary duties, that is, to put the needs of patients or clients first, ahead of their own [2].

In the case of medicine, because the balance of knowledge favors the physician, and patients are vulnerable, patients must be able to trust that physicians will put their needs first and ensure that they can exercise autonomy. Recent emphasis in medical practice on shared medical decision making is predicated on the importance of self-determination. The assumption that physicians will put patients' needs ahead of their own is critical for maintenance of public trust in the profession.

The bar for assessing whether to accommodate objection in health care should be higher than in other domains, as fiduciary duty implies that a clinician should never give higher priority to her/his own conscience than to the patient's needs. However, in practice, it is often lower – and messy – because many countries have laws permitting clinicians to refuse to provide abortions (and sometimes other components of care) on grounds of conscience. Importantly, some countries also specify constraints on the clinician's exercise of conscience, such as mandating that the objector provide the patient with accurate information and timely referrals, and actually provide the contested care in urgent circumstances [10–13].

Many countries other than the USA have national health-care systems that provide publicly funded health care, and the state health-care system has an obligation to provide agreed-on health-care services to its citizens. National health systems in many countries with legal abortion are obligated to assure the provision of free, timely and appropriate abortion care, a task for which they rely on regional health authorities and hospital managers [4].

The duty to provide abortion services therefore rests at the organizational level as opposed to an individual one. This shifts the frame from locating the issue of conscience entirely at the individual level to consideration of obligations at the professional and health system levels. For example, the national health sectors in Norway and Portugal underscore the health-care system's obligation to ensure that care is available by paying for clinicians or patients to travel to provide or receive abortions, only permitting refusal of care if a patient has reasonable access to the contested care [4]. Both countries also permit employers to consider willingness to provide needed services and proficiency as criteria for employment.

Study findings and anecdotal reports from many countries suggest that some clinicians claim conscientious objection for reasons other than deeply held religious or ethical convictions. For example, some physicians in Brazil who described themselves as objectors were, nonetheless, willing to obtain or provide abortions for their immediate family members. A Polish study described clinicians, such as those referred to as the White Coat Underground, who claim conscientious objection status in their public sector jobs but provide the same services in their fee-paying private practices. Other investigations indicate that some claim objector status because they seek to avoid being associated with stigmatized services, rather than because they truly conscientiously object [14].

Moreover, some religiously affiliated health-care institutions claim objector status and compel their employees to refuse to provide legally permissible care [15]. The right to conscience is generally understood to belong to an individual, not to an institution, as claims of conscience are considered a way to maintain an individual's moral or religious integrity. Some disagree, however, and argue that a hospital's mission is analogous to a conscience resembling that of an individual. Others dispute this on the grounds that health-care institutions are licensed by states and often receive public financing, and therefore are reciprocally obligated to put patients' needs and autonomy first, especially if the institution is the sole provider of health-care services in a community.

Various international (the International Federation of Gynecology and Obstetrics [FIGO], the World Health Organization [WHO], the World Medical Association [WMA]) and national medical professional bodies, such as the American College of Obstetricians and Gynecologists (ACOG), have affirmed that the individual clinician has the right to object to performing a component of care that violates his/her conscience BUT that this right is secondary to the obligation to the patient [10–13]. Specifically:

- Providers have a right to conscientious objection and not to suffer discrimination on the basis of their beliefs.
- The primary conscientious duty of health-care providers is to treat or provide benefit and prevent harm to patients; conscientious objection is secondary to this primary duty.

Moreover, the following safeguards must be in place in order to ensure access to services without discrimination or undue delays:

- Providers have a professional duty to follow scientifically and professionally determined definitions of reproductive health services, and not to misrepresent them on the basis of personal beliefs.
- Patients have the right to be referred to practitioners who do not object for procedures medically indicated for their care.
- Health-care providers must provide patients with timely access to medical services, including giving information about the medically indicated options of procedures for care, including those that providers object to on grounds of conscience.
- Providers must offer timely care to their patients when referral to other providers is not possible and delay would jeopardize patients' health.
- In emergency situations, providers must provide the medically indicated care, regardless of their own personal objections.

Few have thought this through in the realm of medical education and post-graduate training, which play essential roles in educating future practitioners. Medical education institutionalizes training in the clinical care, research, social and public health aspects of family planning. When teaching hospitals claim institutional conscientious objection, as do some Catholic hospitals in the USA, for example, they fail to educate their trainees about an essential, potentially life-saving aspect of women's health. How can educational institutions claim institutional objection and yet reconcile the right to conscience of students and residents with the need to ensure that these students and residents are well trained, able to demonstrate competency in all the components of their profession and specialty and clear about their fiduciary duties?

We know very little about the intentions of medical students and residents to participate in training and abortion provision. A convenience sample of Spanish medical and nursing students indicated that most supported access to abortion and intended to provide it [3]. A survey of medical, nursing and physician assistant students at a US university indicated that more than two thirds supported abortion yet only one third intended to provide abortion, with the nursing and physician assistant students evincing the strongest interest in doing so. In the USA, among nearly 1,600 ob-gyn residents, 61% planned to do abortions for all indications after training [16]. A survey of nearly 500 ob-gyn residents in the USA found that 15% had opted out of some portions of their clinical abortion training due to religious or moral reasons, but all benefited from participating in some aspects of abortion care. In order to learn uterine evacuation skills, half of partial *objectors* did at least one abortion during training [17]. A survey of family medicine residents in the USA assessing prevalence of moral objection to 14 legally available medical procedures revealed that 52% supported performing abortion for failed contraception; a recent survey indicated that half supported performing abortion and that all provided medication abortion. Twenty years ago, 52% of a non-random sample of regional consultant ob-gyns in the UK said that insufficient numbers of junior doctors were being trained to provide abortions owing to opting out and conscientious objection [3,15,18,19].

Now in the UK, the General Medical Council's guidance for medical students states that students are entitled to conscientiously object but must meet expected competencies and cannot be exempted from doing so. The Royal College of Obstetricians and Gynaecologists and the Institute of Medical Ethics concur and add detail about conscientious objection, professional obligations and clinical practice. Curricula vary across the UK but a 2018 survey in one medical school in England reported 96% of medical students considered it important to teach about the clinical, legal, ethical and professional concerns related to abortion in medical school, whatever their personal opinions might be. Indeed, 96% endorsed this even though only 87% of students supported the availability of legal abortion. Similar responses were reported by a Scottish medical school Although there is ready access to abortion in England because most procedures are performed by the independent sector in stand-alone clinics, interviewees explained that this had led to a lack of sufficient opportunity for training in abortion care for ob-gyn residents within the NHS. They anticipate that this technical competence gap could prove increasingly problematic, since the need for hospital-based abortion care for women with medical complications may increase

if England's obesity and diabetes epidemics persist [3,21,22].

Norway avoids this problem by relying on ob-gyns in training to provide most in-hospital abortions. While students and ob-gyn residents are allowed to conscientiously object to performing abortion, they are not allowed to object to learning about abortion and contraception and residents may not refuse to perform emergency uterine evacuations and must demonstrate competencies in uterine evacuation, IUD insertion, performance of sterilization and other components of care that are sometimes contested. They are also trained in value free counseling for women requesting abortion and are not allowed to reveal personal opinions [23,24].

8.3 USA

In the USA, training of health-care providers is defined and enforced by professional associations. The training of students and residents takes place in specifically designated teaching hospitals that are accredited by a voluntary private organization to provide specific areas of training. Such training is financed by federal, state and other public and private funds. The objectives of resident training are set and enforced by the Accreditation Council for Graduate Medical Education (ACGME) in the USA. Twenty-two years after abortion had been legalized, the ACGME specifically addressed abortion training, based on agreement by the ob-gyn leadership that such training was a necessary aspect of women's health care and stipulated that a residency program that refused to comply with the mandated training could lose its status. Catholic hospitals objected and received an exemption through a congressional amendment, which allowed them not to do abortions in the hospital but to arrange for training nevertheless (see Chapter 3).

Once the training has been professionally mandated, conscientious objectors have been permitted to opt out of the training, A national initiative, the Ryan Residency Training Program in Abortion and Family Planning, focused on implementation of the abortion training mandate, has conducted intensive studies about the opt-out process and the results on professional perspective and future practice of the resident. (See Chapters 3, 10 and 23.) Findings show that the majority of residents participate in training to some level. Such participation changes their perceptions of the need for and impact of abortion on a woman's and her family's health. Participation also serves to destigmatize both the abortion procedure itself as well as those who provide them. It remains critically important to define which training components constitute "partial participation." While not all residents practice all the aspects of obstetrics and gynecology learned in their four years of training, they nevertheless need to be clinically prepared to make reproductive health care part of their practices.

Although many practitioners of abortions in the USA are trained in family medicine, the leadership of family medicine organizations has thus far failed to issue a training mandate. Mandated training with opt-out provisions is essential both to ensure the clinical competence of future practitioners and to confirm professional agreement that competencies in contraception and abortion are standard aspects of practice. The mandate also requires teaching hospitals to be prepared to offer this training and hence abortion services. National initiatives, such as the Ryan Program, not only ensure institutionalized clinical training, but also add other aspects such as a didactic curriculum and values clarification workshops to help the residents distinguish between their professional obligation as physicians and their personal or religious moral convictions.

8.4 Conscientious Commitment

An alternative framing is provided by the concept of *conscientious commitment*. This term refers to those providers whose conscience requires them to deliver reproductive health services, who place priority on patient care over adherence to religious doctrines or religious self-interest or see their religious/moral obligations as compelling provision of care. This is a significant concern in the USA, where mergers of religiously affiliated hospitals with secular ones have led to struggles as to which worldview and whose rules would prevail. This has emerged as a battleground regarding end-of-life care, stem cell therapies, treatments of LGBTQ populations as well as reproductive health care [20,21]. Half of a stratified random sample of US ob-gyns practicing primarily at religiously affiliated hospitals reported conflicts with the hospital regarding clinical practice; 5%

reported these to center on treatment of ectopic pregnancy [23]. Examples abound from countries with highly restrictive abortion laws of doctors who were in conflict with hospitals because they insisted on providing life-saving medical treatments or terminations of pregnancy to women with ectopic pregnancies, inevitable miscarriages, cancers and other serious health conditions.

8.5 Impact

Refusal to provide abortion and other components of reproductive care has become a significant barrier to access to safe services. In places with many willing providers, although objection may inflict difficulties and delay upon patients, patients are eventually able to procure abortions. However, those with least income or with low levels of information are least likely to be able to negotiate deterrents and, thus, objection can aggravate inequities and health disparities even within resource-rich settings with liberal abortion laws [5].

However, too many women, men and adolescents lack access to essential reproductive healthcare services because they live in countries with restrictive laws, scant health resources, too few providers and slots to train more and limited infrastructure for health care and means to reach care (eg, roads and transport). In such places where services are few, clinician objection can seriously impede access and women may experience delays such that they end up needing more complicated, riskier and later procedures, or are unable to obtain abortions at all because of gestational age limits, or resort to unsafe unofficial options, and risk harm, even death.

8.6 Recommendations for Medical Education

Medical education and residency training offer important opportunities to inform new physicians about the scope of conscientious objection to the provision of components of care. This topic draws on medical ethics and professional obligations, law, society and medicine, and can be tailored so that the discussion is socially and politically contextually specific: the professional community's expectation that such training is necessary to achieve clinical competence, reduce stigma and affirm abortion to be an integrated part of women's health care. When a country legalizes abortion, the government or professional societies have an opportunity to institutionalize abortion and contraception education and training for students and residents. (See Chapters 27 and 29 for Nepal and Ethiopian programs.)

Conscientious objection is relevant to medical students, whatever specialty they end up choosing, as it may arise in infectious disease, public health and pediatrics (vaccination), end-of-life care (palliation, euthanasia), surgical specialties (transfusion), oncology (stem cell therapies) and family medicine and obstetrics-gynecology. Students should learn the origins and diverse applications of conscientious objection and be able to define the core rights of individual freedom of belief, right to have access to legally available services and the pluralist state's obligation to negotiate between these competing rights. Students should become familiar with the limits agreed upon by international covenants. Education about conscientious objection offers the opportunity to teach about fiduciary duties of physicians, a critical crosscutting concept for all in the field. Students should then learn the consensus reached by professional medical societies that stipulate that the physician's primary obligation is to the patient; that only those directly involved in a contested service can object; that these objectors may not refuse to provide care prior to or following the intervention; that the physician must provide accurate information to the patient, a timely feasible referral and care in an emergency if s/he is the only physician available. The objector must also understand that unless he or she has the clinical training, the consequences of not being able to provide the care in urgent situations can be devastating and life threatening for the patient.

While the future practice direction of students is uncertain and may not include family planning, residents must be clinically trained to be proficient in taking care of their patients. This proficiency is particularly relevant to ob-gyns, whose practice includes all aspects of reproductive health.

These residents must be able to demonstrate proficiency in the knowledge and skills required of those providing comprehensive reproductive health care. Thus, even if they decline to perform voluntary terminations, for example, they must be able to insert IUDs and implants, evacuate a uterus, treat ectopic pregnancies and so forth.

For both students and residents, values clarification exercises, anchored in local law and conditions, can stimulate self-awareness and nuanced thinking about one's personal beliefs and that others' beliefs are equally important. Such training can incorporate exercises to generate creative solutions by a health-care team.

8.7 Conclusion

Conscientious objection to the provision of components of legally permitted care is increasingly salient for physicians. Physicians have particular obligations and constraints, as fiduciary duties mandate that they put patients' interests ahead of their own. Physicians can contribute to debates about the effects of conscientious objection because they, more than anyone, are aware of the health effects of denying (or providing) medical care on the basis of physician belief rather than patient need.

References

1. International Covenant on Civil and Political Rights, adopted December 16, 1966, G.A. Res. 2200A (XXI), U.N. GAOR, 21st Sess., Supp. No. 16, at 52, U.N. Doc. A/6316 (1966), 999 U.N.T.S. 171 (entered into force March 23, 1976).

2. Chavkin W, Abu-Odeh D, Clune-Taylor C, Dubow S, Ferber M, Meyer IH. Balancing freedom of conscience and equitable access. *Am J Public Health*. 2018;**108**:1487–1488.

3. Chavkin W, Leitman L, Polin K. Conscientious objection and refusal to provide reproductive healthcare: a white paper examining prevalence, health consequences, and policy responses. *Int J of Gynecol and Obstet*. 2013;**123**(S3):S41–S56.

4. Chavkin W, Swerdlow L, Fifield J. Regulation of conscientious objection to abortion. *Health Hum Rights*. 2017;**19**(1):55–68.

5. Melling L, Lim M, Brighouse R, Aviv NM. Drawing the line: tackling tensions between religious freedom and equality. International Network of Civil Liberties Organizations; 2015. www.cels.org.ar/common/documentos/DrawingtheLine .pdf

6. Raifman J, Galea S. The new US "Conscience and Religious

Freedom Division": imposing religious beliefs on others. *Am J Public Health*. 2018; **108**(7):889–890.

7. US Department of the Interior. Basic obligation of public service. www.doi.gov/ethics/ basic-obligations-of-public-service. Accessed September 26, 2019.

8. California Senate Bill 277: An Act to Amend Sections 120325, 120335, 120370, and 120375 of, to Add Section 120338 to, and to Repeal Section 120365 of, the Health and Safety Code, Relating to Public Health; 2015. https://leginfo.legislature.ca .gov/faces/billNavClient.xhtml? bill_id=201520160SB277

9. New York State Senate Bill S2994A: An Act to Amend the Public Health Law, in Relation to Exemptions from Vaccination Due to Religious Beliefs; to Repeal Subdivision 9 of Section 2164 of the Public Health Law, Relating to Exemption from Vaccination Due to Religious Beliefs; and Providing for the Repeal of Certain Provisions upon Expiration Thereof; 2019. www .nysenate.gov/legislation/bills/ 2019/s2994

10. World Medical Association. Declaration of Helsinki – Ethical principles for medical research involving human subjects. Adopted 1964. www .wma.net/en/30publications/ 10policies/b3/. Accessed September 26, 2019.

11. FIGO Committee for the Ethical Aspects of Human Reproduction and Women's Health. Ethical guidelines on conscientious objection. FIGO Committee for the Ethical Aspects of Human Reproduction and Women's Health. *Int J Gynecol Obstet*. 2006;**92**(3):333–334.

12. American College of Obstetricians and Gynecologists (ACOG) Committee on Ethics. ACOG Committee Opinion Number 385: The limits of conscientious refusal in reproductive medicine; 2007 (reaffirmed 2019). www.acog .org/Clinical-Guidance-and-Publications/Committee-Opinions/Committee-on-Ethics/The-Limits-of-Conscientious-Refusal-in-Reproductive-Medicine. Accessed September 26, 2019.

13. Zampas C, Andion-Ibaniez X. Conscientious objection to sexual and reproductive health services: international human rights standards and European law and practice. *Eur J Health Law*. 2012;**19**:231–256.

14. De Zordo S, Mishtal J. Physicians and abortion: provision, political participation and conflicts on the ground – the cases of Brazil and Poland. *Womens Health Issues*. 2011;**21**(Suppl 3): S32–S36.

15. Charo RA. Health care provider refusals to treat, prescribe, refer or inform: professionalism and conscience. *Journal ACS Issue Groups*. 2007:119–135.

16. Steinauer J, Koenemann K, Coghlan K, Landy U, Turk J. Impact of Ryan Program on resident clinical experience and plans to include abortion in future practice. ePoster presented at the ACOG Annual Clinical Meeting, Nashville, TN; 2019.

17. Steinauer JE, Turk JK, Fulton MC, Simonson KH, Landy U. The benefits of family planning training: a 10-year review of the Ryan Residency Training Program. *Contraception*. 2013;**88**(2):275–280.

doi:10.1016/j. contraception.2013.02.006

18. Harris LH, Cooper A, Rasinski KA, Curlin FA, Lyerly AD. Obstetrician-gynecologists' objections to and willingness to help patients obtain an abortion. *Obstet Gynecol*. 2011;**118**(4):905–912.

19. Frank JE. Conscientious refusal in family medicine residency training. *Fam Med*. 2011; **43**(5):330–333.

20. Srinivasulu S, Maldonado L, Prine L, Rubin SE. Intention to provide abortion upon completing family medicine residency and subsequent abortion provision: a 5-year follow-up survey. *Contraception*. 2019: **100**(3):188–192.

21. Kavanaugh J. What should we teach medical students about abortion. June 4, 2019, webinar.

22. Simpson J. Abortion care: reforming the undergraduate medical curriculum. Paper presented at the meeting of the Faculty of Sexual and Reproductive Healthcare, RCOG, 2019.

23. Stulberg DB, Dude AM, Dahlquist I, Curlin FA. Obstetrician-gynecologists, religious institutions, and conflicts regarding patient-care policies. *Amer J Obstet Gynecol*. 2012;**207**(1):73–75.

24. Norwegian Directorate of Health. Specialist training and authorization for doctors: gynecology. www .helsedirektoratet.no/tema/ autorisasjon-og-spesialistutdanning/ spesialistutdanning-for-leger/ fodselshjelp-og-kvinnesykdommer/ laeringsmal?query=gynekologi. Accessed September 26, 2019.

9

Abortion Training in the USA
Prevalence, Outcomes and Challenges

Jody Steinauer and Jema Turk

9.1 Introduction

In order to meet patients' needs, all clinicians who care for women's reproductive health must be trained in abortion skills. These skills include counseling, preoperative assessment, ultrasound, medication abortion management, uterine evacuation techniques, pain management and postoperative care. With these skills, reproductive health-care clinicians are prepared to provide abortion and early pregnancy loss care. Abortion is common, with a rate of 13.5/1,000 women of reproductive age in the USA in 2017 [1]. Early pregnancy loss is also common, affecting up to 20% of all pregnancies [2]. Additionally, patients sometimes experience a serious pregnancy complication that must be treated immediately to prevent maternal morbidity, such as pre-viable preterm rupture of membranes complicated by chorioamnionitis or acute hemorrhage. National organizations such as the American College of Obstetricians and Gynecologists (ACOG) and the international obgyn organization, International Federation of Gynecology and Obstetrics (FIGO), recommend that all obstetrician-gynecologists (ob-gyns) are skilled in abortion care. For individual physicians who object to abortion, these organizations state that while an individual can opt out of doing abortions, they must be prepared to safely empty a patient's uterus in the setting of an emergency when no one else is available to do the procedure. Thus, training in uterine evacuation skills is critical for all ob-gyns.

Residents (graduate medical education learners) access training based on their program's level of integration, which we will now describe. Training can be fully integrated or "routine," which means that it is routinely included in training. Individual learners who do not want the training can opt out. Training can be "optional," meaning that a learner has to opt in

to and schedule the training. Finally, it can simply not be available in the training program, and a motivated individual would have to learn the skills outside of the program without support. Within programs with routine, scheduled training, the time spent learning abortion care could be in a rotation dedicated to family planning or included in a rotation that already includes other aspects of gynecological care and training.

In the USA, soon after the legalization of abortion across the country, studies demonstrated a steadily decreasing proportion of obgyn residency programs with integrated, "routine" training in abortion over time: between 1978 and 1995, the proportion of programs with routine training decreased from 26% to 12% (see Chapter 3). As described in previous chapters, this led to the Accreditation Council for Graduate Medical Education (ACGME) requirement that all ob-gyn programs include training in abortion, a policy enacted in 1996.

Since 1996, training has increased steadily in order to meet the governing bodies' policies and mandates. Routine training rose to 31% of programs in 1998 and then to 51% in 2004 [3,4]. In the 2004 survey, an additional 39% of residency program directors reported availability of unscheduled, optional training that residents could seek outside of their regular duties, and 10% reported no training options. In 2014, the most recently published study of training found 80% of programs reported routine training when asked to define their training as "routine," "optional" or "not available," the questions being identical to prior studies. However, using a more precise definition of "routine" training, only 64% of programs routinely included training in residents' schedules; another 31% offered optional training, where training was not scheduled but residents could arrange training at the teaching hospital or affiliated clinic; and 5% reported having no

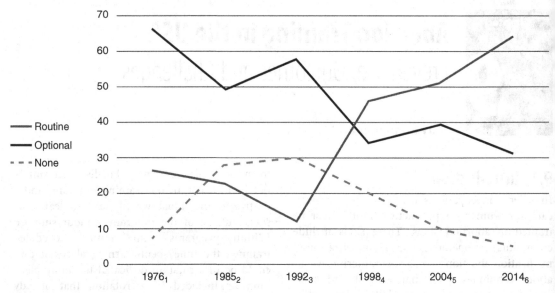

Figure 9.1 Training in US ob-gyn residency programs, 1976–2014

[1] Lindheim BL, Cotterill MA. Training in induced abortion by obstetrics and gynecology residency programs. *Fam Plann Perspect.* 1978;10(1):24–28.

[2] Darney PD, Landy U, MacPherson S, Sweet RL. Abortion training in U.S. obstetrics and gynecology residency programs. *Fam Plann Perspect.* 1987;19(4):158–162.

[3] MacKay HT, MacKay AP. Abortion training in obstetrics and gynecology residency programs in the United States, 1991–1992. *Fam Plann Perspect.* 1995; 27(3):112–115.

[4] Almeling R, Tews L, Dudley S. Abortion training in US obstetrics and gynecology residency programs, 1998. *Fam Plann Perspect.* 2000;32(6):268–271.

[5] Eastwood KL, Kacmar JE, Steinauer J, Weitzen S, Boardman LA. Abortion training in United States obstetrics and gynecology residency programs. *Obst Gynecol.* 2006;108(2):303–308.

[6] Steinauer JE, Turk JK, Pomerantz T, Simonson K, Learman LA, Landy U. Abortion training in US obstetrics and gynecology residency programs. Am J Obstet Gynecol. 2018;219(1):86.e81–86.e86.

training available [5]. We consider these latter proportions to be a more accurate description of the availability of resident training opportunities. Figure 9.1 shows the status of ob-gyn residency training over time. However, in a comparison with a neighbouring country, Canada, only half of obgyn programs have routine training in abortion. This level of training apparently does not meet residents' expectations [6].

This increase in ob-gyn training in the USA was in large part driven by the Kenneth J. Ryan Residency Training Program in Abortion and Family Planning (Ryan Program) [7,8], started in 1999 by Dr. Uta Landy. The Ryan Program was created as a privately funded, national initiative to support departments of obstetrics and gynecology to formally integrate such training. Based at the Bixby Center for Global Reproductive Health at the University of California, San Francisco (UCSF), the Ryan Program had supported 100 ob-gyn residency programs to integrate abortion training by 2019.

The Ryan Program continues to initiate two to four new programs per year. Programs typically have six residents (two to eleven) per year and rotations last an average of one month. Nearly half (94 of 226, 42%) of all US university-based or academic ob-gyn programs have Ryan Programs [9], and more than 6,000 residents have been trained in these programs, through 2019. As we describe the outcomes of training integration, we will reference the Ryan Program data in obstetrics and gynecology.

Obstetrics and gynecology physicians are not the only clinicians who should be trained to do abortions. Family physicians, because they provide the majority of primary care in the USA and often provide gynecologic and obstetric care, should also have abortion care skills. The American Academy of Family Physicians' Core Educational Guideline for Maternity and Gynecologic Care recommends training in abortions up to 10 weeks' gestation as an advanced skill that should be available within training programs for interested residents [10]. The more recent guideline for women's health and gynecologic care also includes abortion training in its advanced skills section and expands the gestation to include surgical and medication abortion in the first trimester [11]. Despite this recommendation, fewer than 40 of the 471 accredited family medicine programs routinely integrate opt-out abortion training. The Reproductive Health Education in Family Medicine (RHEDI) program has supported 28 family medicine programs to integrate abortion training. For more information about family medicine training, see Chapter 15.

Advanced-practice clinicians (APCs) can safely provide abortion care. As of the end of 2019, seventeen states permit APCs to do abortions, with ten states and Washington, DC, permitting them to do uterine aspiration abortion and an additional seven states to provide medication abortion. The American College of Nurse-Midwives Position Statement titled "Midwives as Abortion Providers" [12] recommends that abortion be included in training programs, yet only a minority of training programs includes practical experience in abortion. (See Chapter 16.)

9.2 Impacts of Abortion Training on Skills

Numerous studies have investigated the benefits of abortion training for learners. These include knowledge about and clinical skills in counseling, preoperative assessment, ultrasound, provision of medication abortion, uterine evacuation, pain management and postoperative care [8,13]. These skills are not limited to abortion care and are considered to be transferrable to other settings, such as early pregnancy loss management, intrauterine procedures and pain management, ultrasound assessment of gestational location and duration, placement of local, cervical anesthesia and management of conscious sedation.

In ob-gyn programs, residents gain significant clinical skills during abortion training in programs with routine training. A 2014 study of final-year residents found that those trained in programs with routine training – compared with those in programs with optional or no formal training - did more abortions and reported higher competence in abortion procedures, including manual and electric uterine aspiration and

dilation and evacuation (D&E), and were skilled in uterine evacuation to a later gestational duration [14]. They also had more experience with and competence in pregnancy options and abortion decision counseling. A 2018 study similarly found that residency program directors in departments with routine training reported more resident clinical experience and greater competence in procedural abortion skills than in programs without routine training [5]. Even within programs with routine, integrated training, MacIsaac and Vickery found that residents trained in a rotation dedicated to family planning were more competent in manual uterine aspiration than those trained in unstructured clinical settings or within rotations focused on general gynecology [15].

Family medicine residents who train in an abortion care setting also gain significant skills in ultrasound, uterine aspiration and medication abortion and early pregnancy loss management, as well as increased competency in abortion skills [13]. Similarly, family planning training benefits APCs. With training, APCs can safely provide first-trimester abortions, with complication rates comparably low to ob-gyn counterparts [16]. Training APCs in family planning can potentially help address family planning provider shortages and increase access to abortion care [16–18]. See also Chapter 15 on family medicine training and Chapter 16 on advanced-practice and nursing training.

9.3 Impacts of Abortion Training on Attitudes toward Patients and Abortion Provision

Improved clinical skills are not the only benefits to learners from integrated family planning training. Learners experience changes in attitudes toward patients and in their intentions to provide care in the future. In a qualitative study of ob-gyn residents, for example, those who had planned to only partially participate in the rotation had significant changes in attitudes after training [14]. They described greater acceptance of abortion in general, improved understanding of the reasons for which women sought abortions and greater comfort with abortion counseling. They appreciated that the rotation gave them the opportunity to consider the abortion decision-making process from the patient's perspective. Studies of residents in family medicine have similarly found that exposure to abortion training makes them more likely to consider abortion to be within the scope of family medicine and feel more comfortable counseling patients [19].

Abortion training increases intentions to do abortions after training [8,14]. In one study of ob-gyn residents at training programs supported by the Ryan Program, the proportion of residents who reported their intention to include abortion in their post-residency practice as "certainly yes" increased from 28% to 38% [8] The proportion who planned to do abortions for pregnancy complications was high at 74% and did not change [20]. Exposure to training also clarified intentions for residents who were unsure about doing abortions, with half becoming more likely to intend to do abortions after residency [21].

Family medicine (FM) residents are also more likely to intend to provide abortions after training. Romero et al. in 2013 found a significant correlation between the number of abortion procedures performed in training and intentions to provide abortions in practice. Among those who trained in abortion, 45% planned to do abortion in their post-residency practice [22]. Another study found that of FM residents who did abortions in training, at least 67% said they would probably or certainly provide uterine aspiration abortions after residency [13].

9.4 Impact of Abortion Training on Practice

Abortion training increases intention to provide and the actual performance of abortion. While not all who intend to provide after residency do so, abortion training does increase the likelihood of integrating abortion care after residency. Studies have found that among residents who were trained and intend to do abortions, between 47% and 52% of ob-gyn [21,23] and 42% and 48% of family medicine graduates[24,25] go on to do abortions [19]. Routine, integrated training and a higher number of abortions done in training are independently correlated with future provision [8,24].

Ob-gyn residents who are exposed to abortion training are more likely to do abortions: a study of more than 2,000 ob-gyns [21] in practice found that those who had abortion training in residency

were 1.6 times (95% confidence interval [CI] 1.04–2.3) more likely to do abortions even when controlling for pre-residency intentions and post-training career factors. Having done more abortions in training has also been shown to correlate with future practice. In a study of family physicians, those who did more than one medication abortion training session were more likely to provide medication abortion care than those who had done only one (100% vs. 44%, p<0.01).

However, both ob-gyn and family physicians may experience barriers after training, such as restrictive practice settings and the continuing stigma of abortion. Family physicians report that internal and external barriers to doing abortions include the challenges of incorporating abortions into a large scope of professional services, lack of time to set up services and external barriers such as administrative obstruction and staff resistance to abortion [19,24]. In the large national survey of ob-gyn physicians, working in a rural setting or in a practice or hospital that restricted abortion care negatively correlated with provision. [21]. A more in-depth study of ob-gyn physicians in practice found that practice setting was a common barrier. Forty-eight percent of those trained to do abortions in residency did not do abortions in their practice but would like to, citing practice group restrictions (39%) as the most common "significant" barrier. They also described that doing abortions was logistically difficult (43%), hospital restrictions prohibited abortions (38%) and they lacked community support (26%) [26].

9.5 Training Residents Who Do Not Want to Fully Participate in Training

Ob-gyn residents in the USA can opt out of portions of the family planning rotation if they have personal or religious objections outlined in the ACGME policy. Described more fully in Chapter 23, the proportion of residents who opt out of training components appears to have decreased from an upper estimate of 89% in some individual programs in 1985 [27] to 60% in very few programs in 2019 [5], according to residency program directors. Overall, residency program directors in 50 programs with integrated training, surveyed between 2009 and 2019, reported that 10% of residents partially opted out and 3% completely opted out of training [28]. In routine evaluation of the Ryan Program in which 2,874 residents in 93 programs were asked directly about participation between 1999 and 2019, 17% indicated that they opted out of some portions of the training, and this proportion was stable over time [8,28].

After approximately eight years of supporting ob-gyn departments to meet their abortion training mandates, the Ryan Program switched course to ensure that all residents have a learning experience during their family planning rotation, regardless of their intention to participate in abortion. All residents are expected to participate to some degree, even if it is simply observation or accompanying a woman through intake, counseling and providing post-abortion care including contraception. Rather than considering them "opt-out" we consider them "partially participating" residents because they generally participate in the training to their comfort level and learn highly valuable skills [29,30]. It is important that these partially participating residents learn abortion skills, including pre-abortion counseling and assessment, post-abortion care and uterine evacuation skills that they will use for emergency settings and pregnancy loss. A quantitative study of ob-gyn residents in 2013 found that residents who opted out of at least some portion of the family planning rotation still participated in a range of activities and highly valued the skills they acquired [29]. Some partially participating residents limit their training in uterine evacuation to pregnancy loss only, but many, because they value learning the skills, do abortion procedures. One study found that one third of residents who chose not to fully participate in training did at least one abortion for non-medical reasons, and 84% participated in at least one abortion for pregnancy complications [8]. A qualitative study of partially participating residents found that residents increased their confidence in interacting with patients facing unintended pregnancies, improved their counseling skills and learned to prioritize the care that their patients needed. Residents also reported greater acceptance of women seeking abortions, abortion providers and abortion in general and greater comfort in counseling women about and referring women for abortion [30]. For more details about the benefits of partial participation and how to support partially participating learners, see Chapter 23.

9.6 Benefits of Training as Perceived by Residency Training Leaders

Studies have also looked at the benefits of abortion training from the perspectives of ob-gyn residency program directors. While these data are based on directors' perceived benefits, this view offers an additional, broader assessment of the impacts of family planning training at an institution. The vast majority of residency program directors at Ryan Programs (97%) reported that the addition of formal abortion and family planning training somewhat or significantly improved resident competence in abortion and contraception care. Specifically, directors described the improvement of residents' technical skills, such as improved competence in ultrasound skills (74%), uterine evacuation and pregnancy options counseling (both 93%) [5]. Additionally, 90% of directors reported the family planning rotation improved overall patient care at their institutions, expanding access to abortion care for women in nearby communities. In 2017–2018 interviews with department chairs at Ryan Programs, improving patient care and expanding abortion access were often discussed as significant factors associated with residency training.

Programs with routine training have reported higher levels of institutional support from the obstetrics and gynecology departmental leadership, faculty and residents compared to programs with opt-in or no training [31]. Similarly, programs with opt-in or no training more frequently reported institutional opposition to abortion training [31]. These reports could indicate that having training leads to support or that support leads to training. Certainly, some support from leadership is required to start a program; for example, in the Ryan Program we require formal approval by the department chair and from the dean of the school of medicine prior to receiving support. However, from our experience working with programs, integration of training and providing the care for patients engender additional support. Thus, programs should consider this an additional benefit of integrating training.

We have also collected data about the benefits of integrated abortion training through interviews of faculty and department leaders in Ryan Programs. These data have confirmed the benefits listed throughout this chapter, such as improved resident clinical skills and improved patient care. Leaders often describe that the rotation is one of or the most favorite for residents, as it encompasses much more than simple technical skills, demonstrated in a study comparing residents' evaluations of rotations [23]. In addition, leaders commonly describe that resident applicants prioritize abortion in seeking a residency program, and the presence of training helps them match more attractive applicants. Additionally, looking at the medical school experience, they describe that medical student exposure to abortion training inspires some students to choose ob-gyn or family medicine and some to plan to subspecialize in family planning. In fact, one study has shown that intention to do abortions before residency is the strongest correlate of actual provision after residency training [21]. Thus, medical student exposure is impactful. Finally, leaders report that often residents are inspired by the rotation to do research in family planning, many develop a close personal mentorship relationship with the family planning faculty member due to the apprenticeship nature of the rotation and some are inspired to do family planning as a subspecialty.

While there is little research on family medicine program directors' perceived benefits of abortion training, family medicine physicians have expressed that reproductive health-care training in family medicine programs improves access to family planning and early pregnancy loss care [32]. One study demonstrated that routine and formalized family planning training in family medicine residency programs increases family physicians' skills, thereby expanding patient access to essential health-care services [32]. For more details about family medicine, see Chapter 15.

9.7 Challenges in Abortion Training Integration

Despite the widely reported benefits of training and mandates of governing educational bodies, significant barriers to integration of training exist. A recent national study explored these challenges and found the following [31]: thirty-six percent of ob-gyn residency programs had optional or no training [31]. Even among the 64% (n = 121) of programs with routine training, 57% of directors described some restrictions to the abortion care they can provide based on indications for the abortion (Table 9.1). For example, one quarter could only provide D&E

Table 9.1 Details about US ob-gyn residency programs with routine abortion training, demonstrating restrictions by indication for abortion method, modified from national survey of 190 residency program directors

Type of abortion technique	Indications for which method is available in a program's academic institution	% of US ob-gyn programs with routine training (n = 121)
Medication abortion	All indications	83.5
	Only abnormal pregnancy and pregnancy loss	11.6
	Only early pregnancy loss	4.1
	No training	0.8
First-trimester uterine aspiration	All indications	81.0
	Only abnormal pregnancy and pregnancy loss	9.1
	Only early pregnancy loss	4.1
	No training	5.8
Second-trimester dilation and evacuation	All indications	68.6
	Only abnormal pregnancy and pregnancy loss	24.0
	Only fetal demise	2.5
	No training	5.0
Second-trimester induction termination	All indications	46.3
	Only abnormal pregnancy and pregnancy loss	43.8
	Only fetal demise	7.4
	No training	2.5

Source: Modified from Turk et al., Sources of support for and resistance to abortion training in obstetrics and gynecology residency programs, *Am J Obstet Gynecol*, 2019. [31]

Table 9.2 Reasons for restricted training in 190 US ob-gyn programs, by type of abortion

	Medication abortion	Uterine aspiration abortion	Dilation and evacuation
Hospital policy	56%	54%	58%
State law	27%	22%	26%
University policy	15%	14%	16%
Lack of expert faculty	13%	18%	22%
Nursing concerns	7%	10%	13%

Source: Modified from Turk et al., Sources of support for and resistance to abortion training in obstetrics and gynecology residency programs, *Am J Obstet Gynecol*, 2019. [31]

Table 9.3 Sources of support for and resistance to training in 190 US ob-gyn programs, by type of training

	Routine training, no restrictions	Routine training with restrictions*	Non-routine or not available training
	% Supportive / % Resistant		
Department leadership	90/2	77/15	51/31
Ob-gyn faculty	90/2	70/20	50/30
Residents	90/4	70/19	53/27
University leadership	51/27	28/42	12/42
Hospital administration	52/42	29/61	15/64
Anesthesia faculty	54/40	32/51	15/60
OR/L&D nurses	44/50	15/65	12/70
Clinic nurses	54/40	30/50	8/60

Source: Modified from Turk et al., Sources of support for and resistance to abortion training in obstetrics and gynecology residency programs, *Am J Obstet Gynecol*, 2019. [31]
* Restrictions indicate some limitations on abortion methods to specific indications for the abortion. See Table 9.1.

services for patients with pregnancy complications or demise [5]. Program directors also reported reasons for restrictions in specific abortion procedures (Table 9.2), including hospital and university policies, state law, lack of expert faculty and nursing concerns. The study also explored sources of support for and opposition to training, and while the sources were consistent across programs, the proportion varied by type of training – routine, routine with restrictions and non-routine (Table 9.3) [31].

The Turk et al. study [31] did not separate sources of restrictions and support by location of training. Abortion care and training can take place in a teaching hospital and/or a partner freestanding clinic. Within Ryan Programs, 31% train solely in clinics or surgical centers within the teaching hospital, 2% train solely in partner clinics and 67% in a combination of the two. Programs that train within a hospital may face challenges due to hospital or university policy and individual discomfort with abortion among leaders, faculty, residents, nurses and anesthesia staff. When partnering with a clinic, programs generally do not encounter bias against abortion but may experience unique challenges, such as staff's lack of experience integrating trainees and concerns about training impacts on clinic flow. Programs with training in either or both locations can experience restrictions due to legislative policy. For more information about systems challenges, see Chapter 1.

While there are many challenges that can make provision of abortion care and integration of abortion training difficult, there are also sources of support available to program directors. More directors of programs with routine training and no restrictions cited support from leaders, colleagues and staff than programs with restricted routine trainings, who reported more support than directors of non-routine training programs. One could interpret these findings to mean that greater support allows integration of training, perhaps implying that one should not work to integrate training without strong support. An alternative interpretation, consistent with our experience, is that once training and care are integrated in the program, more people see abortion as a normal component of reproductive health care and become more supportive.

9.8 Conclusion

Training graduate learners in abortion care improves learners' knowledge, attitudes, intentions to do abortions and actual integration of abortion into practice. While there are some obstacles placed in program directors' ways, they should look for sources of support and argue for the many benefits of integrated training to improve resident education and patient care. Integrated training will continue to improve women's access to high-quality, comprehensive, reproductive health care.

References

1. Jones R, Witwer E, Jerman J. *Abortion Incidence and Service Availability in the United States, 2017.* New York: Guttmacher Institute; 2019.

2. ACOG Practice Bulletin No. 200: early pregnancy loss. *Obstet Gynecol.* 2018;**132**(5): e197–e207.

3. Almeling R, Tews L, Dudley S. Abortion training in U.S. obstetrics and gynecology residency programs, 1998. *Fam Plann Perspect.* 2000;**32** (6):268–271, 320.

4. Eastwood KL, Kacmar JE, Steinauer J, Weitzen S, Boardman LA. Abortion training in United States obstetrics and gynecology residency programs. *Obstet Gynecol.* 2006;**108**(2):303–308.

5. Steinauer JE, Turk JK, Pomerantz T, Simonson K, Learman LA, Landy U. Abortion training in US obstetrics and gynecology residency programs. *Am J Obstet Gynecol.* 2018;**219** (1):86.e81–86.e86.

6. Liauw J, Dineley B, Gerster K, Hill N, Costescu D. Abortion training in Canadian obstetrics and gynecology residency programs. *Contraception.* 2016;**94**(5):478–482.

7. Kennth J. Ryan Residency Training Program in Abortion and Family Planning. https://ryanprogram.org/. Accessed 2019.

8. Steinauer JE, Turk JK, Fulton MC, Simonson KH, Landy U. The benefits of family planning training: a 10-year review of the Ryan Residency Training Program. *Contraception.* 2013;**88**(2):275–280.

9. AMA Freida Residency Database of ACGME Accredited Programs.

10. Maternity and gynecologic care. Recommended Core Educational Guidelines for Family Practice Residents. American Academy of Family Physicians. *Am Fam Physician.* 1998;**58**(1):275–277.

11. Recommended curriculum guidelines for family medicine residents: women's health and gynecologic care. American Academy of Family Physicians; 2018.

12. Position statement: midwives as abortion providers. American College of Nurse-Midwives; 2018.

13. Summit AK, Gold M. The effects of abortion training on family medicine residents' clinical experience. *Fam Med.* 2017;**49**(1):22–27.

14. Turk JK, Preskill F, Landy U, Rocca CH, Steinauer JE. Availability and characteristics of abortion training in US ob-gyn residency programs: a national survey. *Contraception.* 2014;**89**(4):271–277.

15. MacIsaac L, Vickery Z. Routine training is not enough: structured training in family planning and abortion improves residents' competency scores and intentions to provide abortion after graduation more than ad hoc training. *Contraception.* 2012;**85**(3):294–298.

16. Levi A, Goodman S, Weitz T, et al. Training in aspiration abortion care: an observational cohort study of achieving procedural competence. *Int J Nurs Stud.* 2018;**88**:53–59.

17. Dermish A, Turok DK, Jacobson J, Murphy PA, Saltzman HM, Sanders JN. Evaluation of an intervention designed to improve the management of difficult IUD insertions by advanced practice clinicians. *Contraception.* 2016;**93**(6):533–538.

18. Patil E, Darney B, Orme-Evans K, et al. Aspiration abortion with immediate intrauterine device insertion: comparing outcomes of advanced practice clinicians and physicians.

J Midwifery Womens Health. 2016;**61**(3):325–330.

19. Greenberg S, Nothnagle M. An "invaluable skill": reflections on abortion training and postresidency practice. *Fam Med.* 2018;**50**(9):691–693.

20. Kenneth J. Ryan Residency Training Program in Abortion and Family Planning, unpublished evaluation data from 1999–2009; 2013.

21. Steinauer J, Landy U, Filippone H, Laube D, Darney PD, Jackson RA. Predictors of abortion provision among practicing obstetrician-gynecologists: a national survey. *Am J Obstet Gynecol.* 2008;**198**(1):39.e31–36.

22. Romero D, Maldonado L, Fuentes L, Prine L. Association of reproductive health training on intention to provide services after residency: the family physician resident survey. *Fam Med.* 2015;**47**(1):22–30.

23. Steinauer JE, Landy U, Jackson RA, Darney PD. The effect of training on the provision of elective abortion: a survey of five residency programs. *Am*

J Obstet Gynecol. 2003; **188**(5):1161–1163.

24. Block A, Dehlendorf C, Biggs MA, McNeil S, Goodman S. Postgraduate experiences with an advanced reproductive health and abortion training and leadership program. *Fam Med.* 2017;**49**(9):706–713.

25. Greenberg M, Herbitter C, Gawinski BA, Fletcher J, Gold M. Barriers and enablers to becoming abortion providers: the reproductive health program. *Fam Med.* 2012; **44**(7):493–500.

26. Turk JK, Preskill F, Landy U, Koenemann K, Steinauer J. Abortion provision among obstetrician-gynecologists who trained at Ryan Programs. Paper presented at the National Abortion Federation annual meeting; 2017.

27. Darney PD, Landy U, MacPherson S, Sweet RL. Abortion training in U.S. obstetrics and gynecology residency programs. *Fam Plann Perspect.* 1987;**19** (4):158–162.

28. Kenneth J. Ryan Residency Training Program in Abortion

and Family Planning, unpublished evaluation data; 2019

29. Steinauer JE, Hawkins M, Turk JK, Darney P, Preskill F, Landy U. Opting out of abortion training: benefits of partial participation in a dedicated family planning rotation for ob-gyn residents. *Contraception.* 2013;**87**(1):88–92.

30. Steinauer JE, Turk JK, Preskill F, Devaskar S, Freedman L, Landy U. Impact of partial participation in integrated family planning training on medical knowledge, patient communication and professionalism. *Contraception.* 2014;**89**(4):278–285.

31. Turk JK, Landy U, Chien J, Steinauer JE. Sources of support for and resistance to abortion training in obstetrics and gynecology residency programs. *Am J Obstet Gynecol.* 2019; **221**(2):156.e151–156.e156.

32. Nothnagle M, Prine L, Goodman S. Benefits of comprehensive reproductive health education in family medicine residency. *Fam Med.* 2008;**40**(3):204–207.

Chapter

10

Starting and Optimizing an Academic Abortion Service

Karen Meckstroth

10.1 What Makes an Abortion Service Unique?

Although abortion is generally a simple, safe procedure or visit, providing abortion in a general academic obstetrics and gynecology (obgyn) or family medicine setting poses unique challenges. This chapter reviews options and considerations and offers resources for starting or optimizing an academic abortion service. Issues for an academic, teaching service include the following:

- *Abortion laws* can be a barrier for those considering adding the service and confusing to medical center leaders.
- *Insurance* has particular restrictions for abortion, which can be imprecise and not aligned with medical terms. It is not unusual to receive inaccurate information about coverage by phone from insurance companies, requiring a second or third inquiry. Because of insurance restrictions, a self-pay option is needed. Insurers require that high-value procedure visits be pre-authorized. Young, healthy women seeking abortion often know little about their own health insurance.
- Seventy-five percent of abortion patients live under 200% of the federal *poverty* level [1] and frequently benefit from specialized financial support options such as the US National Network of Abortion Funds.
- Patients often require urgent appointments, and changes in decisions to terminate pregnancies are common, requiring *frequent schedule revisions*.
- *Teens* are seen in what is otherwise an adult service, requiring staff to know adolescent consent laws and support. These differ by state and national jurisdictions.
- Patients and providers benefit from *trained staff* versed in pregnancy options and decision

making as well as procedure support techniques.
- *Patients regularly travel* long distances and need logistical assistance. Most of the rural USA and many major US cities qualify as abortion "deserts" where most people live more than 100 miles from an abortion provider.
- Patients referred to academic hospital abortion services *are commonly higher risk*, as low-risk patients have the option of care at community abortion clinics.
- *Avoiding multiple visits* helps patients, but requires evaluation and insurance approval prior to the initial visit.
- *Staff refusals* to assist require preemptive planning and awareness of conscientious objection laws and processes [2]. (See Chapter 8.)
- *Residents* have varying comfort levels with abortion and benefit from pre- and post-rotation discussions and opportunities for emotional processing. (See Chapter 25.)
- *Intense emotions, stigma* and relationship issues that patients may experience around abortion often require considerable clinic time and counseling and knowledge of resources; emotions and stigma affect staff, residents, students and other learners in different ways. (See Chapter 23.)
- General ob-gyn *physicians were typically not trained* in second trimester dilation and evacuation (D&E) abortion, which may complicate staffing for urgent cases. This and other chapters in this book describe the programs that accomplish comprehensive abortion training.
- Unlike other services, abortion care may require special consideration and *support for security of staff and patients* from harassment or, in extreme cases, attack.

10.2 Mission

Prioritizing patient-centered care and training is not always aligned with efficient visits. For example, when abortions are done in a typical ambulatory surgical clinic or in an operating room (OR), patients may not have the option for a single visit. Cost is a common reason patients delay abortion to a later gestation; and denial of abortion reduces women's and children's financial security and safety [3]. Abortion patients are more commonly low income and patients of color [4]. Providing an abortion service, particularly for patients who cannot be seen elsewhere, is an issue of health equity.

10.3 Legal Support and Resources

Medical center lawyers may not have specific knowledge of state abortion laws. Details are available on the Guttmacher website and often on state government websites. Other websites that can be helpful include those of the Center for Reproductive Rights and the American Civil Liberties Union (ACLU). Many institutions have benefited from relationships with local law professors or student groups with a particular interest in reproductive rights.

10.4 Facility and Hospital Considerations

Academic medical centers are regulated by federal (Centers for Medicare & Medicaid Services), state (health department) and private (Joint Commission) agencies. Employing the same oversight processes as other clinical services in the hospital allows an abortion service to benefit from institutional experts in health facility regulations. Additional considerations are discussed in the following sections.

10.4.1 Tissue Management

Pregnancy tissue should be examined during the visit to ensure removal of adequate products of conception [5]. If pathologic examination is not required for patient care, it is often not required in clinic procedures. State laws dictate pregnancy tissue management, sometimes under standard biohazard material waste regulation and sometimes with specific laws. In academic medical centers researchers may request to use discarded or sampled pregnancy tissue. We recommend a consent process and form that tells pregnant patients that, as potential tissue donors, tissue given for research is not connected to and will not change their care, and that payment cannot be involved.

10.4.2 Safety

False concerns for patient safety are used as a justification for promoting regulations that specifically target abortion which has similar safety concerns as other office and clinic-based procedures. The American College of Obstetricians and Gynecologists (ACOG), the National Partnership for Women & Families and the American College of Physicians created evidence-informed consensus guidelines [6]. Unfortunately, targeted regulations of abortion providers (TRAP laws) lead to increased workload and increased financial and emotional burden for providers, including those in academic centers [7]. Abortion services should have protocols for emergency procedures, and National Abortion Federation (NAF) clinical guidelines provides detailed recommendations [5]. As D&E requires specialized skills, it is common practice in academic medical centers to evaluate adverse outcomes and abortion statistics in a focused annual morbidity and mortality (M&M) conference in addition to weekly departmental conferences when warranted.

10.4.3 Abortions in a Main OR

As many academic medical centers are referral centers for complex cases, some procedures take place in the general operating rooms. For others, these ORs are the only available sites for surgery of any kind. Relationships with and education for OR leadership and staff are highly beneficial. It is helpful to be familiar with conscientious objection laws and policies and to seek clarity before OR staff decline to participate. Having emergency instruments and medications on the procedure equipment list ensures their availability, even if abortion is routinely provided. In-service education for OR staff that includes information about abortion as well as laws and policies governing abortion, adolescents and conscientious objection can be especially helpful. Although afternoons are not generally a popular OR block time and risk delay from earlier cases, afternoon times allow one-day procedures after cervical ripening. For emergency cases, programs have found benefit from having a contact person in anesthesia who is aware of staff and physician willingness to provide abortion care.

10.4.4 Catholic Hospitals

One out of six US hospital beds are in Catholic hospitals and 11% of US accredited obstetrics and gynecology residency programs are based in Catholic hospitals. These hospitals abide by the Ethical and Religious Directives for Catholic Health Care Services, which all personnel must follow. They conflict with the Accreditation Council for Graduate Medical Education (ACGME) requirements for family planning training. Best practices for these programs include enhanced onsite education with specific abortion didactics and simulations and off-site procedural training [8]. See Chapter 13 for more detail on this topic.

10.4.5 Telemedicine

Abortion care by telemedicine can offer particular advantages. Clinic-to-clinic telemedicine has been studied and found to be beneficial for medication abortion [9]. Gynuity Health Projects studied clinic-to-home telemedicine with evaluation by ultrasound in the community [10], and some providers offer this clinically. Providers have used telemedicine for consent and evaluation prior to abortion. A sample protocol for no-test medication abortion has helped expand access for many programs. This is also possible in states where required waiting periods do not specify an initial in-person visit. Many medical centers have existing telemedicine platforms. Remote evaluation of patient history and results for preparation for an abortion visit is reimbursable if it requires thirty minutes or more. Interprofessional electronic or phone consultation with a written report is reimbursable with new codes.

10.5 Guidelines and Protocols

Protocols are needed for advanced-practice clinicians, nurses, medical assistants and some services. The Fellowship in Family Planning through its listserv exchange with the national community of academic physicians offers the opportunity to use policies and guidelines from other institutions. Reviewing and updating departmental gynecology and obstetrics guidelines and protocols is an important step in creating a new service. Using national guidelines when possible and supplementing those with information specific to the practice can be helpful. NAF requires member clinics, which include academic medical centers, to review and accept the Clinical Policy Guidelines annually, which can serve as the primary guidelines [5]. These organizations have current national and international guidelines with a high level of agreement: Society of Family Planning [11], ACOG, National Institute for Health and Care Excellence [12], Royal College of Obstetricians & Gynaecologists, French College of Gynecologists and Obstetricians [13] and IPAS.

The Department of Obstetrics and Gynecology at the University of California, San Francisco (UCSF), has the following site-specific additions for its two Women's Options Centers (WOCs) (at UCSF Medical Center at Mt. Zion and Zuckerberg San Francisco General [ZSFG] Hospital and Trauma Center):

- Gestational limits for abortion
- Clinic discharge after procedures
- Emergency response
- Post-abortion hemorrhage
- Medications and comfort during clinic procedures
- Cervical preparation
- Ectopic pregnancy and pregnancy of unknown location (required as a NAF clinic)
- Referral and scheduling
- Scheduling when WOC is full
- Telephone call triage

10.5.1 Gestational Limits

State laws dictate gestational limits, but many medical centers have additional restrictions [14]. Like a number of other states, the California Health and Safety Code #123468 does not specify a gestational limit for abortion. Rather, it says that the state cannot interfere with the right to obtain abortion before viability and clarifies that "'viability' means the point in a pregnancy when, in the good faith medical judgment of a physician, on the particular facts of the case before that physician, there is a reasonable likelihood of the fetus's sustained survival outside the uterus without the application of extraordinary medical measures." UCSF and ZSFG do not have a center-wide guideline for abortion limits other than this law, but some services find that having a clearly defined guideline documents department and medical center support for the abortion practice. When medical centers limit abortion beyond state laws, Ryan Residency Training Program directors have found it beneficial to question the origin of the restriction and provide arguments for change. Some programs have extended limits for abortion on request beyond 24 weeks based on the ACOG and the Society for Maternal-fetal Medicine (SMFM) Obstetric Care Consensus on Periviable Birth which places cesarean section (C-section) for fetal indications in the category of "consider" rather than "recommended" until 25 weeks 0 days based on viability statistics which include: 40 to 78% survival at 24+0 to 24+6 gestation with 20 to 45% chance of moderate to severe neurodevelopmental impairment among survivors. Very high-level neonatal care is required to achieve these rates [15]. In the few states without abortion limits for "normal" pregnancies, a few clinics offer uterine evacuations into the third trimester.

In addition to state and hospital restrictions, gestational limits depend on factors specific to each clinic, including the level of anesthesia and emergency care provided and operating room availability. For example, in the UCSF clinic where abortion care is integrated into routine practice, office D&E abortion is offered only to low-risk [16] patients with pregnancies up to 16+ weeks. In hospital-based, ambulatory abortion clinics with full-service anesthesia, however, D&E abortions are accomplished through later in the second trimester.

10.5.2 Cervical Preparation

As cervical preparation is recommended prior to second trimester procedural abortion and used by nearly all clinicians in the later first trimester [17], abortion services must consider type of procedure and timing for scheduling, as well as patient comfort and safety during cervical preparation. Many programs, including both UCSF programs, recommend patients remain in clinic for pre-op misoprostol and regularly employ mifepristone and/or osmotic dilators at home overnight. Cervical preparation at home for patients who present with ruptured membranes is not recommended, but is usually permitted if membranes are inadvertently ruptured at the time of dilator placement. The UCSF WOC has significantly reduced

narcotic medications for home use either pre- or post-operatively, but some patients require a narcotic for comfort with osmotic dilators even with ibuprofen plus acetaminophen.

10.6 Patient Education

Standard patient education materials packaged for electronic medical records rarely address abortion with the details patients need. Taking advantage of the community of practice (Chapter 5), academic abortion clinicians regularly share recommendations, which have included:

- NAF, ACOG and UpToDate Patient Education
- www.reproductiveaccess.org/ Patient and provider information, some in many languages
- www.pregnancyoptions.info/ *Pregnancy Options Workbook, Abortion: Which Method is Right for Me?* and *A Guide to Emotional and Spiritual Resolution after an Abortion*
- www.aheartbreakingchoice.com/, www.nofoottoosmall.org/, https://endingawantedpregnancy.com/ Resources and support for those terminating a wanted pregnancy

10.7 Equipment

Manual uterine aspiration (MUA) syringes, D&E forceps, suction machines and other specialized equipment are available through major medical distributors. Specialized companies often exhibit equipment at conferences such as NAF and the Society of Family Planning. Some items such as Dilapan-S® osmotic dilators are available only from a specialized distributor, which may require opening new accounts for your medical center. The Ryan Residency Training Program maintains comprehensive lists of equipment for those establishing new services.

10.8 Staffing

One of the major issues for starting an academic abortion service is staffing. There may not be an option to hire new staff with an interest in abortion. However, hiring a dedicated practice manager should be considered essential to the success and maintenance of a new service. Some Ryan Programs choose a registered nurse (RN) for this position, though most define it as administrative. A practice manager with strong communication skills can help avoid conflict and provide education throughout the medical center.

Although staff who have moral or religious concerns with abortion are often willing and able to provide care for abortion patients in a respectful manner, patients may nonetheless detect negative emotions. Stressed patients particularly need resilient staff who genuinely support reproductive justice and abortion. Even dedicated staff benefit from empathy training, often called "values clarification," and regular emotional processing and support during "huddles" or staff meetings.

Type of anesthesia will dictate some staffing decisions, as medical centers have staff requirements for moderate or deep sedation. For this reason, a number of centers have dedicated staff for clinic visits and procedures, but use shared procedure or operating rooms for procedures with the patient under sedation. Although it is possible for clinicians and medical assistants (MAs) to staff abortion in a regular ob-gyn clinic (as we do at UCSF), licensed nurses can provide medication and assess and counsel patients, which MAs cannot do. MAs can provide education and information from documented sources, perform limited assessments such as vital signs and pain and help with the myriad of logistical issues. Having knowledgeable MAs perform a fairly extensive phone screening and answer patient questions is extremely beneficial and reduces multiple visits and changes in plans. Institutional staff classification rules can be a barrier to having the same MA perform both clinical and phone/back office activities and is worth creative negotiation. Patients value the continuity of the same person starting with the initial phone contact to the clinic visit.

Staff and clinicians who are familiar with patient language and ethnic backgrounds provide further support and facilitate patient trust and understanding. Since a high proportion of abortion patients are of ethnicities underrepresented in medicine [1], achieving support and trust becomes more difficult and requires dedication. UCSF now considers complex life experience and language skills in hiring decisions and adjusts hiring screening processes to minimize such advantages as prior connections with job interviewers and decision makers.

As clinical abortion expertise may develop in a number of settings, family planning subspecialty training is not required for faculty of an academic abortion service, although it is advantageous if the hospital provides primarily complex abortion procedures, particularly in the second trimester. Studies have demonstrated the safety of medication and surgical abortion in the first trimester by family medicine physicians and advanced-practice clinicians. See Chapter 16 for more on the role of non-physician providers and Chapter 15 on family medicine.

10.9 Scheduling

The decision to terminate a pregnancy is complex and involves many factors. Women may call for an appointment when they first discover an unplanned pregnancy or a possible fetal anomaly, but they often reassess their initial plans, leading to high no-show rates. Since procedure visits are long and essential to sustain a training service, avoiding unused appointment slots is important. As flexible per diem staff scheduling often is difficult for this specialized care, more services request flexibility from patients. For example, some clinics maintain a list of patients who are willing to visit the clinic when called because a scheduled patient fails to appear.

Some services maintain economies of scale by including other gynecological procedures or urgent visits when the schedule permits. Chapter 11 discusses care for early pregnancy loss within or in parallel to an abortion service. Integrating abortion visits into a location where other visits take place supports patient privacy. In locations where significant security is needed to avoid antiabortion harassment and risk, anonymity may be more difficult.

Full clinic days and afternoon OR times allow the option of same-day cervical preparation for later procedures. Often availability of space and clinicians dictate whether same-day procedures can be offered to those needing a few hours of cervical preparation, though a shared decision-making approach is recommended.

10.10 Anesthesia and Comfort

Most US abortion providers use either moderate sedation (38%) or local anesthesia plus oral medication (33%) for early abortion, with deep sedation available if needed or desired [17]. Additional clinical requirements for moderate sedation vary by medical center. Although the American Society of Anesthesiologists (ASA) does not define levels of sedation by types of medications, many medical centers do. ASA guidelines include evaluations, equipment and considerations for moderate sedation [18]. For a low-volume abortion service, offering office sedation usually requires combining with other procedures or services. Offering clinic abortion without sedation has the advantage of improving learner expertise in pain control for other office gynecological procedures.

Unless patients have risk factors other than pregnancy, we generally provide deep sedation without intubation for D&Es after approximately eighteen weeks' gestation and for patients at earlier gestations who desire deep sedation at our medical centers. Traditionally, patients have been considered to be at higher risk for pulmonary aspiration after the first trimester of pregnancy, leading organizations and texts to advise use of general anesthesia with tracheal intubation starting in the mid–second trimester. General anesthesia involving tracheal intubation also has been associated with increased risk of complications, especially hemorrhage, and therefore is not recommended for uterine aspiration or D&E by the World Health Organization [19]. Avoiding intubation allows more comfortable and faster post-operative recovery and earlier discharge. The Ryan Program created a Grand Rounds lecture series by nationally recognized anesthesiologists to end the practice of routine tracheal intubation.

10.11 Integrating Contraception and Sexually Transmitted Infection Evaluation and Care

All reversible contraceptive methods can be started immediately after abortion, and post-abortion is a particularly convenient time to place an intrauterine device (IUD). Insurance reimbursement for the insertion is generally paid with the Current Procedural Terminology (CPT) code -52 modifier for a second procedure. When evaluating insurance coverage for a patient seeking abortion, coverage of long-acting reversible contraception (LARC) methods should be included to inform their consideration. Some patients do not wish to address contraception at the time of abortion for a myriad of reasons, and repetitive requests to do so can be interpreted as disrespectful or paternalistic. Patients can be offered methods in a shared decision-making approach to contraception. (See Chapter 1 regarding integrating education for contraception.)

Since active cervical infection increases the risk for post-abortal infection, high-risk patients should be screened. Some programs choose universal screening based on population prevalence of chlamydia or gonorrhea. For self-pay patients, bundling screening can avoid additional costs that may lead a patient to decline the tests. Some programs also offer routine testing for other sexually transmitted infections (STIs) such as HIV and syphilis.

10.12 Important Relationships

As a service that faces possible stigma and obstruction by other health-care workers with potential antiabortion attitudes, it is especially worthwhile to proactively build relationships, identify others' needs and questions, offer education and provide appreciation to those who facilitate care in this integrated model. Sometimes a single champion or advocate can lead to important opportunities to improve services and training. For example, a particular administrative advocate at UCSF helped our service to be the first to obtain OR block time designated to a specific procedure (abortion) rather than to a department.

See Appendix 10.1 for a comprehensive list describing important relationships that have been vital to the success of the UCSF and other Ryan Programs.

10.13 Fiscal Stability

10.13.1 Building a Financially Sustainable Abortion Practice

Attention to sustainability through billing practices helps garner support from medical center leadership. Understanding billing also helps patients with decisions that may have significant financial implications. Many patients seeking abortion are young and healthy and not familiar with health insurance. Having a patient handout explaining health insurance can save many frustrated phone calls. Patient's insurance can prompt discussions about choices regarding clinical care.

10.13.2 A Self-Pay Option for Hospital Abortion Services

Insurance barriers to abortion payment requires many patients to pay out-of-pocket. Typical hospital charges can be enormous and unaffordable for many patients. All academic medical centers that offer abortion must seek to negotiate a global fee that offers substantial discounts for patients.

Pursuing affordable self-pay options can involve complex negotiations with departments and hospital leadership. Although many Ryan Programs have succeeded, it remains a barrier for many hospital abortion services. For more than half of women seeking abortion without insurance coverage, out-of-pocket costs were found to be equivalent to more than one third of their monthly income [20].

10.13.3 Coding Procedures for Insurance Reimbursement

Abortion services in academic medical centers often serve as the safety net for patients requiring complicated evaluation or procedures. Such referrals increase safety and training opportunities and enhance relationships with community clinics, but can lead to inadequate reimbursement considering the time and resources required. CPT modifier -22 for increased procedural services requires documentation such as:

- Increased intensity or time
- Increased technical difficulty of performing the procedure
- Severity of the patient's condition
- Increased physical and mental effort required

Considering the complexity of care and inadequate reimbursement, some academic abortion services may only be financially sustainable if they obtain general departmental funds, seek grants or philanthropy from private donors for support on the basis of ethics, equity, training and research.

10.14 The UCSF Women's Options Centers

10.14.1 Zuckerberg San Francisco General Hospital's Women's Options Center

10.14.1.1 History

Dr. Philip Darney founded the University of California, San Francisco, Women's Options Center at San Francisco General Hospital as an outpatient training service in 1981. The hospital is a tertiary care and trauma facility and San Francisco's safety-net public hospital.

The WOC was inspired by the abortion service at Harvard's Brigham and Women's Hospital where Darney trained with Kenneth J. Ryan, after whom the Ryan Programs are named. When he joined the faculty at UCSF's San Francisco General Hospital to run the UCSF Family Planning Clinic, Dr. Darney asked to have third-year residents scheduled full-time in the WOC for a six-week rotation block. This resident training became a model for the national Ryan Program initiative in family planning because of its unique features as an outpatient hospital abortion and training service. (See Chapter 3.)

The clinic started with two treatment rooms and a recovery room using couches picked up from curbside discards. Hospital administration was indifferent. But over the years, the service gained respect and recognition because it relieved pressure on the main operating rooms of the busy trauma hospital, garnered hospital facility fee payments and generated many notes from grateful patients, which were sent to the hospital CEO and dean. Accepting complex patients from Planned Parenthood and private abortion clinics and treating their complications in a hospital setting helped create a stellar reputation in the community. Quality clinical care led to frequent referrals from private practitioners and other abortion clinics as well as visits from private patients who sought out the service despite its location in a safety-net hospital for the care of the city's poor.

In the early 1980s ambulatory surgery received professional endorsement, and hospitals began to create specialized ambulatory services within or affiliated with the hospital. Both patients and physicians found that avoiding the hospital OR for surgeries of predictably short duration and not requiring general anesthesia saved turn-around time, freed the OR for longer and more complex cases and avoided long post-operative recovery for patients whose surgery did not require it. Creating an outpatient abortion service requires that hospital and nursing administration recognize that there are advantages to having short cases requiring frequent re-use of the same operating room be separated from the main hospital OR suite when that suite also accommodates emergency cases. Delays of short outpatient procedures can lead to irate patients, surgeons and staff. At this time (and in some hospitals still today), general anesthesia with intubation was a routine hospital OR practice even for simple dilation and curettage.

Since its beginning, the founding director of the WOC sought inspiration from other ambulatory abortion clinics with a long history of providing innovative care to reduce stigma and anxiety for patients and the staff with such small gestures as fresh flowers on the reception desk, a rug in the waiting room, soothing music during the procedure and warm blankets brought to the women in the recovery room.

As the WOC grew and more space was required, architects who specialized in creating serene environments using natural materials redesigned the clinic to create an uplifting space of beauty and serenity for patients and a place where the team would be proud to work. Their goal was a clinic where, at the end of treatment or work, patients and caregivers would feel good about their experience and day. The remodeling was funded by generous San Franciscans, private donors and foundations that wanted to support abortion access and reproductive freedom.

The WOC's national reputation as an exceptional clinical and academic training service attracted medical students and residents from such diverse states as Texas, Alabama, Tennessee and Kentucky and the territory of Puerto Rico seeking elective rotations to learn about abortion care [19].

The WOC and UCSF became the first sites of the Fellowship in Family Planning in 1991. Focus on complex later abortions, research in contraception and abortion conducted at the clinic, and its global reach made it an ideal site for the advanced training of a fellowship in family planning.

Its forty graduates have become leaders in family planning as Ryan Program and

Fellowship directors and with domestic and international organizations. A unique aspect of the training was the close collaboration with the Department of Family Medicine, which led to partnership for resident and fellow training.

10.14.1.2 Services

The UCSF WOC at ZSFG is a private, self-contained unit within the hospital where all related services occur, including eligibility, medical evaluation, counseling, lab work, ultrasound, procedures, recovery and post-abortion contraception. The current space once a labor and delivery unit, includes three procedure rooms, two exam rooms, four counseling rooms and a recovery room accommodating eight patients. Patients move through several rooms within the unit (patient waiting room, ultrasound exam room, counseling room, procedure and then recovery) as they progress through their visits. The family waiting room is outside of the unit, and patients are not accompanied inside past the video phone entrance. On procedure days (Monday, Wednesday and Friday), four nurses and social work associates ("counselors"), an eligibility worker/scheduler, two attending physicians including a fellow in family planning, one anesthesiologist, research staff, a third-year ob-gyn resident and a fourth-year medical student typically staff the clinic. Half as many staff are present on Tuesday and Thursday when patients needing two-day procedures are seen for pre-op and cervical preparation. On these pre-op days, a nurse practitioner or certified nurse-midwife often does pre-op evaluations and dilator placement. On other days, several different faculty physicians and Family Planning fellows rotate as the attendings. The clinic manager is a psychologist renowned for her expertise in abortion counseling; she leads the training of clinic staff, nursing and physicians in this area at both UCSF WOC services. (See Chapter 25.) Nurse salaries and facility fees are subsidized by the city and county of San Francisco as most patients have public (Medi-Cal) insurance or pay a fee that often does not fully cover the cost of providing services.

In our specialized ambulatory unit, nursing staff develop skills in moderate sedation and intraoperative sonography, increasing their own job satisfaction and fostering a team approach to patient care that is rewarding to both staff and patients. This team spirit is encouraged by the "huddle" meeting at the beginning of each day where nurses, counselors, surgeons and anesthesiologists review the scheduled cases, anticipate problems and discuss their probable solutions.

The WOC has served as a model for many abortion services, including the Health and Hospitals Corporation of New York City with its 10 teaching hospitals and for visitors from Vietnam, Nepal, the UK, Mexico, Colombia, El Salvador, Nigeria, Ghana and Mexico City. The total number of abortions reached about 2,000 per year, including a small percentage of patients with miscarriage or requesting medication abortion. Rarely, high-risk cases are moved to the main hospital operating rooms, usually for complex anesthesia or expected hysterectomy. Most patients receive either nurse-administered moderate sedation (first trimester and early second trimester) or "total IV" deep sedation with fentanyl, midazolam and propofol (later-second-trimester patients) without intubation from an experienced anesthesiologist with no other responsibilities for that day. Cervical block with chloroprocaine and vasopressin is routine.

10.14.1.3 Training

The UCSF ob-gyn resident rotation is a dedicated five-week block rotation for third-year residents. Opting out is a rare occurrence. Residents usually rank the "Family Planning Rotation" as the best learning experience of their third year. They particularly value the clinical teachers who consistently receive recognition through student and resident awards and the unique team culture of the abortion service where learners and research are welcomed. As a result, many residents do their required project with the research team in the WOC. This collaborative approach to research has made the WOC one of the worlds' leading contributors to scholarly publications on family planning. As in other Ryan Programs, the availability of abortion and family planning training makes the residency highly desirable during the recruitment process.

10.14.2 UCSF at Mt. Zion Women's Options Center (WOC-MZ)

We started a second model of service and training at UCSF Medical Center at Mt. Zion (WOC-MZ). The impetus was to create additional training opportunities for residents from the other ob-

gyn residency in San Francisco, Kaiser San Francisco, and to care for UCSF and community patients in a setting that also accepts insurance other than Medi-Cal. It is the primarily clinical abortion experience for a large proportion of UCSF medical students. The program is based in a general women's health clinic, across the street from a smaller hospital, which has become an outpatient twenty-three-hour stay facility in recent years. This WOC clinic is unique in its integration with other gynecological outpatient services. For one-day procedures, patients obtain labs and medications a block away just before their visit, and are seen in regular clinic consultation rooms. They remain in the same room for counseling, evaluation, ultrasound, procedure and recovery and may have a support person of their choice for the entire clinic visit. Sedation is minimal; pain relief is achieved with oral medications and lidocaine, bicarbonate and vasopressin local block, with more than the usual 200 mg lidocaine added if discomfort is detected at any time.

The clinic is staffed by one manager and three specially trained practice assistants who do many tasks: detailed phone intake, insurance eligibility, discussions of pregnancy options and what to expect and patient assistance during procedures, followed by discharge information about contraception and post-procedure care. One attending and one resident work together for half of the week and the other half is attended by other faculty without a resident. Since this office model cannot accommodate patients with more advanced gestations or high-risk medical conditions, most second-trimester procedures from fourteen to twenty-four weeks occur in the hospital operating rooms across the street, though some low-risk patients of less than seventeen weeks choose D&E in the clinic. This UCSF campus does not have an emergency department, so the OR usually allows on-time scheduled procedures. Approximately 20% of WOC-MZ procedures are for miscarriage and 12% for medication abortion. Unlike WOC-ZSFG, follow up visits for concerns are scheduled within the WOC. Procedures in the main OR are attended by an anesthesiologist who may or may not have a high level of experience with abortion. Deep sedation without intubation is most common, although some anesthesiologists, as in some other Ryan Programs, choose intubation for D&E for the indication of pregnancy alone.

Residents attend WOC-MZ two days per week during their three-month clinic rotations, which occur twice a year during residency years two, three and four. Over almost twenty years, only a few residents have chosen partial participation and not participated in second-trimester procedures, and none has opted out of providing abortion. The intermittent rotation has allowed special training for residents who specifically plan to include abortion in their own practices after residency.

Our UCSF ob-gyn hub for clinical abortion research is WOC-ZSFG. The WOC-MZ site has collaborated on several studies.

Appendix 10.1 Important Relationship's Starting and Optimizing Academic Abortion Services

Within your department

• Department Chair	Helping the chair understand training, patient care and research benefits of an abortion service is invaluable
• Chief Financial Officer	Modified work relative value unit expectations to offset inappropriately depressed values for aspiration for abortion (3.0) compared to aspiration for miscarriage (4.8)
• Residency Director	Critical relationship to sustain resident training
• Residents	Individuals with an interest in abortion training can be a potent voice of support.
• Maternal-fetal Medicine	Attendings and fellows have done additional training in order to provide D&E to inpatients and others.
• Genetics Counselors & Fetal Treatment Center	Helpful to coordinate discussions of fetal anomalies, further testing and procreative issues
• Labor & Delivery	At UCSF and ZSFG, induction termination is performed on L&D as well as occasional D&Es. Nursing support is critical to this option.
• Call Center	Directs calls for abortion to a detailed intake with a knowledgeable medical assistant

Other departments and health-care areas

• Anesthesia Department	The Chief at both centers helps coordinate which faculty will participate for routine and emergent cases and distributed education around deep sedation without intubation for D&Es
• Emergency Medicine Department	Many programs have found MUA in the ED preferable to waiting for an OR or rescheduling for patients with miscarriage or retained tissue, and occasionally for induced abortion
• Pathology Department	Pathology technicians who receive D&E specimens check information about desire to obtain fetal remains to a mortuary and requests for detailed autopsy-like evaluation; created a lower cost "quick" evaluation for routine abortion in the hospital. (We rarely send specimens from the clinic)
• Pharmacy	Helped develop a closed system for mixing local anesthetic, vasopressin and bicarbonate that optimizes single-use meds and meets standards for point-of-care mixing; meds on formulary such as mifepristone, misoprostol and cabergoline
• Operating Room, Preoperative Care Unit & Post-anesthesia Care Unit	Have appreciated in-services on abortion and discussions to cultivate empathy
• Surgery Department	Emergency assistance for complications
• Interventional Radiology Department & Care Units	Recommend preparatory discussions to prepare for emergency uterine artery embolization

• Social Work Services	Identified someone with specific interest who reserved a visit each week for abortion patients
• Clergy Services	Administrator queries clergy to identify supportive individuals

Medical Center

• Hospital Administration	Recognized the lack of options for poor, medically complicated women seeking abortion and agreed to a highly subsidized self-pay option
• Sterile Processing Unit	We found assembly of autoclaved MUA syringes better left to trained MAs, so they are processed as a package
• Infection Control Teams	Provides guidance for tissue management and gross evaluation in clinic
• Nursing Administration	Identified alternatives for non-procedure visits to help cluster uterine aspiration visits
• Patient Relations Team	Communicates with mortuaries and facilitates transfer of fetal remains when desired
• Risk Management Team	Provides guidance for contacting patients who experience complications and documentation
• Billing and Coding Unit	Modified practice to expect payment for all procedures, as all are preauthorized
• Human Resources Team	Included interest in providing abortion care in descriptions of jobs specifically for abortion
• Security Department	We notify them when there is a planned antiabortion action in the area

Medical Education

• Clerkship directors	Include discussions of abortion in student orientation
• Clerkship administrators	Missing a transition in this role led to a significant breakdown in the routine scheduling of medical students
• Graduate Medical Education team	Need to know the process and timeline for visiting residents

Surrounding Community

• Other abortion services	Helpful to have current information about criteria and limits for referrals
• Prenatal Diagnosis Centers & Obstetric Providers	Recommend sending referral information and summaries and results after referred procedures
• City & County Lawyers and Administrators	Stood up for patient and provider privacy at WOC-ZSFG and refused to provide abortion records at federal request
• Community Pharmacies	Conversations with nearby small pharmacies who desire to provide confidential, respectful care have allowed many patients to avoid the risk of condescending and stigmatizing interactions when obtaining medications
• Mental Health Providers & Emergency Services	Helpful to know hours of operation, locations and insurance
• Domestic Violence & Sexual Assault resources	Both are up to three times more common for patients having abortion compared to those continuing a pregnancy and pregnancy in general is a risk factor [21]
• Volunteer or private doulas	May be helpful for medication abortion (MAB) or in-clinic abortion [22]

References

1. Jerman JJ, Rachel K, Onda T. *Characteristics of U.S. Abortion Patients in 2014 and Changes since 2008*. New York: Guttmacher Institute; 2016. www.guttmacher.org/report/characteristics-us-abortion-patients-2014

2. Arthur JH, Fiala C. The FSRH guideline on conscientious objection disrespects patient rights and endangers their health. *BMJ Sex Reprod Health*. 2018;**44**(2):145.

3. Foster DG. *The TurnAway Study*. San Francisco: Advancing Standards in Reproductive Health, University of California, San Francisco; 2019. www.ansirh.org/research/turnaway-study

4. Induced abortion in the United States. Fact sheet. 2019. www.guttmacher.org/fact-sheet/induced-abortion-united-states. Accessed April 7, 2020.

5. *Clinical Policy Guidelines for Abortion Care*. Washington, DC: National Abortion Federation; 2018.

6. Levy BS, Ness DL, Weinberger SE. Consensus guidelines for facilities performing outpatient procedures: evidence over ideology. *Obstet Gynecol*. 2019;**133**(2):255–260.

7. Mercier RJ, Buchbinder M, Bryant A. TRAP laws and the invisible labor of US abortion providers. *Crit Public Health*. 2016;**26**(1):77–87.

8. Guiahi M, Teal S, Kenton K, DeCesare J, Steinauer J. Family planning training at Catholic and other religious hospitals: a national survey. *Am J Obstet Gynecol*. 2020; **222**(3):273.e1–273.e9.

9. Upadhyay UD, Grossman D. Telemedicine for medication abortion. *Contraception*. 2019;**100**(5):351–353.

10. Raymond E, Chong E, Winikoff B, et al. TelAbortion: evaluation of a direct to patient telemedicine abortion service in the United States. *Contraception*. 2019;**100**(3):173–177.

11. Society of Family Planning. *Clinical Guidance*.

12. National Institute for Health and Care Excellence. Abortion care. In *National Institute for Health and Care Excellence: Clinical Guidelines*. London: National Institute for Health and Care Excellence; 2019.

13. Vayssiere C, Gaudineau A, Attali L, et al. Elective abortion: clinical practice guidelines from the French College of Gynecologists and Obstetricians (CNGOF). *Eur J Obstet Gynecol Reprod Biol*. 2018;**222**:95–101.

14. Zeldovich V, Rocca CH, Langton C, Landy U, Ly ES, Freedman LR. Abortion policies in United States teaching hospitals: formal and informal parameters beyond the law. *Obstet Gynecol*. 2020;**135**(6):1296–1305.

15. ACOG Obstetric Care Consensus No. 3 summary: periviable birth. *Obstet Gynecol*. 2015;**126**(5):1123–1125.

16. ACOG Practice Bulletin No. 135: second-trimester abortion. *Obstet Gynecol*. 2013;**121**(6):1394–1406.

17. White KO, Jones HE, Lavelanet A, et al. First-trimester aspiration abortion practices: a survey of United States abortion providers. *Contraception*. 2019;**99**(1):10–15.

18. Practice guidelines for moderate procedural sedation and analgesia 2018: a report by the American Society of Anesthesiologists Task Force on Moderate Procedural Sedation and Analgesia, the American Association of Oral and Maxillofacial Surgeons, American College of Radiology, American Dental Association, American Society of Dentist Anesthesiologists, and Society of Interventional Radiology. *Anesthesiology*. 2018;**128**(3):437–479.

19. Aksel S, Lang L, Steinauer JE, et al. Safety of deep sedation without intubation for second-trimester dilation and evacuation. *Obstet Gynecol*. 2018;**132**(1):171–178.

20. Roberts SC, Gould H, Kimport K, Weitz TA, Foster Greene D. Out-of-pocket costs and insurance coverage for abortion in the United States. *Womens Health Issues*. 2014;**24**(2):e211–218.

21. Mainey L, Taylor A, Baird K, O'Mullan C. Disclosure of domestic violence and sexual assault within the context of abortion: meta-ethnographic synthesis of qualitative studies protocol. *Syst Rev*. 2017;**6**(1):257.

22. Chor J, Lyman P, Ruth J, Patel A, Gilliam M. Integrating doulas into first-trimester abortion care: physician, clinic staff, and doula experiences. *J Midwifery Womens Health*. 2018;**63**(1):53–57.

The Role of Early Pregnancy Loss Care in Ensuring Competence in Uterine Evacuation

Sarah Ward Prager and Erin McCoy

11.1 Early Pregnancy Loss Background

Early pregnancy loss (EPL), also called spontaneous abortion or miscarriage, is defined as a nonviable, intrauterine pregnancy with either an empty gestational sac or a gestational sac containing an embryo or fetus without cardiac activity before thirteen weeks' gestation [1]. The most common complication of early pregnancy, EPL occurs in up to 31% of all clinically recognized pregnancies [2,3,4]. In the USA, this incidence of EPL is approximately equivalent to that of abortion, about one million of each annually [5,6]. As with abortion, accepted management options for EPL include medication management using misoprostol or a combination of misoprostol and mifepristone, and uterine aspiration using a manual vacuum aspirator (MVA) or electric vacuum aspirator, both of which have been shown to be reasonably effective and accepted by patients. EPL may also be managed expectantly if preferred by the patient. No management approach has been shown to result in different long-term outcomes [1]. Given the similarity in outcomes in stable patients, informed choice should dictate the management decision.

To date, EPL in the USA has largely been managed by uterine aspiration in hospital operating rooms [7,8], likely due to concerns about hemorrhage and infection as well as physician preference, With patients often receiving general anesthesia [7,9]. However, all three forms of miscarriage management can be offered in other appropriately equipped settings [10], including in the office and emergency room (ER). Office-based management of EPL using manual vacuum aspiration has the potential to improve access to comprehensive health care and the quality and satisfaction with care that patients receive from

their providers [11,12]. Patients with vaginal bleeding as a result of EPL often seek care in emergency departments (EDs) owing to lack of prenatal care or occurrence of symptoms during non-business hours [13]. ER management may decrease delays in obtaining care, facilitate ED efficiency by avoiding long waits for transfers to operating rooms, and decrease costs [14,15].

11.2 Miscarriage in Mainstream Medical Education

Despite good evidence that outpatient management of miscarriage is safe, effective, and acceptable to patients, it is not routinely offered as a standard component of medical education to the many providers of early pregnancy care, including advanced-practice clinicians, family medicine physicians and emergency medicine (EM) physicians.

Obstetrician-gynecologists (ob-gyns) routinely learn aspiration EPL management in an operating room. While frequently offered training in outpatient management, many ob-gyns do not ultimately employ it due to concern that others may think they are performing abortions, or due to their own discomfort with the similarity of the procedure to an abortion. Others may choose not to offer aspiration management in the outpatient setting due to concerns about inadequate pain relief or over sedation; perceived resistance from colleagues, nurses, and administration; and perception that it is difficult to provide due to the emotional aspects of the patient experience [12,16,17]. Another concern may be cost, although there is evidence that office-based aspiration management results in significant time and cost savings compared to operating room management [18,19,20].

Family medicine residents do not routinely receive education in EPL management despite recommendations that residents who plan to practice in regions without easy access to ob-gyns should learn this skill. In urban areas, referral to a specialist is often easier than in rural areas, though potential advantages to avoiding referral still exist, including the ability to provide continuity of care to patients, expansion of access to the procedure especially for underserved patients and decreased costs. In addition, the skills learned in MVA training in the office setting can be translated to other procedures, including uterine hemorrhage, IUD placement, endometrial biopsies and abortion [12].

EDs are often the first place patients with bleeding in pregnancy go for care, accounting for approximately 1.6% (500,000) of emergency room visits annually [2,3,4,21,22]. The American College of Emergency Physicians' clinical policy on EPL focuses primarily on recognition and treatment of ectopic pregnancy, and does not address stabilization of uterine hemorrhage from pregnancy loss or management of evolving, though stable, pregnancy loss [23]. Similar to the office setting, barriers to providing miscarriage care in the ED include physician preference for providing care in the operating room, the similarity of miscarriage management and abortion procedures, limited availability of support staff, difficulties integrating miscarriage management into patient flow and uncertainty about responding to women's emotional needs [15]. However, there has been recent momentum to integrate options for these patients in the ED setting as a way to decrease OR wait time, improve throughput, decrease costs and return ED visits, and increase patient satisfaction. The skills learned in MVA training in the ED setting can be translated to other procedures, including intracervical and paracervical regional nerve blockade useful for decreasing cervical pain from cervical dilation, cervical laceration repair and other potentially painful conditions of the cervix. Vaginal sonography skills may also be developed [13,24,25].

11.3 Miscarriage Training as an Introduction to Abortion Training

The delivery of quality EPL care achieved in offering patients options other than aspiration management in an operating room is a worthwhile goal. In addition, training in EPL management is a valuable way to ensure competence in uterine evacuation for learners, a skill that is also applicable to abortion. It is difficult to overstate the stigma often attached to the termination of a viable pregnancy. This stigma exists regardless of the indication for abortion, though stigma is often less pronounced when reasons of fetal anomalies (especially lethal ones) are involved. In these pregnancies, if nothing were done, the pregnancy would continue to develop and grow (at least at that point) without intervention. This contrasts clearly with EPL, where the pregnancy has already stopped progressing, and regardless of intervention would not have the capacity to continue to term. Since the pregnancy has at that point already terminated, intervention via uterine evacuation does not change the status of the pregnancy. Thus, training in EPL care creates an opportunity for talking about uterine evacuation management techniques separate from any value assigned to pregnancy continuation.

In both EPL and abortion, patients and clinicians are resolving pregnancies that have adverse health effects. These could be due to pregnancy loss, a lethal fetal anomaly, a significant maternal morbidity, a social situation that does not allow for parenting at that moment, or any of the many reasons for both pregnancy loss and abortion. However, it is clear that for some people, the embryo or fetus holds at least equivalent importance to the pregnant person: EPL allows the embryo or fetus to essentially be removed from consideration. Now, a discussion can be simply about how to manage this process most safely and effectively for each patient. Since the management options are exactly the same, even providers who are uncomfortable managing abortion are able to gain experience with both medication management and uterine aspiration.

One arena in which we very clearly see this benefit is in teaching residents. While uterine evacuation training is most readily available in abortion clinics due to the generally high volume of cases from which to learn, not all residents feel comfortable providing abortion care, and some of them choose to opt out of learning how to perform abortions. Furthermore, in highly restrictive settings, uterine evacuation training with abortion indications may not even be possible. Uterine aspiration for an indication of EPL can provide these "opt-out" residents an opportunity to learn the skills necessary to provide this service despite their discomfort with abortion. Additionally, many of these physicians feel a strong sense of obligation to help their patients and recognize the value of competency to manage an emergency situation, even when there is still a viable fetus. If they have been trained to manage EPL, and have practiced uterine aspirations in situations with non-viable pregnancies, they will still be able to act urgently or emergently when the need arises. Some Ryan and other abortion training programs approach trainees in an all-or-nothing manner – a resident must be interested in learning and performing all aspects of abortion care or they are reassigned and do not participate in the family planning rotation. We recommend more of a "comfort continuum" option, which allows residents to participate to the extent they are comfortable in abortion care. (See Chapter 23.) This may involve only diagnosis and counseling, or may also include learning about medication management and uterine aspiration in cases of EPL. It may take a resident longer to reach competence in uterine aspiration if the only cases they feel comfortable managing are EPL, but this approach provides an important opportunity.

Focusing on EPL can expand the sites where uterine aspiration and evidence-based medication management can occur, which creates options for patients. The seminal article by Schreiber et al. [26] demonstrating improved efficacy in EPL management using mifepristone and misoprostol as compared to misoprostol alone provides an excellent example of this option. It is too soon for survey information, but clinics and hospitals that previously could or did not have access to mifepristone now report having convinced their hospital pharmacies to stock it, given its proven use in treating EPL. Additionally, outpatient EPL management, both surgical and medical, is now possible at several Catholic hospitals.

11.4 Miscarriage Management Training in the Office Setting (the TEAMM Project)

The Resident Training Initiative in Miscarriage Management (RTI-MM) was created in 2008 to bridge a critical gap between the needs of patients to access patient-centered comprehensive EPL care and the technical training and practice integration assistance required by health-care teams to change practice [12]. The inception of the project was an intensive, multidimensional intervention designed to facilitate implementation of office-based management of spontaneous abortion using MVA in family medicine residency settings in the WWAMI region, which includes Washington, Wyoming, Alaska, Montana, and Idaho. This initiative, funded by the Washington Department of Health, began in 2008 and ended in 2010.

The format of the intervention from its inception was interdisciplinary, aimed at not only physician providers, but the entire health-care team including key administrative and clinical support staff. The literature on practice change suggests that interactive and mixed (passive and interactive) and multilevel (individual and team) approaches can impact practice, and that systems change approaches that target multiple levels within a system to achieve change are also successful [27,28]. Development of the RTI-MM program model was guided by these principles; its cornerstone is on addressing systems barriers and identifying motivated champions and stakeholders from the entire care delivery team to facilitate change. The intervention includes a didactic component, a hands-on Papaya Workshop to simulate the MVA procedure, and participatory discussion. The didactic session gives an overview of the epidemiology, etiology, diagnosis and management options for EPL. The hands-on session using the papaya to mimic the uterus allows participants an opportunity to practice the MVA technique. (See Chapter 22.) All training participants are encouraged to practice on a papaya irrespective of role, since understanding the procedure can facilitate invaluable awareness of the simplicity and expediency involved in the procedure, and can help give team members the knowledge needed to provide the support their patients desire. The discussion portion of this session is focused on systems change and includes an exercise designed to help participants self-reflect with their colleagues on their values surrounding support of pregnant patients. It also includes a "hopes and hesitations" discussion in which participants are invited to share perceived barriers and facilitators to integration of the service in their own setting and begin to create an action plan together.

After the completion of the singular residency program focus of the project, the name of the program was changed to Training, Education, & Advocacy in Miscarriage Management (TEAMM). From 2009 to 2015, with continued funding from the Washington Department of Health and the addition of funding from a private family foundation, the program evolved to shift its audience to ob-gyn residencies, private practices, federally qualified health-care centers, advanced-practice clinician training programs and military sites in Washington, Montana, Alaska, South Carolina and Oklahoma. The format of the intervention remained the same.

By providing EPL service delivery training and disseminating EPL information and research, the TEAMM project works to increase knowledge and provision of patient-centered EPL care in all settings to which patients of reproductive age present throughout the health-care system. The goal of the TEAMM project is to increase access to all forms of EPL management in locations where women access health care for pregnancy loss. TEAMM operates in areas where comprehensive EPL management services are not offered or are incompletely integrated and/or where access to training in abortion and spontaneous abortion is restrictive.

One example of how the TEAMM training has been instrumental in leading to expansion of abortion care is at several rural hospitals in Washington State. Washington has the Reproductive Privacy Act, a law passed by voter initiative in 1991. One element of this law mandates that if a hospital that receives any state funding provides obstetric care, it also has to provide equivalent abortion care. Many rural hospitals that receive state funding were not providing any abortion care, necessitating the patients in those areas to travel far distances to access this care. The Washington State American Civil Liberties Union (ACLU) sent notices to these hospitals that they were not in compliance with this law, and several decided they should change their policies and provide abortion care. The challenge to provision of services was training the clinicians, nurses and clinic staff to integrate this service. TEAMM was asked to provide these trainings, using the context of EPL management, to help facilitate this transition to providing a new service. We provided standard EPL management training, and then also opened up the discussions

to abortion management. All but one of these rural hospitals are now successfully providing abortions for their patients.

11.5 Integration of EPL Management into the ED Setting

Through a combination of casual polling and conversations in the first phase of the project, it became clear that many ob-gyn departments in major urban academic medical centers had challenges offering comprehensive outpatient EPL management, despite the fact that these locations often had one or more family planning subspecialty trained physicians on faculty. This finding, combined with a documented high incidence of ED presentations of EPL [22] and lack of options for these patients, made clear that change in EPL (and abortion) practices might come more quickly if we focused on these academic medical programs that were often the source of trained providers in their regions. (See Chapter 1.)

As a result, in 2015 TEAMM piloted an intervention in a joint, interdepartmental and interprofessional ob-gyn and EM setting, leveraging lessons learned from the history of the project. The immediate success of this pilot and convergence of ob-gyn and EM understanding led to an expansion of interdepartmental training. In partnership with an ob-gyn champion and an EM champion at each site, TEAMM began focusing on these sites to help them define their service integration goals over a period of time, leading up to on-site trainings. These trainings followed the same general structure of our prior trainings: didactic review of EPL, papaya uterine simulation workshop to give participants a chance to use the equipment and practice the procedure and time for discussion on values and integration of services specific to the site. Each session is interprofessional whenever possible and includes a hybrid of topics ranging from development of protocols, equipment and supplies, ER and/or clinic triage and flow, development of patient education materials and support of the emotional needs of patients. Training sessions prioritize thinking together as a team about the entire patient encounter. Participants engage in professionalism exercises that facilitate thinking through supporting patients needs and prioritizing patient-centered care.

We also added a key additional component to our training sessions – an integration meeting between stakeholders in both the ob-gyn and EM departments to talk though the characteristics of this practice change and come together to make a detailed plan for integration of services. Having clinician, nursing and administrative leaders meet together and formulate action items for integration has been valuable in achieving sustainable success. This interprofessional, interdepartmental and multidimensional approach is in line with prior findings about practice integration that establish that clinical evidence is necessary, but not sufficient, for practice change to occur [12,29].

The ob-gyn champion at every TEAMM site was capable of managing EPL from a technical standpoint, and often already has created relationships with leaders in the ED. There is an intangible benefit of having TEAMM, as a group of outside experts, come to each of these sites with suitcases full of manual uterine aspirators and papaya to facilitate change. Part of that benefit is that leaders in both departments are motivated to carve out time to do the persistent and often tedious work required at their institution to integrate change by preparing for TEAMM's training visit. The time together, as described above, is really one of the most valuable components of the project. Another key element, in our opinion, is the universal tendency to hold higher regard for a "visiting expert" than for a local one, no matter the topic and including EPL management.

11.6 Other Miscarriage Management Training Programs

In addition to the TEAMM project, there are several other groups contributing to the important work of helping individuals and sites train in EPL care and integrate services. Some of these groups include the Miscarriage Care Initiative, an effort by the Reproductive Health Access Project [30], which specifically focuses on supporting family physicians and clinic administrators to integrate

all three forms of miscarriage management into their outpatient clinical practice. The support offered to their clinical champions include technical advice, start-up funds for equipment and supplies, ultrasonography training, conference attendance and development of a long-term sustainability plan.

Another important program contributing to EPL education is the Innovating Education in Reproductive Health group at the University of California, San Francisco, Bixby Center for Global Reproductive Health [31]. This program generates, curates and disseminates free, open-source curricula and learning tools about sexual and reproductive health, including abortion and miscarriage. The learning tools for EPL include several video modules on EPL topics that can be used to train people in an online platform.

The American College of Obstetricians and Gynecologists recently made a commitment to providing abortion training. One of the ways they are executing this commitment is by providing a menu of trainings in abortion-restrictive settings that includes EPL technical and practice change assistance. By putting their name on abortion and EPL education, they are able to increase the importance of including these services as a standard component of reproductive health care.

11.7 Conclusion

There is no technical difference between the management used to empty a uterus for the indication of EPL or unplanned pregnancy. However, the emotions, stigma and rhetoric associated with those indications are often very different. The value of providing technical training to a broad group of clinicians around the indication of EPL has the added benefit of broadening the application of these skills to the indication of abortion. This education is a critical component of achieving competence for a much wider audience, which can only lead to better access for patients to skilled care.

References

1. ACOG Practice Bulletin No. 200 summary: early pregnancy loss. *ObstetGynecol.* 2018;**132**(5):1311–1313.

2. Wilcox AJ, Weinberg CR, O'Connor JF, et al. Incidence of early loss of pregnancy. *N Engl J Med.* 1988;**319**(4):189–194.

3. Wang X, Chen C, Wang L, Chen D, Guang W, French J. Conception, early pregnancy loss, and time to clinical pregnancy: a population-based prospective study. *Fertil Steril.* 2003;**79**(3):577–584.

4. Zinaman MJ, Clegg ED, Brown CC, O'Connor J, Selevan SG. Estimates of human fertility and pregnancy loss. *Fertil Steril.* 1996;**65**(3):503–509.

5. Jones RK, Jerman J. Abortion Incidence and service availability in the United States, 2014. *Perspect Sex Reprod Health*. 2017;**49**(1):17–27.

6. Curtin S, Abma J, Ventura S, Henshaw S. Pregnancy rates for U.S. women continue to drop. *NCHS Data Brief*. 2013; (136):1–8.

7. Harris LH, Dalton VK, Johnson TRB. Surgical management of early pregnancy failure: history, politics, and safe, cost-effective care. *Am J Obstet Gynecol*. 2007;**196**(5):445.e1–5.

8. Dalton VK, Harris LH, Gold KJ, et al. Provider knowledge, attitudes, and treatment preferences for early pregnancy failure. *Am J Obstet Gynecol*. 2010;**202**(6):531.e1–8.

9. Nanda K, Peloggia A, Grimes D, Lopez L, Nanda G. Expectant care versus surgical treatment for miscarriage. *Cochrane Database Syst Rev*. 2006;(2):CD003518.

10. Jauniaux E, Johns J, Burton GJ. The role of ultrasound imaging in diagnosing and investigating early pregnancy failure. *Ultrasound Obstet Gynecol*. 2005;**25**(6):613–624.

11. Nothnagle M, Sicilia JM, Forman S, et al. Required procedural training in family medicine residency: a consensus statement. *Fam Med*. 2008;**40**(4):248–252.

12. Darney BG, Weaver MR, Stevens N, Kimball J, Prager SW. The family medicine residency training initiative in miscarriage management: impact on practice in Washington State. *Fam Med*. 2013;**45**(2):102–108.

13. Quinley KE, Chong D, Prager S, Wills CP, Nagdev A, Kennedy S. Manual uterine aspiration: adding to the emergency physician stabilization toolkit. *Ann Emerg Med*. 2018;**72**(1):86–92.

14. Kinariwala M, Quinley KE, Datner EM, Schreiber CA. Manual vacuum aspiration in the emergency department for management of early pregnancy failure. *Am J Emerg Med*. 2013;**31**(1):244–247.

15. Dennis A, Fuentes L, Douglas-Durham E, Grossman D. Barriers to and facilitators of moving miscarriage management out of the operating room. *Perspect Sex Reprod Health*. 2015; **47**(3):141–149.

16. Darney BG, Weaver MR, VanDerhei D, Stevens NG, Prager SW. "One of those areas that people avoid": a qualitative study of implementation in miscarriage management. *BMC Health Serv Res*. 2013;**13**:123.

17. Darney BG, VanDerhei D, Weaver MR, Stevens NG, Prager SW. "We have to what?": lessons learned about engaging support staff in an interprofessional intervention to implement MVA for management of spontaneous abortion. *Contraception*. 2013;**88**(2):221–225.

18. Dalton VK, Harris L, Weisman CS, Guire K, Castleman L, Lebovic D. Patient preferences, satisfaction, and resource use in office evacuation of early pregnancy failure. *Obstet Gynecol*. 2006;**108**(1):103–110.

19. Rocconi RP, Chiang S, Richter HE, Straughn JM. Management strategies for abnormal early pregnancy: a cost-effectiveness analysis. *J Reprod Med*. 2005; **50**(7):486–490.

20. Blumenthal PD, Remsburg RE. A time and cost analysis of the management of incomplete abortion with manual vacuum aspiration. *Int J Gynaecol Obstet*. 1994;**45**(3):261–267.

21. Marx J, Hockberger R, Walls R. (Eds.). *Rosen's Emergency Medicine: Concepts and Clinical Practice*. Philadelphia: Elsevier; 2014.

22. Wittels KA, Pelletier AJ, Brown DFM, Camargo CA. United States emergency department visits for vaginal bleeding during early pregnancy, 1993–2003. *Am J Obstet Gynecol*. 2008;**198**(5):523. e1–6.

23. ACEP Clinical Policies Committee and Clinical Policies Subcommittee on Early Pregnancy. American College of Emergency Physicians. Clinical policy: critical issues in the initial evaluation and management of patients presenting to the emergency department in early pregnancy. *Ann Emerg Med*. 2003;**41**(1):123–133.

24. Tangsiriwatthana T, Sangkomkamhang US, Lumbiganon P, Laopaiboon M. Paracervical local anaesthesia for cervical dilatation and uterine intervention. *Cochrane Database Syst Rev*. 2013;(9): CD005056.

25. Renner R-M, Nichols MD, Jensen JT, Li H, Edelman AB. Paracervical block for pain control in first-trimester surgical abortion: a randomized controlled trial. *Obstet Gynecol*. 2012;**119** (5):1030–1037.

26. Schreiber CA, Creinin MD, Atrio J, Sonalkar S, Ratcliffe SJ, Barnhart KT. Mifepristone pretreatment for the medical management of early pregnancy loss. *N Engl J Med*. 2018;**378**(23):2161–2170.

27. Davis D, O'Brien MA, Freemantle N, Wolf FM, Mazmanian P, Taylor-Vaisey A. Impact of formal continuing medical education: do conferences, workshops, rounds, and other traditional continuing education activities change physician behavior or health care outcomes? *JAMA*. 1999;**282** (9):867–874.

28. Grol R, Grimshaw J. From best evidence to best practice:

effective implementation of change in patients' care. *Lancet*. 2003;362(9391): 1225–1230.

29. Dopson S, FitzGerald L, Ferlie E, Gabbay J, Locock L. No magic targets! Changing clinical practice to become more evidence based. *Health Care Manage Rev*. 2010;35 (1):2–12.

30. Miscarriage Care Initiative. Reproductive Health Access Project. www .reproductiveaccess.org/ programs/mci/.

Accessed August 12, 2019.

31. Early Pregnancy Loss. Innovating education in reproductive health. www .innovating-education.org/ category/early-pregnancy-loss/. Accessed August 12, 2019.

Academic Family Planning and Sexual and Reproductive Health Collaborations

Training and Advocacy with Community Partners

David Turok and Sarah Ward Prager

12.1 Introduction

A great deal of energy and attention has been directed toward stigma, controversy and isolation of abortion providers; the care they provide; and, most important, those who seek their care. It appears less common that abortion providers, advocates and those seeking abortion services focus on the universal nature of abortion that links all humans. Globally, 25% of all pregnancies end in abortion and approximately 56 million abortions occurred annually from 2010 to 2014 [1], which means that nearly everyone knows, and likely loves, someone who has had an abortion. At the intersection of stigma and universality exist opportunities for comradery and collaboration. Like many marginalized communities, this creates a real sense of fellowship between abortion providers and broader connections with a diverse array of academic and community partners. Such connections extend much more broadly beyond just those who provide abortions and work in abortion and reproductive health clinics. Thus, we broadly define community here to include all internal and external ties to supporters of the work. This includes the local, institutional academic community; the national community of family planning and sexual and reproductive health (FPSRH) academics and advocates; and community organizations.

12.2 Opportunities for Collaboration within the Academic Center

Large universities offer enormous partnership opportunities. These exist in clinical training, education, research and advocacy. Even after two decades at our respective institutions we continue to expand our collaborations. Critical to expanding connectivity is being a reliable partner making broad contributions to your institution's academic mission. Throughout this chapter we use the term *family planning* when referring to academic entities that currently use that name such as the national fellowship program in the USA and individual sites executing the mission of the "Fellowship in Complex Family Planning." More broadly, we use the term *family planning and sexual and reproductive health* (FPSRH) when referring to activities because this label includes a broader scope of interests around sex beyond just managing fertility. Ideally, FPSRH programs have roles that demonstrate this by providing timely, competent and compassionate clinical care; delivering meaningful educational content across the health-care training spectrum; being timely and impactful research collaborators and mentors; and serving as reliable advocates.

12.2.1 University-Based FPSRH Care Delivery and Training

Assuring access to the full range of FPSRH care means working with providers across disciplines. This means constantly working to train providers and coordinate care. Clinical care delivery and training are considered together in this section because they are closely intertwined. We recommend a very broad definition of FPSRH providers to include all who deliver sexual and reproductive health care. Even abortion providers can extend broadly across health-care specialties. Providers are found among obstetrician-gynecologists (ob-gyns), family medicine physicians, physicians from other specialties (an especially important opportunity for provision of medication abortion, which requires less training), advanced-practice clinicians, anesthesiologists and nurse anesthetists, medical assistants, counselors, nurses and administrative staff in an FPSRH clinic or setting. It may also include abortion doulas, naturopaths and non-traditional, community abortion providers who are assisting with patients to manage their abortions outside of a clinic or hospital setting [2] (these are non-physician and sometimes non-clinician people who have an interest in FPSRH and are motivated to help people obtain access to abortion – usually medication abortion – even if the person doesn't want to have care in a clinic or hospital). People in every position who choose to work in abortion care are often very proud of that work and should be recognized for their roles as critical participants in this care.

Frequently, integrating clinical care provision and training personnel expands clinical services. For example, clinical teaching stimulates interest in FPSRH by providing positive clinical experiences for students, residents and fellows. For ob-gyns, this traditionally has meant teaching medical students on their ob-gyn clinical rotation, training ob-gyn residents during their FPSRH rotation and working together on other services and more focused training for family planning fellows. However, to build a web of clinical support we see great utility in fostering interest beyond this traditional approach. Family medicine, family and women's health nurse practitioners and certified nurse midwives are the most obvious source of clinical allies. Significant opportunities to provide backup for clinical care in obstetrics and complicated contraceptive care can form durable relationships and bidirectional referrals, depending on level of complexity. Depending on local abortion practice and training requirements, some or all of these groups create potential contributors to the abortion care pool, and all medical providers need to be aware of the availability of abortion services and referral patterns.

Additional clinical training requests come from residents in other specialties. We have devoted considerable energy to improving miscarriage management by emergency medicine residents (see Chapter 11 on how early pregnancy loss [EPL] management improves training in uterine aspiration) [3,4]. This relationship has been important as we seek to expand medical treatment for miscarriage and incorporate new findings, such as adding mifepristone to increase efficacy for medical management [5]. Working with emergency medicine departments and residents has also led to opportunities to expand training in ultrasound and contraceptive care.

For example, in Utah, emergency medicine residents rotate on the obstetrics service. These residents learn contraceptive implant insertion while providing immediate postpartum placement, and that experience has motivated them to work on providing that service in the emergency department. We have also seen interest from pediatrics and internal medicine residents to broaden their experience with contraceptive care. Again, implant insertion and removal are simple skills to learn that they can bring back to their programs. We make sure to include interested family medicine, pediatric and internal medicine trainees when providing implant training to our ob-gyn residents. All of these relationships ease the comfort of these care givers when referring their patients for more complicated FPSRH scenarios, especially abortion services and contraception for those with medical complexities.

12.2.2 University Educational Opportunities

We both work in academic medical centers associated with large state universities where we often discover new intra-institutional partners and collaborators. Several obvious clinical training opportunities are addressed in the preceding section. In addition, schools of medicine, nursing, law and social work can bring extremely motivated students and faculty who are eager to collaborate on educational and research projects. We attempt to stimulate that interest by lecturing on various FPSRH topics to these students and create future colleagues who will support preservation and expansion of reproductive health care, rights and justice. On a smaller scale, we also offer lectures and educational experiences for students in the college of pharmacy and the genetic counseling programs. These educational efforts yield important results when students become clinicians and can work with FPSRH faculty respectively on increasing contraceptive access in pharmacies when new legislation permits it or easing the process for abortions for fetal indications when students become clinicians. In addition, students can create novel educational opportunities such as the alliance formed between Medical Students for Choice and Law Students for Reproductive Justice at the University of Utah that collectively sponsored a symposium on abortion access focused on targeted regulation of abortion providers (TRAP) laws. Similarly, at the University of Washington, a conference on the Human Right to Family Planning was planned and held in collaboration between the departments of ObGyn, Pediatrics, Family Medicine, School of Law, School of Pharmacy and Department of Global Health.

12.2.3 University Research Partnerships

Faculty and students in public health programs are other obvious sources of collaborators focused in the research realm. It is critical to cultivate these relationships, as often these partners will have expertise in epidemiology, biostatistics and research methodology that the clinician researcher may need to develop and conduct research projects.

The department of global health is another critical partner. Many universities have already merged the talents of their FPSRH and global health faculty. The University of Michigan has created the Center for International Reproductive Health Training (CIRHT), in which family planning faculty play a critical role. Johns Hopkins family planning faculty and JHPIEGO are also closely linked, as is family planning and global health at the University of California, San Francisco (UCSF) and the University of North Carolina, to name two. Conducting research in global settings is challenging, and departments of global health have often found solutions to conduct successful studies. Partnership can save countless hours of needless frustration and work, especially when beginning one's career.

Less obvious but highly productive partnerships can also be found within the departments of sociology, anthropology, gender studies, history, psychology, philosophy, law and likely many others. We are continually astonished by how many people in disparate fields share interests in sexual and reproductive health at our own institutions. We strongly encourage people to read the course catalogue for the undergraduate and graduate schools to get a broad sense of which other faculty share similar interests.

12.2.4 Advocacy and Administrative Contributions

Circling back to the medical community, many people we speak with describe the benefits of being overall good citizens within the broader medical system. Other specialists often do not think they need FPSRH expertise until they have a patient who critically needs safe contraception or abortion. When we provide this expertise quickly and professionally, it is meaningful, and our colleagues remember. Abortion stigma often results in abortion providers being seen as less competent physicians, and by always doing our jobs well, we can help change this opinion. Members of the national FPSRH community hold administrative positions beyond heading academic divisions or sections; they also serve as department chairs, research and education program directors, deans and higher-level university administrators.

12.3 Opportunities for Collaboration Outside of the Academic Center

12.3.1 Clinical Partnerships

In many communities, important multidimensional collaborations exist between academic medical centers, local hospitals and outpatient reproductive health clinics. For example, the University of Utah FPSRH faculty provide abortion services for the Planned Parenthood Association of Utah. A single clinic serves as the training site for medical students, the Ryan Residency Training Program, Fellowship in Complex Family Planning, Medical Students for Choice externs and a wide variety of students and trainees from the university. We have collaborated with the Planned Parenthood Association of Utah (PPAU on research projects that have yielded more than two dozen publications in scientific journals including extensive efforts on use of IUDs for emergency contraception [6–11], yielding practice change through National Institutes of Health–funded research. This continues with a current non-inferiority randomized controlled study of the copper versus levonorgestrel IUD for emergency contraception (ClinicalTials.gov Identifier: NCT02175030). PPAU also collaborated with the University of Utah family planning team to conduct the HER Salt Lake Contraceptive Initiative [12]. This project provided no-cost contraceptive care for 7,402 Salt Lake County residents, 4,425 of whom enrolled in a 3-year prospective study assessing many aspects of contraceptive care. All of these participants enrolled in the study via PPAU staff who served as research staff and clinical assistants. After enrollment, follow-up occurred through university research staff to avoid burdening clinical staff with this chore. The data from this project support research collaborations with university faculty in a wide variety of disciplines and multi-institutional partnerships with faculty from outside Utah [13–16]. In addition, qualitative and quantitative research generated from the project will be used to improve care at participating clinics [17]. The research partnership with PPAU grew from our relationship with the staff and administration as providers of medical care.

In Seattle, we are fortunate to have a plethora of abortion providers. The Cedar River Clinics, a collective of three feminist women's health clinics around the Puget Sound, have a long history of training students, residents (ob-gyn and family medicine) and now family planning fellows. We have an abortion elective for first- and second-year medical students, where we introduce students to abortion, and there is a fourth-year elective for students who want to learn to perform abortions. We also have a productive research collaboration with Cedar River, using their data to evaluate various abortion questions. The local Planned Parenthood affiliate also trains family medicine residents and family planning fellows.

12.3.2 Legal Partnerships

Beyond clinical relationships, legal organizations such as the American Civil Liberties Union (ACLU) often have local chapters and can provide partnerships with significant benefit to both parties and the community. Abortion providers have the first contact with the patients, and often are the first to hear of situations in which infringement of patients' rights or obstruction of their health care access occurred. Patients often do not know how or even that they can discuss their cases with lawyers, and through partnerships we can guide our patients to them. We can also provide legal expertise and testimony to support evidence-based, patient-centered care. Without our participation in legal efforts, abortion cases could never be won. Additionally, these experts in reproductive health law can guide us to make sure we are practicing firmly within our legal rights, and to support us if our rights as providers are being violated.

12.3.3 Other Community Partnerships

Other community groups can serve as important allies for advocacy efforts. For example, when legislation is presented that can influence reproductive health, rights and justice, the voices of collaborators from health-care associations, government (department of health, the state Medicaid program), service groups (YWCA) and community agencies can impact legislation and policy decisions. Because FPSRH affects so many people at critical moments, it can be a focus for advocacy efforts. For example, when educating lawmakers about a family planning Medicaid waiver in the 2018 Utah state legislature, we combined efforts with organizations addressing decreasing the gender-based wage gap, education, homelessness and opioid dependency.

12.3.4 Reproductive Justice Framework and Organization Partnerships

Finally, we find collaborations with reproductive justice partners critical to our efforts to provide equitable care and to maintain a firm stance that progress is not being made unless marginalized populations are positively impacted. Women of color developed the reproductive justice framework specific for the USA [18], which does not currently legally acknowledge the human right to health, let alone reproductive health. The USA was founded on the dual atrocities of genocide of Indigenous peoples and slavery. This history requires acknowledgment of the intersection of those practices with sexual and reproductive health. For example, associated reproductive injustices began with children of slaves being the property of the slave owner, not the women who carried and delivered them, even when they were raped by their slave owners. In the twentieth century, US policy supported sterilizing poor women and women of color without consent [19], which occured at academic and community hospitals, and more recently courts have required some women to use a long-acting contraceptive method in order to receive government benefits [20]. So now, we must exercise extreme caution when simultaneously addressing the reproductive options and access to care for people of color and those with limited resources, balancing easy access to all reproductive options and removal of barriers to care with enough checks in the system that coercion is not occurring, especially to marginalized people [21,22].

Reproductive Justice is a framework that asserts that basic human rights include three principles around reproduction: that everyone has the human right *to* have a child, to *not have* a child and to parent their children in safe and healthy environments [18]. Our interactions with local communities must be guided by Reproductive Justice principles. We want to acknowledge the work of women of color led by Loretta Ross and her co-founders who created the framework for Reproductive Justice, and to the current cadre continuing to lead this work. Sister Song, a collective activist organization dedicated to reproductive justice for women of color, provided the original language and framework for Reproductive Justice, and they continue to be critical allies, providing an annual conference and other resources from which we can all learn. Many communities have organizations doing this work locally; in Seattle, Surge Northwest is the organization that has supported the efforts of the University of Washington Family Planning Division in making sure we keep equity and justice at the forefront of our work. In Salt Lake City, Utah, this work is led by the Reproductive Justice Community Advisory Board. When academic family planning programs support Reproductive Justice organizations in our communities, we can play a role in correcting prior wrongs rather than compounding them.

It is time to collectively embrace Reproductive Justice and focus on increased opportunities when all are able to receive high-quality FPSRH care and have the rights to access these important services. Reproductive Justice also includes the opportunity to address a broad spectrum of issues including infertility treatment, safe pregnancy care, educational opportunities, police violence and environmental injustices that have been traditionally seen beyond the scope of FPSRH. Though Reproductive Justice is a framework used specifically in the USA, it has relevance worldwide. Many other countries in the world acknowledge that health is a human right, and it is critical, both in the USA and globally, to incorporate this concept into any and all trainings on FPSRH. We have the power to shift the ugly, mean-spirited, shaming and blaming around FPSRH we are seeing in many parts of the world with examples that demonstrate what real pro-women, pro-family, pro-autonomy reproductive health care, rights and justice looks like. Collaborations in FPSRH care and rights – both expected and unexpected – are an important way to accomplish this.

12.4 Conclusion

Family planning and sexual and reproductive health care derive many benefits from collaborations with other organizations and groups, be they advocates or other health care providers and organizations. (See Chapters 3 and 4.) FPSRH has never belonged solely within the purview of physicians or clinicians. Healers, midwives, female elders and other women in a community commonly provided care for women, most especially reproductive health care (pregnancy, its prevention and its termination). The advent of science in medicine led to its institutionalization, but as is evident from the examples of our academic, hospital-based family planning programs, collaborations enhance the quality and humanity of care and training. They lead to new, scientifically based findings, which in turn lead to new evidence in changing policy. (See Chapter 4.) Encouraging and nurturing these collaborations expand the tent under which we all stand in support of FPSRH and reproductive rights and justice.

References

1. Sedgh G, Bearak J, Singh S, et al. Abortion incidence between 1990 and 2014: global, regional, and subregional levels and trends. *Lancet.* 2016;**388** (10041):258–267. doi:10.1016/S0140-6736(16)30380-4

2. Foster AM, Arnott G, Hobstetter M. Community-based distribution of misoprostol for early abortion: evaluation of a program along the Thailand-Burma border. *Contraception.* 2017;**96** (4):242–247. doi:10.1016/j.contraception.2017.06.006

3. Darney BG, Weaver MR, VanDerhei D, Stevens NG, Prager SW. "One of those areas that people avoid": a qualitative study of implementation in miscarriage management. *BMC Health Serv Res.* 2013;**13**:123. doi:10.1186/1472-6963-13-123

4. Darney BG, Weaver MR, Stevens N, Kimball J, Prager SW. The family medicine residency training initiative in miscarriage management:

impact on practice in Washington State. *Fam Med.* 2013;**45**(2):102–108.

5. Schreiber CA, Creinin MD, Atrio J, Sonalkar S, Ratcliffe SJ, Barnhart KT. Mifepristone pretreatment for the medical management of early pregnancy loss. *N Engl J Med.* 2018;**378**(23):2161–2170. doi:10.1056/NEJMoa1715726

6. Sanders JN, Moran LA, Mullholand M, Torres E, Turok DK. Video counseling about emergency contraception: an observational study. *Contraception.* 2019;**100**(1):54–64. doi:10.1016/j.contraception.2019.02.014

7. Sanders JN, Turok DK, Royer PA, Thompson IS, Gawron LM, Storck KE. One-year continuation of copper or levonorgestrel intrauterine devices initiated at the time of emergency contraception. *Contraception.* 2017;**96**(2):99–105. doi:10.1016/j.contraception.2017.05.012

8. Turok DK, Sanders JN, Thompson IS, Royer PA, Eggebroten J, Gawron LM. Preference for and efficacy of oral levonorgestrel for emergency contraception with concomitant placement of a levonorgestrel IUD: a prospective cohort study. *Contraception.* 2016;**93**(6):526–532. doi:10.1016/j.contraception.2016.01.009

9. Turok DK, Jacobson JC, Dermish AI, et al. Emergency contraception with a copper IUD or oral levonorgestrel: an observational study of 1-year pregnancy rates. *Contraception.* 2014;**89**(3):222–228. doi:10.1016/j.contraception.2013.11.010

10. Turok DK, Gurtcheff SE, Handley E, et al. A survey of women obtaining emergency contraception: are they interested in using the copper IUD? *Contraception.* 2011;**83**(5):441–446. doi:10.1016/j.contraception.2010.08.011

11. Turok DK, Gero A, Simmons R, Kaiser J, Stoddard GJ, Sexsmith CD, Gawron LM, Sanders JN. The Levonorgestrel vs. Copper Intrauterine Device for Emergency Contraception: a Non-inferiority Randomized Controlled Trial. *N Engl J Med.* 2021 Jan 28;**384**(4):335–344. doi:10.1016/j.contraception.2010.06.001

12. Sanders JN, Myers K, Gawron LM, Simmons RG, Turok DK. Contraceptive method use during the community-wide HER Salt Lake Contraceptive Initiative. *Am J Public Health.* 2018;**108**(4):550–556. doi:10.2105/AJPH.2017.304299.

13. Geist C, Aiken AR, Sanders JN, et al. Beyond intent: exploring the association of contraceptive choice with questions about Pregnancy Attitudes, Timing and How important is pregnancy prevention (PATH) questions. *Contraception.* 2019;**99**(1):22–26. doi:10.1016/j.contraception.2018.08.014

14. Sanders JN, Higgins JA, Adkins DE, Stoddard GJ, Gawron LM, Turok DK. The impact of sexual satisfaction, functioning, and perceived contraceptive effects on sex life on IUD and implant continuation at 1 year. *Womens Health Issues.* 2018;**28**(5):401–407. doi:10.1016/j.whi.2018.06.003

15. Everett BG, Sanders JN, Myers K, Geist C, Turok DK. One in three: challenging heteronormative assumptions in family planning health centers. *Contraception.* 2018;**98**(4):270–274. doi:10.1016/j.contraception.2018.06.007

16. Higgins JA, Sanders JN, Palta M, Turok DK. Women's sexual function, satisfaction, and perceptions after starting long-acting reversible contraceptives. *Obstet Gynecol.* 2016;**128**(5):1143–1151. doi:10.1097/AOG.0000000000001655

17. Simmons RG, Sanders JN, Geist C, Gawron L, Myers K, Turok DK. Predictors of contraceptive switching and discontinuation within the first 6 months of use among Highly Effective Reversible Contraceptive Initiative Salt Lake study participants. *Am J Obstet Gynecol.* 2019;**220**(4):376 e1–e12. doi:10.1016/j.ajog.2018.12.022

18. Ross LJ, Solinger R. *Reproductive Justice: An Introduction.* Oakland: University of California Press; 2017.

19. Committee on Ethics. Committee Opinion No. 695: sterilization of women: ethical issues and considerations. *Obstet Gynecol.* 2017;**129**(4): e109–e16. doi:10.1097/AOG.0000000000002023

20. Roberts D. *Killing the Black Body: Race, Reproduction, and the Meaning of Liberty.* New York: Pantheon; 1997.

21. Moaddab A, McCullough LB, Chervenak FA, et al. Health care justice and its implications for current policy of a mandatory waiting period for elective tubal sterilization. *Am J Obstet Gynecol.* 2015;**212**(6): 736–739. doi:10.1016/j.ajog.2015.03.049

22. Darney PD. New kinds of injustice for women? *Am J Obstet Gynecol.* 2015;**212**(6):693–694. doi:10.1016/j.ajog.2015.04.021

Family Planning Training at Catholic and Other Faith-Based Hospitals

Maryam Guiahi

13.1 Training Requirements for Obstetrics and Gynecology Residents at Catholic and Other Faith-Based Hospitals

Residency training in obstetrics and gynecology (ob-gyn) is aimed at developing physicians with expertise in all aspects of women's health care. Since 1996, the Accreditation Council for Graduate Medical Education (ACGME) has recognized that family planning and abortion training are essential components of ob-gyn training and has set forth the expectation that all ob-gyn residency programs provide such training. In 1996, the requirement specified: "If a residency program has a religious, moral, or legal restriction that prohibits the residents from providing abortions within the institution, the program must ensure that the residents receive satisfactory education and experience in managing the complications of abortion" [1]. More recently, ACGME updated the ob-gyn program requirements in 2017 to say, "All programs must have an established curriculum for family planning, including for complications of abortions and provisions for the opportunity for direct procedural training in terminations of pregnancy for those residents who desire it" [2]. Accordingly, exceptions for residency programs that face institutional barriers, including those at religious hospitals, are not warranted. These recommendations are also in line with those of the American College of Obstetricians and Gynecologists (ACOG) [3].

13.2 Institutional Barriers to Provision of Family Planning Services at Catholic and Other Faith-Based Hospitals

Programs that primarily train at Catholic and other faith-based hospitals face significant institutional barriers to the provision of family planning services and consequently face barriers to training their ob-gyn residents. Specifically, Catholic hospitals are expected by the United States Conference of Catholic Bishops to follow the *Ethical and Religious Directives for Catholic Health Care Services* (hereafter referred to as "the directives"), which only allows natural family planning counseling for married heterosexual couples and otherwise restricts contraceptive services and abortion care [4,5]. As of 2016, 14.5% of acute care hospitals were Catholic owned or affiliated [6]. A recent review of available studies on the topic of reproductive health-care provision in Catholic settings demonstrated that provision of family planning services is lower at Catholic hospitals, often secondary to adherence to the directives [7]. This review also acknowledged that when nonadherence to the directives occurs, it is often with respect to provision of less controversial services like prescription of oral contraceptives [7]. In contrast, contraceptive services that require on-site administration, including provision of long-acting reversible contraception and sterilization, were more likely to be restricted [7]. These findings present a significant barrier to training residents in these programs. Additionally, the directives describe concerns about potential "scandal" when associated with actions deemed by the Church to be immoral, including abortion, and cautions about collaboration with institutions that perform such services; such guidelines may cause concerns about off-site collaborations [5].

Less is known about family planning practices at other religious hospitals. Formal contraceptive teachings differ across Buddhist, Protestant, Hindu, Muslim and Jewish faiths, with certain methods promoted over others [8]. Additionally, teachings about when life begins and in what circumstances abortion is acceptable vary across faiths [7]. At present, there do not appear to be clear institutional recommendations for medical care based on religious teachings implemented across religious hospitals that are non-Catholic. Complicating our understanding of this is that at an institutional level, there are comparatively few non-Catholic religious hospitals; other religious non-profit hospitals accounted for 4.0% of all US hospitals in 2016, with significant heterogeneity in this category [6]. Indirect data obtained from residents and program directors in Christian settings (eg, Protestant, Methodist) suggest that restrictions to abortion care exist, but that significant barriers to provision of contraceptive methods do not [9]. In contrast, there does not appear to be evidence that substantial restrictions to abortion care exist at Jewish hospitals.

13.3 Prevalence of Catholic and Other Restrictive Faith-Based Hospitals That Are Associated with Obstetrics and Gynecology Training Programs

The exact proportion of ob-gyn residency training programs that are located at religious hospitals that restrict family planning services is not well known and varies year to year as the number of accredited programs vary. Complicating this understanding is that many programs rely on several hospital sites to achieve adequate training. Thus, the experience of ob-gyn residents who only or mainly train at a Catholic hospital is likely different from the experience of ob-gyn residents who primarily train at secular sites and spend limited training at a Catholic site. At present, the Fellowship and Residency Electronic Interactive Database (FREIDA) available from the American Medical Association does not specify whether hospitals are religious, and many such hospitals fall under the description of "community hospital(s)."

Prior program director surveys provide some understanding of the proportion of hospitals that primarily train ob-gyn residents and are religiously affiliated, but are limited by response rates. A 1991 survey reported that 31 of the 268 ob-gyn residency programs (11.5%) were Catholic; no other religious hospitals were specified [10]. In a 1998 survey of the 261 accredited US residency programs, there was a 69% response rate (179/261) for which 10% had a primary affiliation with a "Private, Church" hospital; no other categories

suggested a religious affiliation [11]. A 2004 survey of 252 existing accredited US residency ob-gyn programs had 183 respondents (73% response rate), of which 74% (n = 137) reported as nonreligious, 8.6% (n = 16) reported as Catholic, 3.2% (n = 6) reported as Protestant, 6.5% (n = 12) reported as Jewish and 4.9% (n = 9) reported as other [12]. The most recent national survey of the 2013 US ob-gyn residency programs had 190 of 242 programs respond (79% response rate), of which 26 (14%) reported any faith affiliation [13].

Recently, an ob-gyn program leader survey was conducted during the 2017–2018 academic year and aimed to better estimate the proportion of programs that train at faith-based hospitals with restrictions to family planning [9]. These investigators excluded Jewish hospitals, as prior data did not suggest a correlation with restrictions and because we were not aware of institutional restrictions [12]. The investigators examined all ob-gyn programs listed in the FREIDA online site as part of the American Medical Association database [14], which at the time of review (2016) acknowledged religious ownership of training hospitals. They cross-referenced the primary hospital websites to understand if they were religiously affiliated and also relied on other educational stakeholders. Only programs that reported at least 70% of resident training at a restrictive, faith-based hospital(s) were included. Using this approach, they found 30 eligible programs, which accounted for 10.8% of the 278 accredited 2017–2018 ob-gyn accredited programs. Among these 30 programs, 76% were Catholic hospitals.

13.4 Family Planning Training at Catholic and Other Restrictive Faith-Based Hospitals That Are Associated with Obstetrics and Gynecology Training Programs

13.4.1 Selection of Training at Catholic and Other Restrictive Faith-Based Hospitals

Many hypothesize that residents who want training in line with religious institutions choose to go to such training hospitals. Based on limited data, this does not appear to be the case. In a 2008–2009 survey of ob-gyn residents at

20 Midwest programs, 232 of 340 eligible residents responded (68% response rate) from 7 faith-based and 10 nonfaith-based training programs [1]. Most respondents, regardless of program type, were female, Roman Catholic and prochoice, and planned on practicing general ob-gyn. In this cohort, plans to provide family planning procedures did not differ across groups, suggesting similar intentions for family planning training [1]. Between 2018 and 2019, ob-gyn residents from 5 ob-gyn programs affiliated with Catholic hospitals were surveyed. Among 41 respondents, only 5 residents (12.2%) reported selecting a Catholic program based on its religious affiliation and 6 residents (14.6%) reported that their personal views on reproductive care were in line with their institution [15].

13.4.2 Report of Obstetrics and Gynecology Training Experience by Residents at Catholic and Other Restrictive Faith-Based Hospitals

Data regarding the experiences of ob-gyn residents at faith-based hospitals are limited, but demonstrate that institutional restrictions to on-site procedures are a significant barrier to training to competency in family planning procedures. A 2008–2009 survey of ob-gyn residents at 20 Midwest programs had a response rate of 68% (232 of 340 eligible residents responded) across 17 programs (85% program response rate) [1]. In this survey, 7 programs were faith based. Baseline characteristics were similar across training programs, except residents at non-faith-based programs were 3.4 times more likely (95% confidence interval, 1.9–6.2) to report feeling completely satisfied with their family planning training compared to residents at faith-based programs [1]. Respondents were queried about self-rated competency for performance of a range of family planning procedures. Compared to residents at faith-based programs, those at non-faith-based programs reported higher rates of competency for most family planning procedures. Table 13.1 highlights these comparisons and indicates whether a dedicated family planning rotation existed and whether or not the program was a Ryan Residency Training Program. These differences persisted after controlling for year of training, gender and career plans.

Between 2014 and 2015, 15 graduates from 10 different ob-gyn training programs affiliated with Catholic hospitals throughout the USA participated in qualitative interviews [16]. Participants graduated between 2008 and 2013, were mostly female (14 of 15, 93%) and were mostly employed in private practice (11 of 15, 73%). Many participants reported a lack of awareness regarding limitations of family planning training at their institutions, particularly with respect to contraceptive and sterilization services. Participants reported varying experiences, with most providing short-acting contraceptive methods with more variations with respect to procedures that require on-site administration including injectable contraception and long-acting reversible contraception. Most commented on sterilization limitations, especially when performed in the immediate postpartum period. All reported that they did not have any on-site abortion training. Many explained that "elective" training required resident initiative to obtain it, and that routine off-site experiences improved training. Overall, participants reported dissatisfaction with their family planning training, despite satisfaction with other aspects of their training. Many reported delayed competency with certain procedures like IUD insertion and laparoscopic sterilization, and others reported inability to provide certain family planning procedures like postpartum sterilization and dilation and evacuation (D&E) [15]. A conceptual model highlighting these findings is demonstrated in Figure 13.1.

13.4.3 Report of Obstetrics and Gynecology Training Experience by Program Leaders at Catholic and Other Restrictive Faith-Based Hospitals

Data from program directors and other relevant stakeholders at religious hospitals generally match resident experiences. In a 2013 national survey of ob-gyn residency programs, program directors at religiously affiliated programs were more likely to report abortion training restrictions, often secondary to hospital policies [8]. Recently, an ob-gyn program director survey was conducted during the 2017–2018 academic year and only included hospitals that trained residents at a Catholic or other faith-based hospital with family

Table 13.1 Residents reporting they "understand and can perform on their own" by program type [1]

Family planning skill	Total residents, n = 232 (%)	Non-faith-based, n = 166 (%)	P*	Dedicated rotation, n = 123 (%)	P*	Ryan Program, n = 105 (%)	P*
Long-acting reversible contraception							
Contraceptive implant insertion	100 (43.1)	79 (47.6)	.04	61 (49.6)	.05	47 (44.8)	.69
Intrauterine device insertion	187 (80.6)	142 (85.5)	<.01	107 (87)	.01	90 (85.7)	.10
Interval sterilization							
Laparoscopic sterilization	135 (58.2)	105 (63.3)	.02	78 (63.4)	.11	66 (62.9)	.23
Hysteroscopic sterilization	103 (44.4)	78 (47)	.24	55 (44.7)	1	49 (46.7)	.60
First-trimester uterine evacuation techniques							
Suction curettage	179 (77.2)	129 (77.7)	.73	99 (80.5)	.21	83 (79)	.64
Manual vacuum aspiration	105 (45.3)	90 (54.2)	<.001	70 (56.9)	<.001	60 (57.1)	.001
Electric vacuum aspiration	113 (48.7)	86 (51.8)	.15	66 (53.7)	.12	56 (53.3)	.24
Paracervical block	162 (69.8)	132 (79.5)	<.001	103 (83.7)	<.001	87 (82.9)	<.001
Second-trimester uterine evacuation techniques							
Laminaria insertion	113 (48.7)	97 (58.4)	<.001	71 (57.7)	<.001	63 (60)	<.001
Dilation and evacuation	62 (26.7)	57 (34.3)	<.001	43 (35)	<.01	40 (38.1)	.001

Data are in (%)>

* P values were calculated using the Fisher exact test.

planning restrictions (Jewish hospitals excluded) for at least 70% of resident time [9]. Among 30 programs, 25 responded (83%) and the majority of respondents were program directors (84%) and represented Catholic hospitals (76%). All reported adequate contraceptive training. Sixty percent reported concerns about inadequate sterilization training, particularly postpartum tubal ligations (53% of Catholic respondents vs. 0% of non-Catholic respondents, p = 0.02). Catholic sites were also more likely than other religious programs to report poor abortion training (47% vs. 0%, p = 0.04). Approximately half (56%) of all of the programs offered abortion training as part of the curriculum ("routine"), 32% offered

residents the opportunity to arrange training ("elective") and 12% did not offer such training. Five Catholic programs (26% of Catholic programs) reported their residents did not meet the graduate training requirement for completion of 20 dilation and curettage (D&Cs) [9].

13.4.4 Innovative Ways of Accomplishing Comprehensive Family Planning Training at Catholic and Other Restrictive Faith-Based Hospitals

Prior investigations and reports have highlighted ways in which ob-gyn residency programs,

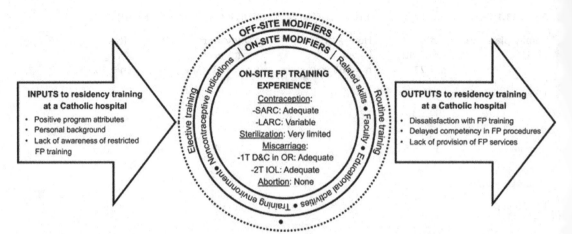

Figure 13.1 Conceptual framework for inputs, outputs and family planning training experiences of residency training at Catholic institutions [15]

FP, family planning; SARC, short-acting reversible contraceptives; LARC, long-acting reversible contraceptives; 1T, first trimester; D&C, dilation and curettage; OR, operating room; 2T, second trimester; IOL, induction of labor.

Note: Central wheel: Inner circle is the reported experience in family planning methods at Catholic hospitals. Middle circle demonstrates modifiers that affected family planning training within Catholic hospitals. Outer circle demonstrates strategies used at off-site centers to supplement family planning training.

particularly those at Catholic sites, overcome institutional limitations to family planning training.

13.4.4.1 Educational Interventions

Many graduates from Catholic programs have described educational activities that were often initiated by faculty who were supportive of their educational needs [16]. Improving on-site education with didactics and simulations have proved successful in these settings. A one-day session at Loyola University Medical Center in Illinois that incorporated family planning lectures and simulation sessions resulted in improved knowledge, both immediately and ten months later [17]. A contraceptive simulation lab, which included a postpartum tubal ligation simulation developed at Saint Joseph Hospital in Denver, Colorado, similarly resulted in improved knowledge [18]. Many graduates have also commented on how procedural training for other interventions helped build related skills for family planning procedures [16]. For example, many reported how laparoscopic training made the transition to laparoscopic sterilizations easier in practice.

13.4.4.2 Non-contraceptive Indications and Workarounds

Graduates and program directors from Catholic programs have highlighted better contraceptive and sterilization training exposure when family planning interventions are applied for non-contraceptive indications [1, 9,16]. In many Catholic institutions, levonorgestrel IUDs can be inserted based on US Food and Drug Administration labeling for heavy menstrual bleeding, whereas copper IUD insertions are rarely available based on the Church's concern that it is an abortifacient [1,9,16]. In some locations, use of risk-reducing salpingectomy for the indication of ovarian cancer reduction has been used to justify salpingectomies [9]. Some graduates and stakeholders have described directive counseling specifically to elicit possible non-contraceptive indications from patients desiring contraception, exaggeration of non-contraceptive indications in documentation to help patients achieve family planning goals and/or institutional cultures that tend to be permissive with such indications [1,16]. Informants from Catholic settings have also described ethics committee approval in cases of medically complex patients who desire sterilization, even when these indications do not necessarily meet the criteria set forth by the directives [16].

13.4.4.3 Off-Site Training

Many Catholic and other faith-based programs rely on off-site locations to accomplish family planning training; 47% reported reliance on off-site locations for contraception training and 72% reported reliance on off-site locations for sterilization training [9]. Graduates and program leaders from Catholic programs often describe reliance on off-site community health clinics or private practice offices to accomplish contraceptive training [9,16]. Many Catholic programs accomplish interval tubal ligation training by affiliating with nearby surgical centers and community hospitals [9,14].

Among program stakeholders at Catholic and other faith-based hospitals, 84% reported relying on a family planning–specific clinic for abortion training. Despite this, only 58% of Catholic respondents and 50% of other faith-based institutions provide routine abortion training, as recommended by ACGME [9]. When off-site training occurred, residents were more likely to obtain first-trimester compared to second-trimester training [9]. Graduates of Catholic programs that relied on elective time to individually pursue off-site training opportunities vocalized frustrations over how such arrangements were logistically difficult; that often there was no elective time or they had competing interests; and that when established relationships with an off-site facility did not exist, it was difficult to arrange an ad hoc rotation [14]. Other programs have found off-site collaborations to accomplish routine abortion training for all of their residents; in Denver, Colorado, a unique collaboration was formed between the Saint Joseph residency program (a Catholic hospital) and the University of Colorado program (a nearby secular hospital) with the assistance of a Kenneth J. Ryan Residency Training Program in Abortion and Family Planning training grant [19].

13.4.4.4 Residency Review Committee Evaluations

One third of Catholic and other faith-based programs have reported a prior Residency Review Committee family planning citation(s) [9]. Many of these respondents endorsed that these citations actually helped provide leverage for improved training among other stakeholders.

13.5 Conclusion

At least 10% of ob-gyn residency programs are based at religiously affiliated hospitals, and of these at least two thirds are Catholic affiliated. Given that Catholic-affiliated hospitals have demonstrated recent expansion within the US health-care market [6] and that more religiously affiliated osteopathic programs may be transitioning to ACGME status, it is possible that this proportion will increase. Religiously affiliated programs face significant barriers to training residents in abortion care given restrictions. Additionally, Catholic programs face additional limitations with respect to contraceptive and sterilization services. Many Catholic programs have developed off-site collaborations for contraceptive and laparoscopic sterilization training, while training in postpartum tubal ligation remains insufficient. Approximately half of religiously affiliated training programs have developed off-site collaborations to accomplish abortion training. Catholic institutions in particular are faced with conflicting guidelines about institutional restrictions to reproductive care and expectations for comprehensive family planning training and likely warrant additional support to develop adequate didactic and simulation training and off-site collaborations.

References

1. Guiahi M, Westhoff CL, Summers S, Kenton K. Training at a faith-based institution matters for obstetrics and gynecology residents: results from a regional survey. *J Grad Med Educ.* 2013;**5**(2):244–251.

2. Accreditation Council for Graduate Medical Education Review Committee for Obstetrics and Gynecology Clarifications of Program Requirements. ww.Acgme.Org/Portals/0/Pfassets/ Programresources/220_ Obgyn_Abortion_Training_ Clarification.Pdf. Accessed July 23, 2019.

3. Committee on Health Care for Underserved Women. ACOG Committee Opinion No. 612: abortion training and education. *Obstet Gynecol.* 2014;**124**(5):1055–1059.

4. Guiahi M. Catholic health care and women's health. *Obstet Gynecol.* 2018;**131**(3):534–537.

5. United States Conference of Catholic Bishops. *Ethical and Religious Directives for Catholic Health Care Services.* 2018. www.usccb.org/about/ doctrine/ethical-and-religious-directives/upload/ethical-religious-directives-catholic-health-service-sixth-edition-2016-06.pdf. Accessed July 23, 2019.

6. Uttley L. Growth of Catholic hospitals and health systems: 2016 update of the Miscarriage of Medicine Report. 2016. http://static1.1.sqspcdn.com/ static/f/816571/27061007/ 1465224862580/MW_Update-2016-MiscarrOfMedicine-

report.pdf?token=rf3rsQaaC
VCzLV9hKOIHuFcaWiU%3D.
Accessed June 4, 2019.

7. Thorne NB, Soderborg TK,
Glover JJ, Hoffecker L, Guiahi
M. Reproductive health care in
Catholic facilities: a scoping
review. *Obstet Gynecol.*
2019;**133**(1):105–115.

8. Turk JK, Landy U, Chien J,
Steinauer JE. Sources of
support for and resistance to
abortion training in obstetrics
and gynecology residency
programs. *American J Obstet
Gynecol.* 2019;**221**(2):P156.
E1–156.E6.

9. Guiahi M, Teal S, Kenton K,
Decesare J, Steinauer J. Family
planning training at Catholic
and other religious hospitals: a
national survey. *American
J Obstet Gynecol.* 2020;
222(3):273.e1–273.e9.

10. MacKay HT, MacKay AP.
Abortion training in obstetrics
and gynecology residency
programs in the United States,
1991–1992. *Fam Plann
Perspect.* 1995;**27**(3):112–115.

11. Almeling R, Tews L, Dudley S.
Abortion training in U.S.
obstetrics and gynecology
residency programs, 1998. *Fam
Plann Perspect.* 2000;
32(6):268–271, 320.

12. Eastwood KL, Kacmar JE,
Steinauer J, Weitzen S,
Boardman LA. Abortion
training in United States
obstetrics and gynecology
residency programs. *Obstet
Gynecol.* 2006;**108**(2):303–308.

13. Steinauer JE, Turk JK,
Pomerantz T, Simonson K,
Learman LA, Landy U.
Abortion training in US
obstetrics and gynecology
residency programs. *Am
J Obstet Gynecol.* 2018;
219(1):86 e81–86 e86.

14. American Medical Association
FREIDA™, the AMA Residency
& Fellowship Database® 2015;
https://freida.ama-assn.org/
Freida/#/. Accessed March 7,
2019.

15. Guiahi M, Wilson C, Claymore
E, Simonson K, Steinauer J.
Influence of a values

clarification workshop on
residents training at Catholic
Hospital programs. *Contracept
X.* 20212021 Jan 20;3:100054.

16. Guiahi M, Hoover J, Swartz M,
Teal S. Impact of Catholic
hospital affiliation during
obstetrics and gynecology
residency on the provision of
family planning. *J Grad Med
Educ.* 2017;**9**(4):440–446.

17. Guiahi M, Cortland C,
Graham MJ, et al. Addressing
ob/gyn family planning
educational objectives at a
faith-based institution using
the TEACH program.
Contraception. 2011;
83(4):367–372.

18. Wollschlager K, White K.
A contraception simulation lab
developed for ob/gyn residents
in Catholic hospitals. *Obstet
Gynecol.* 2016;**12**:58S.

19. Fennimore R, Guiahi M,
Gottesfeld M, Ricciotti, H.
Enhancing family planning
training at a Catholic obgyn
residency program. *Obstet
Gynecol.* 2017;**130**:56S.

Chapter 14

The Importance of Including Abortion in Undergraduate Medical Education

Jody Steinauer and Teresa DePiñeres

14.1 Introduction

Medical educators have a responsibility to train medical students in the competencies needed to improve the sexual and reproductive health (SRH) of their communities [1]. Abortion is not only a core component of SRH care; it is also common. Annually, approximately 56 million abortions occur worldwide [2]. Induced abortion by trained clinicians is very safe, with a case fatality rate of 0.7 per 100,000 abortions in the USA [3]. Worldwide, almost half (45%) of abortions are practiced under unsafe conditions [4], leading to an estimated 7 million complications and account for 8% of maternal deaths [5] each year. According to the World Health Organization (WHO), unsafe abortion can be prevented by giving women access to legal abortion by trained, competent practitioners and timely emergency treatment of complications [6]. One global survey estimated that approximately 60% of the world's population lives in countries where abortion is officially legal. However, despite its legality, barriers to obtaining a safe abortion remain. Significant barriers to implementing abortion laws in these settings are the lack of properly trained health personnel [7,8], physician misunderstanding of laws and lack of abortion training in medical schools [9]. WHO states, "The availability of facilities and trained providers within reach of the entire population is essential to ensuring access to safe abortion services" [10]. Providing abortion care at the primary care level and through outpatient services in higher-level settings is not only safe but also reduces costs while maximizing access [11].

This chapter begins with an overview of medical education standards and their relevance for sexual and reproductive health. It then reviews the literature on medical student education about abortion and includes a sample of regional and national organizational recommendations. It finally describes opportunities for inclusion of abortion in medical education, using the educational objective standards set by the World Federation for Medical Education.

14.2 Medical Education Overview

The goal of medical education is to improve the health of all peoples by preparing physicians to meet the health needs of a country's populations [12]. The structures and governance of undergraduate medical education, as well as the number of medical schools and annual graduates, vary by country. In this chapter, we focus on undergraduate medical education (UME, or "medical school"), defined as the first stage of educating students to become physicians. This education occurs after high school or after university depending on the country's education system; includes didactic and clinical components; and usually consists of classroom time in the beginning and clinical rotations for the last few years. The structures and governance of undergraduate medical education, as well as the number of medical schools and graduates, vary by country.

The World Federation for Medical Education (WFME) recommends standards for medical education worldwide. It is a not-for-profit organization established by the World Medial Association (WMA) and the WHO, and its mission is to support health care through promoting high-quality medical education and offering an accreditation program for medical schools. In the WFME's *Global Standards for Quality Improvement*, all medical schools must define educational outcomes for graduation, in relation to, among other factors, the health needs of the community, the needs of the health-care delivery system and other aspects of social accountability [12]. The WFME recommends that educational outcomes and competencies must include documented knowledge and understanding of (a) the basic biomedical sciences, (b) the behavioural and social sciences, (c) medical ethics, human rights and law related to medical practice, (d) the clinical sciences, and (e) life-long learning and professionalism. The WFME also specifies that the clinical sciences include the content of the specialty of obstetrics and gynecology (ob-gyn).

While countries often have a governing body that issues guidance on the required medical school curriculum content, this guidance is often general and sexual and reproductive health are only indirectly covered [1]. Similarly, many medical schools' guidelines do not explicitly address abortion care. Moreover, even if these objectives and competencies exist, many medical schools are individually governed and not regulated by a single enforcing body.

Accreditation is one formal process by which an institution is able to grant degrees, based on the quality of training, allowing its graduates to achieve licensing for practice [13]. There is great global diversity in how and whether accreditation is completed, who oversees this process and how it is enforced. Subsequently, there is also great diversity in the curricular content of medical schools.

After graduation, some physicians continue their education to a medical specialization, such as obstetrics and gynecology, others are required to work as a general practitioner (GP) for a specified time before specializing, and many, and in some countries, the majority, work as GPs for their entire career. These graduates who will practice as GPs need a broad, high-quality medical education in SRH to prepare them to provide competent care.

14.3 Medical Student Knowledge about and Medical School Inclusion of Abortion

14.3.1 Medical Student Knowledge about Their Country-Level Legal Restrictions for Abortion

Studies [14–18] have documented lack of medical student knowledge about the legal rights of women who seek abortion care and to what gestational limit and for what indications it is legal. For example, Al-Amoudi et al. [17] published in 2017 that students did not know the health rights of women in Saudi Arabia; 25% thought abortion was completely forbidden in Islam, and only 50% knew that it is available in specific circumstances. An interview study of medical students in India found that many confused the legal regulation of abortion with the law governing gender-biased sex selection, and incorrectly concluded that abortion was illegal in Maharastra [18]. In Turkey, one study found that only 52% [16] knew the federal gestational limit for abortion, and while another found that more students (73%) [14,19] knew about the gestational limit, 88% incorrectly thought adult women needed consent from their partners [14]. A survey of students [16] in Argentina found that while more final-year students correctly answered questions about the abortion law than first-year students, their knowledge was not complete; for example, 57% incorrectly thought abortion was legal for fetal malformations. In contrast, only a few studies, for example, in Brazil [20] and Pakistan [21], have documented that medical students had adequate knowledge of which indications for abortion were legal.

14.3.2 Medical Student Knowledge about and Skills in Abortion Clinical Care

Studies indicate that medical students commonly have inadequate clinical knowledge and lack skills in abortion [22–25,14,18,26,9,27]. For example, in a study of 209 students at 3 medical schools in Turkey, only three quarters knew of surgical abortion as a method to induce abortion (medication abortion is not currently available in Turkey), and did not have an understanding about complications of abortion [14]. In India, students at 6 medical schools demonstrated knowledge gaps about medication abortion, for example, confusing it with emergency contraception [18], and only 13% of 2,000 senior students at 27 colleges had been exposed to a clinical abortion experience [28]. In a study of new medical graduates in Thailand published in 2013, despite the Thai Medical Council stipulating that experience in manual uterine aspiration (MUA) is a requirement for a medical license, a significant minority of new graduates (43–44%) had seen but never used MUA. [29]

In the USA, students at one medical school lacked knowledge about abortion care and patients' challenges accessing abortion [27]. Students described that they felt efforts by faculty to promote opportunities for training and exposure were minimal and that the onus was largely on students to seek out clinical training. Veazey et al. [26] described that half of students who chose to do a final-year elective course in abortion care did so to obtain knowledge not available during their core clerkships. Proficiency in contraception and pregnancy options counseling was a top competency these students desired and gained.

14.3.3 UME Curricular Inclusion of Abortion

Studies of curricular content have confirmed that abortion is often not included in the regular medical school curriculum. A recent publication by Mihciokur et al. [14] in Turkey describes the challenge. They wrote, "... while guidelines are available to ensure medical students meet specified women's health care competencies, fixed learning objectives and curriculum requirements do not exist on reproductive health care, family planning education or abortion care. Although it is expected that all the medical schools include abortion in their curriculum, most do not even have lectures with abortion as a primary focus."

Similarly, a 2017 study of Colombian physicians found that only 1 of 35 medical schools included abortion training in the curriculum. In the other Colombian medical schools, outdated uterine evacuation techniques were taught, such as dilation and curettage without suction, and only in the context of early pregnancy failure [9]. Espey at al. [30] conducted a cross-sectional study of faculty responsible for medical student education at all US medical schools in 2003. They found that 44% of the 78 responding medical schools had no pre-clinical education about abortion, and that during the obstetrics and gynecology clerkship only 45% of programs offered clinical experiences in abortion care and 23% had no formal didactic education [30]. Also in the USA, one third of medical students reported that their pre-clinical education included no mention of abortion. When it was mentioned, it was often discussed for less than a total of 30 minutes

and often only the context of ethics rather than in clinical content [31].

14.3.4 Medical Student Beliefs about and Satisfaction with Abortion Training

Medical students throughout the world believe abortion should be included in medical education [31–34]. Among medical students in Malaysia [32], 90% believed that general knowledge on and legal aspects of abortion and pre- and post-abortion counseling should be included in their education, and 80% felt they should be trained in doing surgical and medication abortions. Among students in Chile, 70% believed their universities should provide abortion training for medical students [33]. In Ireland, 76% believed it should be included as mandatory in medical education [34], 19% thought it should be optional and only 3% thought it should not be included. Medical students have advocated for inclusion of abortion in their medical education throughout the world [35–37]. (See Chapter 21.)

Additionally, studies demonstrate that medical students who have participated in clinical training in abortion found it valuable. For example, the vast majority (84%) of US medical students who participated in abortion care during their clerkship thought it was beneficial [38]. Many students have articulated disappointment in their inadequate training, for example, in medical schools in North Ireland [39], the USA [22,40] and the UK [41].

14.4 Examples of Regional and National Organizational Recommendations for Undergraduate Medication Education in Abortion

Regional and national obstetrics and gynecology organizations have made recommendations and created guidelines about abortion in medical education. These recommendations have included specific content areas that should be included in medical education, as well as specific competencies.

Regional guidance includes the Federación Latinoamericana de Sociedades de Obstetricia y Ginecologia (Latin American Federation of Societies of Obstetrics and Gynecology,

FLASOG), which represents societies in 19 countries. FLASOG recommends that all medical schools include sexual and reproductive health, specifically human rights and gender, laws related to SRH in each country, prevention of unsafe abortion and management of abortion complications, legal abortion, post-abortion counseling and contraception and bioethics in SRH.

Country-specific, organizational guidelines also exist. For example, the Royal College of Obstetricians and Gynaecologists publishes the national undergraduate curriculum in obstetrics and gynaecology: "Students must understand and demonstrate appropriate knowledge, skills and attitudes in termination of pregnancy. It is recognised that there may be conscientious objection to the acquisition of knowledge and skills within the ... abortion components; however, it is essential that undergraduates are familiar with the issues and with the management options. Even though they may choose not to practice electively in this area, they must be aware of and able to recognise complications that may arise from this area of practice to be competent to provide appropriate emergency care in their careers" [42]. The curriculum mentions specific competencies.

1. As a clinical competency, students must have visited a family planning clinic and be able to take a history related to unplanned pregnancy.
2. As a knowledge competency, students must know the methods, indications, contraindications and complications of abortion.
3. Students must also demonstrate an understanding of the relevance to clinical practice of the Abortion Act.

In the USA, the Association of Professors of Gynecology and Obstetrics (APGO), publishes *Educational Objectives*, currently in its eleventh edition, revised in 2019 [43], which they consider to be the core women's health knowledge for all medical students regardless of their future medical specialization plans. According to APGO, upon graduation, students must have a thorough understanding of abortion and have met the following five learning objectives: the ability to provide non-directive pregnancy counseling to patients, list surgical and nonsurgical methods of pregnancy termination, identify potential complications and patient safety implications of pregnancy terminations, describe the public health

impact of the legal status of abortion, and discuss how health policy impacts access to abortion. For each of these objectives, they include the level of competence the medical student should have achieved at graduation, instructional methods to teach and methods to assess the objective, which type of Accreditation Council for Graduate Medical Education (ACGME) competency it is considered, which resources the organization makes available to teach that objective and to which Entrustable Professional Activity (a task that an individual can be trusted to perform in a given health-care context, once sufficient competence has been demonstrated) [44] it maps.

14.5 Sample Curricular Content Using the WFME Educational Outcomes

The WFME recommends that medical educational outcomes and competencies must include documented knowledge and understanding of the domains discussed here. Abortion content is suggested below, organized by each domain. At the time of this chapter's publication, 169 of the 195 (86%) countries of the world have at least one indication for legal abortion [2]. The legal status has implications for curricular content: medical educators in countries with an indication for legal abortion should consider how to educate medical students about abortion as part of SRH. Medical educators in countries with no legal exceptions, and throughout the world where some women cannot access safe abortion care due to restrictive policies and costs, should consider how to prepare medical students to care for women who have accessed abortion care outside of the clinical system, including management of complications.

The basic biomedical sciences:

- Pharmacology: medication abortion methods – misoprostol and mifepristone, as well as misoprostol alone, in the event that mifepristone is not available
- Reproductive physiology: menstruation, ovulation, fertilization, pregnancy physiology, pregnancy loss, abnormal pregnancy, medical illness that can be negatively affected by pregnancy, abnormal fetal development, abortion as a pregnancy outcome

The behavioural and social sciences, including public health and population medicine:

- Safe abortion as a public health and human rights priority
- Unsafe abortion as a public health problem, morbidity and mortality, evaluation of "risk" of health as defined by the WHO as extending beyond the risk of death [45]
- Social and structural determinants of health as complex factors that affect health, health-care access and health-care decision making, related to undesired pregnancy and abortion
- Cultivating compassion and empathy toward patients who make decisions with which physicians are uncomfortable or disagree, including reflecting on beliefs or values about patients' family planning and pregnancy decision making

Medical ethics, human rights and medical jurisprudence relevant to the practice of medicine:

- Review of local, regional and national laws about abortion
- Ethical principles involved in abortion care: patient autonomy, confidentiality, primacy of patient welfare, social justice, principles of informed consent and human rights
- The limits of conscientious objection in abortion care

The clinical sciences, including clinical skills with respect to diagnostic procedures, practical procedures, communication skills, treatment and prevention of disease, health promotion, rehabilitation, clinical reasoning and problem solving:

- Counseling about pregnancy options, pre- and post-abortion counseling
- Pregnancy decision making, including abortion as a choice that pregnant women might make
- Pregnancy complications such as fetal abnormalities or maternal health conditions that might make a woman with a desired pregnancy choose to terminate
- Pre-abortion and post-abortion care
- Abortion safety, techniques (including medication and procedural), complications, management
- Counseling and management of pregnancy loss, including methods of uterine evacuation
- Management of obstetric emergencies that require urgent uterine evacuation skills
- Managing complications of unsafe abortion
- The ability to undertake lifelong learning and demonstrate professionalism in connection

with the different roles of the doctor, also in relation to the medical profession.

- The importance of promoting social justice as a core professionalism value of medicine defined by the global Charter on Professionalism for the New Millennium [46], which includes advocating for access to health care services
- Reflection about reconciling personal beliefs with supporting patient autonomy and the primacy of patient welfare [46], both core pillars of professionalism

14.5.1 Clinical Learning Opportunities to Meet These Objectives

Many of the above objectives could be met in preclinical courses. Given that the WFME [12] also recommends content knowledge in and exposure to obstetrics and gynecology, we describe what can also be learned during the clinical learning experiences. While working in ob-gyn clinical spaces, students can participate in didactic teaching about topics listed above, such as reproductive physiology and clinical care knowledge. In addition, students should participate in the clinical care of women considering and choosing to have an abortion. This includes counseling women before abortion, and following women through the pre-abortion, abortion and post-abortion care processes. Students could observe abortion procedures, and more advanced students are able to learn the techniques of uterine aspiration. They may also gain knowledge and competence in medication abortion during and after the first trimester.

The same could be included in all clinical rotations in reproductive health care. In some settings, reproductive health care is provided in family medicine, for example. In addition, Emergency Medicine could include the workup of women who have possibly taken medication to induce an abortion or who have sought abortion care outside of a safe, clinical environment. This could also include the indications for legal abortion, as well as the rights of patients to confidential health care, to prevent reporting to law enforcement.

A key component of clinical education is establishing opportunities for medical students to work with clinicians who do abortions. Thus, medical schools could ensure achieving these learning objectives by allowing students to spend time in an abortion care setting. The vast majority (93%), for example, of US ob-gyn residency programs with abortion training supported through the Ryan Program have created formal rotation time for medical students to spend time in an abortion clinic, either within the primary teaching hospital or in a partner clinic, side by side with the graduate medical education learners [47]. (For more details about Ryan Programs, see chapters throughout this book, especially Chapters 3 and 9.)

14.6 Conclusion

While abortion is a critical component of primary sexual and reproductive health care worldwide, the literature suggests that it is not routinely included in medical schools globally. Governmental bodies and professional organizations should adopt the WFME standards and articulate specific content, learning objectives and competencies in abortion care. Given the charge of undergraduate medical education – to train physicians who are socially accountable and prepared to meet the needs of people in their community – and the importance of safe abortion as a component of primary sexual and reproductive health, topics for medical school education should include the laws in local settings, the public health framework of abortion, how women can safely access care (including counseling and referral), provision of safe abortion services and the management of patients who experience the rare complications of safe abortions and the more common complications of unsafe abortions. Ensuring that all physicians are trained in these dimensions of abortion care will increase access to safe abortion and decrease morbidity and mortality related to unsafe abortion.

References

1. Haslegrave M, Olatunbosun O. Incorporating sexual and reproductive health care in the medical curriculum in developing countries. *Reprod Health Matters*. 2003; 11(21):49–58. doi:10.1016/s0968-8080(03)02177-3

2. Singh S, Remez L, Sedgh G, Kwok L, Onda T. *Abortion Worldwide 2017: Uneven Progress and Unequal Access*. Washington, DC: Guttmacher Institute; 2018.

3. Zane S, Creanga AA, Berg CJ, et al. Abortion-related mortality in the United States: 1998–2010. *Obstet Gynecol*. 2015;126(2):258–265. doi:10.1097/aog.0000000000000945

4. Ganatra B, Gerdts C, Rossier C, et al. Global, regional, and subregional classification of abortions by safety, 2010–14: estimates from a Bayesian hierarchical model. *Lancet*. 2017;390(10110):2372–2381. doi:10.1016/s0140-6736(17)31794-4

5. Singh S, Maddow-Zimet I. Facility-based treatment for medical complications resulting from unsafe pregnancy termination in the developing world, 2012: a review of evidence from 26 countries. *BJOG*. 2016; 123(9):1489–1498. doi:10.1111/1471-0528.13552

6. World Health Organization. *Preventing Unsafe Abortion: Evidence Brief*. Geneva: World Health Organization Department of Reproductive Health and Research.

7. Benagiano G, Pera A. Decreasing the need for abortion: challenges and constraints. *Int J Gynaecol Obstet*. 2000;70(1):35–48. doi:10.1016/s0020-7292(00)00228-9

8. Dickson-Tetteh K, Billings DL. Abortion care services provided by registered midwives in South Africa. *Int Perspect Sex Reprod Health*. 2002;28(3):144–150.

9. Stanhope K, Rochat R, Fink L, Richardson K, Brack C, Comeau D. Physician opinions concerning legal abortion in Bogota, Colombia. *Cult Health Sex*. 2017; 19(8):873–887. doi:10.1080/13691058.2016.1269365

10. World Health Organization. *Safe Abortion: Technical and Policy Guidance for Health Systems*. 2nd ed. Geneva: WHO; 2012. https://apps.who.int/iris/bitstream/handle/10665/70914/9789241548434_eng.pdf?sequence=1.

11. Shearer JC, Walker DG, Vlassoff M. Costs of post-abortion care in low- and middle-income countries. *Int J Gynaecol Obstet*. 2010;108(2):165–169. doi:10.1016/j.ijgo.2009.08.037

12. *WFME Global Standards for Quality Improvement: Basic Medical Education*. London: World Federation for Medical Education; 2015.

13. Frenk J, Chen L, Bhutta ZA, et al. Health professionals for a new century: transforming education to strengthen health systems in an interdependent world. *Lancet*. 2010;376(9756):1923–1958. doi:10.1016/s0140-6736(10)61854-5

14. Mihciokur S, Akin A, Dogan BG, Ozvaris SB. The unmet need for safe abortion in Turkey: a role for medical abortion and training of medical students. *Reprod*

Health Matters. 2015;**22**(44 Suppl 1):26–35. doi:10.1016/s0968-8080(14)43790-x

15. O'Grady K, Doran K, O'Tuathaigh CM. Attitudes towards abortion in graduate and non-graduate entrants to medical school in Ireland. *J Fam Plann Reprod Health Care.* 2016;**42**(3):201–207. doi:10.1136/jfprhc-2015-101244

16. Provenzano-Castro B, Oizerovich S, Stray-Pedersen B. Future healthcare professionals' knowledge about the Argentinean abortion law. *Int J Med Educ.* 2016;**7**:95–101. doi:10.5116/ijme.56e0.74be

17. Al-Amoudi SM, Al-Harbi AA, Al-Sayegh NY, et al. Health rights knowledge among medical school students at King Abdulaziz University, Jeddah, Saudi Arabia. *PLoS One.* 2017;**12**(5):e0176714. doi:10.1371/journal.pone.0176714

18. Sjostrom S, Essen B, Gemzell-Danielsson K, Klingberg-Allvin M. Medical students are afraid to include abortion in their future practices: in-depth interviews in Maharastra, India. *BMC Med Educ.* 2016;**16**:8. doi:10.1186/s12909-016-0532-5

19. Luleci NE, Kaya E, Aslan E, Senkal ES, Cicek ZN. Marmara University medical students' perception on sexual violence against women and induced abortion in Turkey. *Balkan Med J.* 2016;**33**(2):173–180. doi:10.5152/balkanmedj.2015.15230

20. Medeiros RDd, Azevedo GDd, Oliveira EAAd, et al. Opinião de estudantes dos cursos de Direito e Medicina da Universidade Federal do Rio Grande do Norte sobre o aborto no Brasil. *Revista Brasileira de Ginecologia e Obstetrícia.* 2012;34:16–21.

21. Kumar R, Malik S, Qureshi A, et al. Comparative analysis of knowledge, attitudes and perceptions about induced abortions among medical and non-medical students of Karachi. *J Pak Med Assoc.* 2002;**52**(10):492–494.

22. Tocce K, Sheeder J, Vontver L. Failure to achieve the association of professors in gynecology and obstetrics objectives for abortion in third-year medical student curriculum. *J Reprod Med.* 2011;**56**(11–12):474–478.

23. Cessford TA, Norman WV. Making a case for abortion curriculum reform: a knowledge-assessment survey of undergraduate medical students. *J Obstet Gynaecol Can.* 2011;**33**(6):580. doi:10.1016/s1701-2163(16)34905-2

24. Fernandes KG, Camargo RP, Duarte GA, et al. Knowledge of medical abortion among Brazilian medical students. *Int J Gynaecol Obstet.* 2012;**118**(Suppl 1):S10–S14. doi:10.1016/j.ijgo.2012.05.004

25. Fayers T, Crowley T, Jenkins JM, Cahill DJ. Medical student awareness of sexual health is poor. *Int J STD AIDS.* 2003;**14**(6):386–389. doi:10.1258/095646203765371268

26. Veazey K, Nieuwoudt C, Gavito C, Tocce K. Student perceptions of reproductive health education in US medical schools: a qualitative analysis of students taking family planning electives. *Med Educ Online.* 2015;**20**:28973. doi:10.3402/meo.v20.28973

27. Smith KG, Gilliam ML, Leboeuf M, Neustadt A, Stulberg D. Perceived benefits and barriers to family planning education among third year medical students. *Med Educ Online.* 2008;**13**:4. doi:10.3885/meo.2008.Res00250

28. Hogmark S, Klingberg-Allvin M, Gemzell-Danielsson K, Ohlsson H, Essen B. Medical students' knowledge, attitudes and perceptions towards contraceptive use and counselling: a cross-sectional survey in Maharashtra, India. *BMJ Open.* 2013;**3**(12):e003739. doi:10.1136/bmjopen-2013-003739

29. Suphanchaimat R, Boonthai N, Tangthasana S, Putthasri W, Tangcharoensathien V, Chaturachinda K. A survey of manual vacuum aspiration's experiences among the new medical graduates in Thailand. *Reprod Health.* 2013;**10**:49. doi:10.1186/1742-4755-10-49

30. Espey E, Ogburn T, Chavez A, Qualls C, Leyba M. Abortion education in medical schools: a national survey. *Am J Obstet Gynecol.* 2005;**192**(2):640–643. doi:10.1016/j.ajog.2004.09.013

31. Steinauer J, LaRochelle F, Rowh M, Backus L, Sandahl Y, Foster A. First impressions: what are preclinical medical students in the US and Canada learning about sexual and reproductive health? *Contraception.* 2009;**80**(1):74–80. doi:10.1016/j.contraception.2008.12.015

32. Tey NP, Yew SY, Low WY, et al. Medical students' attitudes toward abortion education: Malaysian perspective. *PLoS One.* 2012;**7**(12):e52116. doi:10.1371/journal.pone.0052116

33. Biggs MA, Casas L, Ramm A, Baba CF, Correa SV, Grossman D. Future health providers' willingness to provide abortion services following decriminalisation of abortion in Chile: a cross-sectional survey. *BMJ Open.* 2019;**9**(10):e030797. doi:10.1136/bmjopen-2019-030797

34. Fitzgerald JM, Krause KE, Yermak D, et al. The first survey of attitudes of medical students in Ireland towards termination of pregnancy. *J Med Ethics.* 2014;**40**(10):710–713. doi:10.1136/medethics-2013-101608

35. Joffe C. The crisis in abortion provision and pro-choice medical activism in the 1990s. In *Abortion Wars: A Half Century of Struggle, 1950–2000.* Berkeley: University of California Press; 1998:320–334.

36. Evans ML, Backus LV. Medical students for choice: creating tomorrow's abortion providers. *Contraception.* 2011;**83** (5):391–393. doi:10.1016/j. contraception.2011.01.019

37. O'Shea M. Education in abortion care in Ireland: Medical Students for Choice (MSFC) taking a lead. *TSMJ.* 2017;**35**(41).

38. Espey E, Ogburn T, Leeman L, Nguyen T, Gill G. Abortion education in the medical curriculum: a survey of student attitudes. *Contraception.* 2008;77(3):205–208. doi:10.1016/j. contraception.2007.11.011

39. Steele R. Medical students' attitudes to abortion: a comparison between Queen's University Belfast and the University of Oslo. *J Med*

Ethics. 2009;**35**(6):390–394. doi:10.1136/jme.2008.026344

40. Guiahi M, Maguire K, Ripp ZT, Goodman RW, Kenton K. Perceptions of family planning and abortion education at a faith-based medical school. *Contraception.* 2011;**84** (5):520–524. doi:10.1016/j. contraception.2011.03.003

41. Burton R. UK medical students should be taught how to manage unwanted pregnancy. *BMJ.* 2018;**362**:k3800. doi:10.1136/bmj.k3800

42. *Undergraduate Training in O&G.* London: Royal College of Obstetricians & Gynaecologists; 2020. rcog.org. uk/en/careers-training/ specialty-training-curriculum/ undergraduate-training-in-og/

43. APGO. *APGO Medical Student Educational Objectives.* 2019. https://cdn.ymaws.com/apgo .site-ym.com/resource/resmgr/ apgo-11th-ed-mso-book.pdf

44. Obeso V, Brown D, Aiyer M, et al. (Eds.). *Core Entrustable Professional Activities for*

Entering Residency; Toolkits for the 13 Core EPAs. Washington, DC: Association of American Medical Colleges; 2017.

45. Gonzalez Velez AC. "The health exception": a means of expanding access to legal abortion. *Reprod Health Matters.* 2012;**20**(40):22–29. doi:10.1016/s0968-8080(12) 40668-1

46. ABIM Foundation, ACP-ASIM Foundation, European Federation of Internal Medicine. Medical professionalism in the new millennium: a physician charter. *Ann Intern Med.* 2002;**136**(3):243–246. doi:10.7326/0003-4819-136-3- 200202050-00012

47. Pomerantz T, Turk J, Simonson K, Steinauer J, Landy U. Integrated training for residents in family planning and abortion – do medical students benefit? Involvement in Ryan Residency Program Family Planning and Abortion Training. Poster presentation. 2014.

15

Integrating Sexual and Reproductive Health-Care Training into Family Medicine

Emily M. Godfrey and Christine Dehlendorf

15.1 Background

Family medicine physicians have the highest number of office visits of any medical specialty in the USA, with more than 200 million annually [1]. During these visits, family physicians deliver a broad range of acute, chronic and preventive medical services for patients across all ages and genders, including gynecological, obstetrical and other reproductive health services. This includes contraceptive care, as indicated by the National Ambulatory Medical Care Survey, which found that family planning provision is one of the top health services provided by family physicians to women aged 15–44 years [1]. Evidence suggests that close to 70% of female patients aged 18–44 years seen by family physicians have two or more chronic medical or mental health conditions, making family medicine physicians critical players in providing the family planning services to medically complex patients of reproductive age. Family physicians also provide abortion services, with a recent nationally representative survey of ambulatory care centers, physician offices and hospital-based clinics finding that family physicians make up 20% of clinicians providing first-trimester abortion services and 10% of those providing second-trimester services [2]. The National Academies of Sciences, Engineering, and Medicine recently issued evidence-based guidelines for the safety and quality of abortion care in the USA, noting family medicine physicians routinely provide safe and effective medication and aspiration abortions [3].

Unique aspects of family medicine training make the specialty particularly well-situated to contribute to meeting patients' family planning needs. First, family medicine residency training focuses on providing integrated, full-person care, including preventive health services, and uses a continuity of care model. Family medicine training also emphasizes the need to consider patients' overall health and social context when providing care. These aspects of family medicine care means that the reproductive health services provided by family medicine providers can be integrated with knowledge gained from the continuity of care across the life course about an individual's medical and social situation [4]. In fact, studies have shown that many patients would prefer to have their abortion performed by their own family physician within their primary care medical home and are highly satisfied with their care when early abortion is provided in this setting [5,6].

Further, the practice of family medicine is guided by principles related to giving access for persons of any and all backgrounds regardless of life circumstances. This makes family physicians important players in meeting the unmet need for family planning services in the USA [7]. Family medicine clinics and physicians are often the only source of care in rural and underserved areas. For example, the physician workforce in Community Health Centers, which provide basic health services to 28 million mostly lower income and rural people throughout the USA, is composed of 46% family physicians and only 10% obstetrician-gynecologists [8]. This is particularly important, given that most abortion services are concentrated in cities and almost 90% of counties in the USA lack an abortion provider [9]. Family medicine has also contributed to abortion service access through its role in the availability of medication abortion, including many of the early research studies that led to the US Food and Drug Administration (FDA) approval of mifepristone in 2000 and to US FDA labeling changes since its approval. For example, in academic departments of family medicine, researchers authored key studies that helped increase the gestational age limits from 49 to 63 days' gestation, shortened the interval between taking mifepristone and misoprostol, promoted the home use of miso-prostol and simplified follow-up visits after medication abortion [10].

The unique contribution of family physicians to family planning services, and particularly abortion – based on their broad knowledge of their patients and their families, as well as their commitment to providing care needed by their patients – is illustrated by the story of Dr. George Tiller. Dr. Tiller, a family physician, was, for much of his career before his assassination in 2009, one of only three US physicians providing abortions as late as the early third trimester. Dr. Tiller's entry into and lifelong dedication to providing safe abortion care was rather coincidental. With his eye set on being a dermatologist, Dr. Tiller took over his father's family medicine practice after his father's untimely death in an airplane accident in 1970. To Dr. Tiller's surprise, patients approached him asking if he was going to provide abortions like his father had done (his father began doing so only after having turned away a pregnant patient who later sought an illegal abortion and died). This need expressed by his patients led to a career in which Dr. Tiller committed himself to meeting women's needs for abortion care, an embodiment of the commitment of family physicians being willing to care for any type of problem or assure care is provided by an appropriate source.

As new legal restrictions to accessing contraceptive and abortion care flourish, and attempts to suppress pregnancy options counseling increase throughout the USA, family physicians have the potential to play an even more crucial role in providing comprehensive and compassionate patient-centered reproductive health care within their own primary care practices. In this chapter, we discuss the landscape of training for family physicians in contraception and abortion, including unique components of this training. We note that as the practice of contraceptive and abortion care does not change according to the specialty or discipline of the practitioner, other content in this volume is also relevant to the training of those in family medicine. We particularly call attention to the following chapters as having content that is relevant to the training of family physicians in contraception and abortion:

– Academic family planning and sexual and reproductive health collaborations: training

and advocacy with community partners (Chapter 12)
– Creating and implementing a curriculum for reproductive and sexual health training programs (Chapter 18)
– The benefits of and strategies for supporting residents' partial participation in abortion training (Chapter 23)
– Assessing competence in family planning skills through milestones (Chapter 19)

15.2 Family Medicine Contraception and Abortion Training Programs

The Accreditation Council for Graduate Medical Education (ACGME) requires that family medicine residents have either 100 hours or 125 patient encounters in gynecological care, which should include family planning, miscarriage management, contraceptive services and options counseling for unplanned pregnancy. The American Academy of Family Physicians (AAFP) has more specific, competency-based guidelines, which include training to care for people who are pregnant, to provide comprehensive contraceptive method counseling and pregnancy options counseling, to evaluate gestational age and to perform women's health office-based procedures such as endometrial biopsy, subdermal and intrauterine contraceptive device insertions and removals. Further, the Society of Teachers of Family Medicine Group on Hospital and Procedural Training issued a consensus statement that during residency, every family medicine resident should be exposed and given the opportunity to train to competence for independent provision of first-trimester aspiration abortion [11].

Fewer than 40 of the 471 accredited family medicine residency programs in the USA, however, specifically offer integrated, "opt-out" contraception and abortion training. These opt-out programs share similar components, including didactics and clinical training in contraception and options counseling skills, medication abortion, miscarriage management, and procedural training in long-acting contraceptive method placement, early pregnancy ultrasound and first-trimester uterine aspiration. Resident training typically occurs within a gynecology or procedural rotation over a period of 1 to 3 months with a

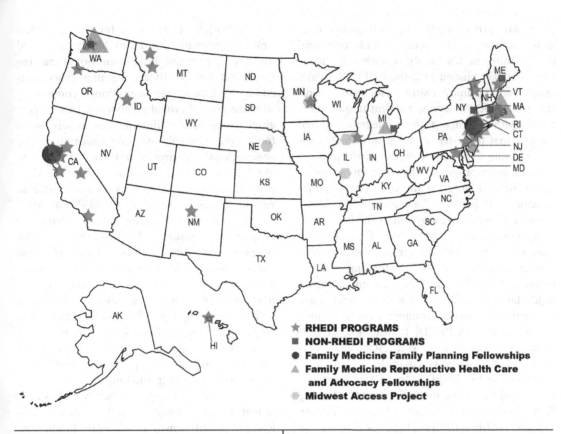

Figure 15.1 Selected family medicine residency and fellowship programs offering abortion training in the USA

Residency Training Programs

★ **RHEDI PROGRAMS**
Pawtucket, RI
Lewiston, ME
Martinez, CA
Boise, ID
Kalispell and Missoula, MT
Seattle, WA
Bronx, NY
New York, NY
Salinas, CA
Portland, OR
New Brunswick, NJ
Santa Rosa, CA
Sacramento, CA
Boston, MA
Sacramento, CA
Irvine, CA
San Francisco, CA
Fresno, CA
Mililani, HI
Chicago, IL
Baltimore, MD

Minneapolis, MN
Albuquerque, NM
Philadelphia, PA
Burlington and Milton, VT

■ **NON-RHEDI Training Sites**
Albany, NY
Detroit, MI
Vallejo, CA
Augusta, ME
Worcester, MA
Seattle, WA

● **Midwest Access Project**
Chicago, IL
Minneapolis, MN
Eastern Nebraska
Aurora, IL
Granite City, IL

Post-residency Training Programs

● **Family Medicine Family Planning Fellowships**
San Francisco, CA
New York City, NY

▲ **Family Medicine Reproductive Health Care and Advocacy Fellowships**
New York City, NY
Boston, MA
Seattle, WA
Rutgers, NJ
Ann Arbor, MI

Midwest Access Project
(refer to the "Residency Training Programs" section)

total of 2 to 8 days of training during the 3-year residency [12]. Trainers are usually family physicians, but can also include obstetrician-gynecologists, adolescent health pediatricians and physician assistants. Many of these programs adjust their training based on the learner's goals, beliefs and desired level of involvement [13] (Figure 15.1).

The Reproductive Health Education in Family Medicine (RHEDI) Program is the most prominent program offering high-quality integrated, comprehensive abortion and contraception training in US family medicine residency programs. Established in 2004, RHEDI provides funding and technical assistance for family medicine residencies to develop resident training programs, with the intent to fully integrate required opt-out first-trimester abortion and contraception training into the three-year curriculum. At each residency program, a faculty member serves as the RHEDI program director. The program director is responsible for generating a family planning primary care curriculum and is involved with direct clinical supervision of trainees. To date, there are twenty-six family medicine residencies that received RHEDI funding and are considered RHEDI sites. There are an additional eight family medicine residencies that have incorporated abortion training into their programs but are not RHEDI funded, and an additional two residencies with established local training opportunities (rhedi.org).

Several of the RHEDI sites in San Francisco, Seattle and New York also include the Continuing Reproductive Education for Advanced Training Efficacy (CREATE) program, which is an advanced training program for family medicine residents who have already completed the basic training in abortion (www.teachtraining.org). CREATE consists of three fundamental components: participation in at least four advanced clinical training sessions at high-volume clinics; participation in evening workshops focusing on essential skills for becoming a reproductive health provider and advocate; and completion of an independent reproductive health project with faculty mentorship. Through this additional clinical exposure, CREATE residents also gain more hands-on experience and competence with long-acting reversible contraceptive methods. The yearlong CREATE program includes instruction in early abortion complication cases, advocacy training and negotiation skills aimed at overcoming integration of abortion care within family medicine clinics post-residency graduation. The CREATE participants who pursue independent projects contribute to ongoing efforts related to education, quality improvement or advocacy.

There are additional training programs that support an opt-in option for family medicine residents whose programs do not integrate abortion training. Established in 2007, the Midwest Access Project (MAP) has an Individual Clinical Training program that trains highly motivated individuals who can leave their home training institution for short-term learning experiences and then return to their institution or community with the goal of providing abortion care in geographic areas of need. Rotations are usually two to four weeks in length and offer hands-on and/or observational experiences; trainees can return to MAP for additional rotations as desired. MAP pairs trainees with trainers, who are located in various places throughout the Midwest. MAP is responsible for ensuring trainees have the appropriate licensure, liability insurance, health screening and education to be in family planning training settings. MAP maintains formal agreements with trainers and, where needed, with the trainees' home training institutions. MAP works with trainers to optimize the trainees' experiences, assists with giving feedback to trainees and helps them progress to the next level of becoming independent reproductive health providers (midwestaccessproject.org).

Post-residency fellowship training offers additional clinical training for family medicine physicians in comprehensive reproductive health care, as well as training related to research, teaching and advocacy. The Fellowship in Family Planning (FFP), which is also available to obstetrician-gynecologists, has two programs housed in family medicine departments, the University of California, San Francisco (UCSF) and Albert Einstein College of Medicine. The overall goal of the FFP is to develop leaders in clinical care, science, education and advocacy to ensure all people have access to the abortion and contraception they want and need. The family medicine FFP programs specifically focus on that goal within the primary care setting, in addition to focusing on raising the profile of family planning within family medicine and bringing a family medicine perspective to the family planning community. The FFP is a two-year post-residency academic fellowship program that provides advanced longitudinal training in research, teaching and clinical practice of abortion and contraception. FFP fellows receive training in clinical family planning and family planning educational methods, and complete an independent research project. In addition, FFP fellows are also expected to partially train in a global or domestic low-resource setting and acquire advocacy skills.

Additionally, the Reproductive Health Care and Advocacy Fellowship is a separate fellowship through the Reproductive Health Access Project (RHAP) (www.reproductiveaccessorg). The RHAP fellowship is a one-year post-residency intensive clinical training program to train family physicians to provide, teach and lead the integration of abortion into primary care. The curriculum entails didactic topics that cover evidence-based contraceptive and abortion care, trauma-informed gynecological exam, early pregnancy complications, common gynecological complaints and reproductive justice and advocacy. Fellows teach residents and students how to perform abortion procedures in the clinical setting, as well as in simulation trainings at their institutions and at regional and national conferences. Fellows are expected to create a resolution for the AAFP and participate in advocacy leadership training. Another post-residency training program for family medicine, called Training in Early Abortion for Comprehensive Healthcare (TEACH) Leadership Fellowship is offered through UCSF. It is a one-year fellowship focused on developing primary care leadership, advocacy skills, teaching and research capacity. It assists with advanced clinical practice in early abortion and comprehensive reproductive and sexual health care (www.teachtraining.org). Some family medicine departments are incorporating comprehensive contraception and early abortion training into their obstetrical, women's health or faculty development fellowship programs, but these opportunities are not widely publicized.

For family physicians who are either in training or have completed their training, RHAP offers a network of more than 2,500 family physicians throughout the USA who wish to expand access to abortion services in their clinical and teaching settings. The network has local "Clusters" for networking, peer-to-peer support, training, advocacy and leadership development. RHAP also has training opportunities and technical support for practicing family physicians to incorporate comprehensive contraceptive care, miscarriage management or abortion services into their practices (www.reproductiveaccess.org) (Figure 15.2).

15.3 Challenges and Opportunities with Contraception and Abortion Training in Family Medicine

Training family medicine physicians specifically in contraception and abortion has unique characteristics, as well as some challenges, related to the context and structure of family medicine residency programs. One consideration in the procedural training of family physicians should be whether the program offers the opportunity to provide abortion training in the primary care

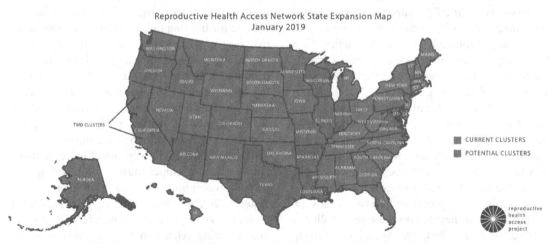

Figure 15.2 Map describing US network of family physicians who wish to expand abortion services, indicating local clusters

context. Training family physicians to provide at least medication abortion, and ideally also uterine aspiration abortion, within the primary care context is recognized as an effective strategy to enhance access to services. This is especially beneficial in remote rural areas with less access to health-care providers. Providing this training in the primary care setting also can help to normalize abortion care. This integration is feasible, given the simplicity of early abortion services, and its similarity to other reproductive health services, such as endometrial biopsies, which are commonly provided in the primary care setting. Providing abortion care in this context requires a different model of care than that in high-volume, specialized abortion settings, with attention given to different workflows and availability of support staff. This training prepares family physicians to provide abortion care in primary care settings and meet the reproductive health needs of their patients who prefer to receive abortion care in this setting.

Unfortunately, many family medicine primary care practices do not currently provide abortion services. That makes it even more important that training programs prepare family medicine trainees in the necessary practice management skills, so they in turn acquire the ability to initiate training and new services within family medicine practices. One example of how family medicine training programs have addressed this need includes having a teaching session that includes review of an "Office Practice Integration" chapter in a widely used family medicine abortion workbook [14]. In addition, some training programs, such as CREATE and RHAP have incorporated components specifically related to practice change into their curricula, with sessions related to developing negotiation skills and practice. This helps prepare trainees to be successful at advocating for integrating abortion training in their practice settings following graduation.

The inclusion of training in primary care settings has also provided the motivation to develop new, simplified approaches to delivering abortion care that better match the services and technologies in non-specialty contexts. This includes the development and use of protocols for identifying patients who are appropriate to have medication abortion without having an ultrasound or Rhesus (Rh) factor testing first, and by doing follow-up using serum human chorionic gonadotropin

(hCG) testing or low-sensitivity urine pregnancy testing, as opposed to ultrasound [15,16]. By providing this training in this way, family medicine programs enhance the flexibility of trainees to provide care in diverse settings.

The emphasis of family medicine training on patient-centered care also provides opportunities to integrate patient-centered counseling into family planning care. Family medicine researchers have led the movement toward an increasingly patient-centered, nonjudgmental approach to counseling in this area, in which trainees learn how to inquire about the patient's needs and preferences regarding pregnancy prevention and contraceptive options [17,18]. This is especially important for family physicians who, compared to those in other medical specialties, are more likely to provide care within clinics that serve low-income and/or racially/ethnically diverse communities, where patients may feel vulnerable to their community's long-standing history with reproductive coercion and abuse.

A significant challenge to providing comprehensive reproductive health-care training for family physicians includes the fact that many training programs are not able to provide abortions on-site due to religious or other policy restrictions. Even when abortion provision is present in primary care training sites, it is often necessary to augment this exposure with additional training in high-volume family planning clinics. As a result, family medicine programs are more likely to become reliant on off-site training in high-volume clinics, compared to similarly situated obstetrics and gynecology programs. While this is most likely to be an issue for abortion training, there may also be inadequate volume for training to competency for contraceptive care overall. This is particularly related to procedural training of subdermal implant and intrauterine device (IUD) insertion and removal, in which research suggests the number of IUD insertions performed during residency correlates with likelihood of providing IUDs once in practice [19]. The need to orchestrate off-site training can also create barriers as unaffiliated, outside family planning clinics must be both willing and able to incorporate trainees into their clinical systems [20]. Residency training programs must therefore take a proactive approach to identifying and fostering relationships with these sites. To make these collaborations work, it is important that the high-volume family planning clinics near the family medicine residency programs recognize that helping to train family physicians to provide abortion or contraceptive care enhances the shared mission of meeting patient's reproductive health needs, and at the same time helps to maintain their own pipeline of future providers.

An additional contextual factor for consideration when training family physicians in abortion care, as compared to obstetrician-gynecologists, is the fact that family doctors generally do not have the same surgical experience as it relates to intrauterine procedures. Focusing attention to the basics of anatomy and procedural skills at the outset of training can help to ensure that family physician trainees acquire the necessary foundation to provide skilled abortion care and procedural skills related to IUD insertion. The fact that family physicians have less surgical training can also be a factor when developing training in managing complications. Given the safety of aspiration and medication abortion and the resulting infrequency in which complications occur [3], many family physician trainees may not have observed or experienced complications such as perforation or hemorrhage at the point in their training when they have achieved procedural competency. Innovative approaches to training around complication management, including the use of simulations (Chapter 22) and case studies, can help to ensure that family physicians are equipped to manage complications on the rare occasions when they do occur.

15.4 Establishing Family Medicine Training Programs

Given the distinct context in which family medicine training programs are implemented, establishing these programs requires attention to barriers to and facilitators of their implementation. The literature on this topic highlights the importance of having support from stakeholders both inside and outside the residency program [20]. Obstetrician-gynecologist colleagues are particularly influential in serving as facilitators of successful programs. Unfortunately, sometimes they have also been a barrier to this process. Dedicating limited resources to faculty time and, in some cases, making payments to outside high-volume training sites have been observed as prominent barriers. Even programs that have worked hard to establish training within residency clinics themselves have found logistical and operational barriers, such as issues related to billing and hospital regulations. Lack of support from clinical, administrative and support staff; difficulty in obtaining equipment and supplies; difficulty in scheduling patients; interference with clinic flow; scope of practice limitations; and challenges in reimbursement for services have also been noted to be issues when establishing new, on-site abortion services [20]. Successful approaches to overcoming these barriers have included stepwise procedures in which integration of medication abortion was followed by the introduction of manual vacuum aspiration. The use of surveys to elicit concerns from staff and other stakeholders followed by educational forums were also effective in addressing these issues [20].

Other models of training include assistance from change agents to implement new clinical services at multiple organizational levels in order to accelerate the uptake of care offered to patients. Upstream USA (www.upstream.org) is an example of a change agent that has trained practicing family medicine physicians and other providers who already provide clinical services within a larger health-care clinic or system. Their implementation process entails a one-day simulation training for clinicians as well as didactic teaching for administrators and staff, followed by post-training, data-driven quality-improvement activities.

Overall, previous experiences with establishing these training programs underscore the need for intentional approaches to overcoming commonly encountered barriers, a focus on stakeholder engagement, and ensuring adequate resources to support the new training initiative. In addition, developing and leveraging relationships with obstetrician-gynecologist colleagues can be key to the success of these programs. While some family physicians and obstetrician-gynecologists may experience tension related to the overlapping scope of their practices, by focusing on the shared interests in meeting women's reproductive health needs, they can help to foster positive collaborations together that enhance the training and practice of both specialties [21].

15.5 Impact of Family Medicine Training Programs

Although initiating family planning training programs can be challenging, the benefits these programs offer to resident education and experience is substantial. In fact, most family medicine residents who are trained in family planning services report an intention to provide these services in their future practice [22] (Figure 15.3).

A substantial proportion of residents who had the opportunity to participate in comprehensive reproductive health training provided a variety of reproductive health services, including, in one study, 72% providing IUDs, 52% miscarriage management and 27% abortions [23]. These proportions are substantially higher than for residents from the same programs who did not participate in the training and for family physicians overall. Trainees reported an array of other benefits of training, including improved knowledge about and technical skills related to providing reproductive health services. They also reported improved comfort caring for women with an unwanted pregnancy, including patient-centered counseling, options counseling, active listening, support related to obtaining an abortion and improved knowledge of system-based practice [25,24]. Residents also reported that learning how to provide abortion services was a valuable contribution to their overall ability to provide continuity of care across the life course, consistent with family medicine values. While most of this literature has historically focused on programs that include abortion training as part of comprehensive reproductive health training, a recent initiative described the results of a training initiative created specifically for management of early pregnancy loss [26]. Evaluation of this initiative revealed that engagement in the training was associated with improved knowledge and attitudes about management of early pregnancy loss, as well as an increase of 43% in the proportion of family physicians providing uterine aspiration for miscarriage management in their regular practice.

15.6 Fulfilling Family Medicine's Potential

Training in contraception and abortion care in family medicine training programs has increased over the past two decades, yet the vast majority of

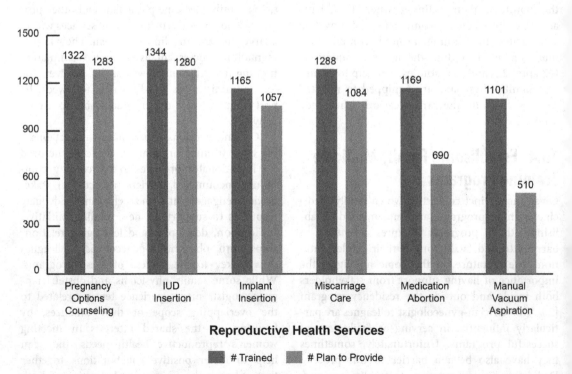

Figure 15.3 Family medicine residents trained and planning to provide reproductive health care in their future practice, 2008–2018 (n=1,417)

residency programs do not currently provide an integrated approach to contraception and abortion training. Lack of training in this essential area prevents family physicians from fulfilling the specifically stated goal of their specialty to provide integrated care across the life course. One barrier to expanding this training is that about 30% of the family medicine program directors polled think that family medicine residencies should not include first-trimester abortion training, although most (56%) agree that first-trimester abortion is within the scope of family medicine [25]. In addition, lack of experience among family medicine educators is a barrier, as one survey of this group identified an overall lack of experience in abortion care and comprehensive management of early pregnancy failure [27]. Therefore, to be effective, efforts to expand abortion and contraceptive training in family medicine require an intentional approach that emphasizes the importance of providing this training among family medicine educators. Family medicine educators who wish to enhance their skills can connect with any of the organizations mentioned earlier in this chapter, with the most relevant resource being RHAP's Reproductive Health Access Network, which connects primary care clinicians in their own communities.

Quality family planning training in family medicine residency programs is paramount, and care needs to be taken to ensure teaching is evidence based. A recent review of family medicine textbooks identified critical deficiencies in reproductive health content, including having inaccurate information about IUDs and their use, and a failure to include adequate information about early abortion methods and management of early pregnancy failure [28]. Incorporating evidence-based guidelines such as the *US Medical Eligibility Criteria (US MEC) for Contraceptive Use* from the Centers for Disease Control and Prevention into family medicine training programs can help overcome these deficiencies and ensure that the best available evidence is highlighted within each program. As discussed, collaboration with obstetrician-gynecologist colleagues can be of benefit when establishing this training. Family medicine residency faculty should also consider joining forces with advocates who work to improve access to primary care services within the larger health-care system, including supporters of point-of-care testing,

which would increase access to obstetrical ultrasounds in primary care, and single-payer national health insurance, which provides coverage for all medically necessary health-care services, including reproductive health care. Clinic-wide training models implemented by organizations like Upstream USA should also be considered to expand high-quality services and training in family medicine programs.

One powerful voice that can potentially enhance motivation to provide training in abortion and contraception is family medicine's professional organization, the AAFP. Other organizations, such as the American College of Obstetricians and Gynecologists (ACOG) and the American Academy of Pediatrics (AAP), have already published policy statements addressing the importance of the safety and efficacy of long-acting contraceptives and access to confidential, safe and legal abortion services for teens and women. If the AAFP were to follow the ACOG and AAP and provide its own policy statements related to contraceptive and abortion services, it would institutionalize and strengthen the recognition of the need to provide the highest level of training for comprehensive contraceptive and abortion training for all family physicians. Ultimately, widespread family planning training in family medicine residency programs would substantially improve reproductive health access and care for the communities and patients that family physicians serve.

External factors affecting abortion and contraception training in family medicine residencies – including the FDA's Risk Evaluation and Mitigation Strategies (REMS) for mifepristone and the location of residency programs within religious institutions, federally funded community centers and health clinics that accept federal Title X Family Planning funding – are also necessary to consider. REMS is a designation given by the FDA to certain medications with serious safety concerns to help ensure that benefits of the medication outweigh risks [29]. The US FDA REMS mandate for mifepristone requires health-care providers to register in a centralized database, and for their facility to store and dispense their own supply of mifepristone to patients. This can serve as a barrier to both training in family medicine residency programs and the provision of medication abortion by trained residency graduates. This requirement is unnecessary [30] and makes it impossible for a physician to write a prescription for the abortion pills for a patient to discretely fill the prescription. Instead, the pills are dispensed on site and many decision makers within a larger health-care system must agree that abortion services will be offered "on-site," even though the patient will actually pass the pregnancy outside the clinical setting. Such restrictions lead to misperceptions about the complexity and safety of medication abortion provision.

Perceptions that Federally Qualified Health Centers cannot offer abortion services provides another barrier. These centers are frequently the training sites for family medicine residencies in the USA because of the Teaching Health Center Graduate Medical Education program of the 2010 Affordable Care Act (ACA). The confusion exists because of the Hyde Amendment, which prohibits use of federal funds "to pay for any abortion or to cover any part of the costs of any health plan that includes coverage of abortion" except in cases of rape, incest or danger to the life of the pregnant woman. Although programs located within federally funded clinics can offer abortion services, provided the finances for this care are kept separate from other services provided in the clinic, mechanisms to accomplish this are not widely known. Abortion care in these settings is further complicated when family

medicine residency faculty are employed by the clinic, rather than the residency program, and have medical liability coverage under the federal tort insurance plan, which excludes malpractice coverage for abortion-related cases. Additional barriers for family physicians include working for residencies that reside within religiously affiliated clinics or Catholic-owned health-care facilities. As the ability to provide comprehensive reproductive health-care training in these institutions varies depending on the details of contracts and affiliation agreements, finding approaches to optimize training and care requires ongoing attention and advocacy.

15.7 Conclusion

Family medicine physicians in the USA have a critical role to play in ensuring that all patients have access to safe, patient-centered abortion and contraceptive care. This is particularly important, as the current political and regulatory climates increasingly limit access to family planning counseling and care. In light of the abundance of challenges facing family planning training today, achieving comprehensive, quality training in family medicine will require coordinated efforts by those in family medicine, as well as support from those in other specialties, and the greater family planning and abortion community alike.

References

1. Hsiao CJ, Cherry DK, Beatty PC, Rechtsteiner EA. National Ambulatory Medical Care Survey: 2007 summary. *Natl Health Stat Report.* 2010:(27) 1–32.

2. White KO, Jones HE, Lavelanet A, et al. First-trimester aspiration abortion practices: a survey of United States abortion providers. *Contraception.* 2019;**99**:10–15.

3. National Academies of Sciences, Engineering, and Medicine. The safety and quality of abortion care in the United States. http://nationalacademies.org. Accessed November 4, 2019.

4. Carek PJ, Anim T, Conry C, et al. Residency training in family medicine: a history of innovation and program support. *Fam Med.* 2017;**49**:275–281.

5. Rubin SE, Godfrey EM, Shapiro M, Gold M. Urban female patients' perceptions of the family medicine clinic as a site for abortion care. *Contraception.* 2009;**80**:174–179.

6. Wu JP, Godfrey EM, Prine L, Andersen KL, MacNaughton H, Gold M. Women's satisfaction with abortion care in academic family medicine centers. *Fam Med.* 2015;**47**:98–106.

7. Force T, Green L, Graham R, et al. Task Force 1. Report of the Task Force on Patient Expectations, Core Values, Reintegration, and the New Model of Family Medicine. *Ann Fam Med.* 2004;**2**:S33–S50.

8. National Association of Community Health Centers. *Community Health Center Chartbook.* www.nachc.org. Accessed November 4, 2019.

9. Jones RK, Jerman J. Abortion incidence and service availability, In the United States, 2014. *Perspect Sex Reprod Health.* 2017;**49**:17–27.

10. Schaff EA. Mifepristone: ten years later. *Contraception.* 2010;**81**:1–7.

11. Nothnagle M, Sicilia JM, Forman S, et al. Required procedural training in family medicine residency: a consensus statement. *Fam Med*. 2008;**40**(4):248–252.

12. Brahmi D, Dehlendorf C, Engel D, Grumbach K, Joffe C, Gold M. A descriptive analysis of abortion training in family medicine residency programs. *Fam Med*. 2007;**39**:399–403.

13. Nothnagle M. Benefits of a learner-centred abortion curriculum for family medicine residents. *J Fam Plann Reprod Health Care*. 2008;**34**:107–110.

14. Training in Early Abortion for Comprehensive Healthcare. *Early Abortion Training Workbook*. www.teachtraining.org. Accessed November 4, 2019.

15. Clark W, Panton T, Hann L, Gold M. Medication abortion employing routine sequential measurements of serum hCG and sonography only when indicated. *Contraception*. 2007;**75**:131–135.

16. Costescu D, Guilbert E, Bernardin J, et al. Medical abortion. *J Obstet Gynaecol Can*. 2016;**38**:366–389.

17. Dehlendorf C, Levy K, Kelley A, Grumbach K, Steinauer J. Women's preferences for contraceptive counseling and decision making. *Contraception*. 2013;**88**:250–256.

18. Carvajal DN, Gioia D, Mudafort ER, Brown PB, Barnet B. How can primary care physicians best support contraceptive decision making? a qualitative study exploring the perspectives of Baltimore Latinas. *Womens Health Issues*. 2017;**27**:158–166.

19. Rubin SE, Fletcher J, Stein T, Segall-Gutierrez P, Gold M. Determinants of intrauterine contraception provision among US family physicians: a national survey of knowledge, attitudes and practice. *Contraception*. 2011;**83**:472–478.

20. Dehlendorf C, Brahmi D, Engel D, Grumbach K, Joffe C, Gold M. Integrating abortion training into family medicine residency programs. *Fam Med*. 2007;**39**:337–342.

21. Steinauer J, Dehlendorf C, Grumbach K, Landy U, Darney P. Multi-specialty family planning training: collaborating to meet the needs of women. *Contraception*. 2012;**86**(3):188–190.

22. Romero D, Maldonado L, Fuentes L, Prine L. Association of reproductive health training on intention to provide services after residency: the family physician resident survey. *Fam Med*. 2015;**47**:22–30.

23. Goodman S, Shih G, Hawkins M, et al. A long-term evaluation of a required reproductive health training rotation with opt-out provisions for family medicine residents. *Fam Med*. 2013;**45**:180–186.

24. Kumar V, Herbitter C, Karasz A, Gold M. Being in the room: reflections on pregnancy options counseling during abortion training. *Fam Med*. 2010;**42**:41–46.

25. Herbitter C, Greenberg M, Fletcher J, Query C, Dalby J, Gold M. Family planning training in US family medicine residencies. *Fam Med*. 2011;**43**:574–581.

26. Darney BG, Weaver MR, Stevens N, Kimball J, Prager SW. The family medicine residency training initiative in miscarriage management: impact on practice in Washington State. *Fam Med*. 2013;**45**:102–108.

27. Herbitter C, Bennett A, Schubert FD, Bennett IM, Gold M. Management of Early Pregnancy Failure and Induced Abortion by Family Medicine Educators. *The Journal of the American Board of Family Medicine*. 2013;**26**(6):751–758.

28. Schubert FD, Akse S, Bennett AH, Glassman NR, Gold M. A review of contraception and abortion content in family medicine textbooks. *Fam Med*. 2015;**47**:524–528.

29. US Food and Drug Administration. Risk Evaluation and Mitigation Strategies | REMS. www.fda.gov/drugs/drug-safety-and-availability/risk-evaluation-and-mitigation-strategies-rems. Accessed November 4, 2019.

30. Raymond EG, Blanchard K, Blumenthal PD, et al. sixteen years of overregulation: time to unburden Mifeprex. *N Engl J Med*. 2017;**376**:790–794.

Chapter 1

Integrating Abortion Training into Advanced-Practice Clinician Programs

Katherine Simmonds, Amy Levi and Joyce Cappiello

16.1 Introduction

This book is focused on training specialist physicians to become clinical and advocacy leaders in family planning, but in most countries obstetrician-gynecologists (ob-gyns) are not the primary providers of abortion care. Many nations' laws require that abortions be done only by physicians. Everywhere, however, nurses are critical to abortion access. Even if they are not direct providers of abortion, they make referrals, organize the service and influence their health systems with regard to abortion.

In the USA, most states passed physician-only abortion laws that precluded nurse practitioners (NPs), certified nurse-midwives (CNMs) and physician assistants (PAs) from providing abortions. Mounting evidence has demonstrated that these advanced-practice clinicians (APCs) are safe and effective abortion providers, and patients are satisfied with their care. In recent years, several more states have enacted legislation and attorneys general have issued opinions allowing NPs, CNMs and PAs to do abortions. Nevertheless, currently they are not able to provide either uterine aspiration or medication abortion in most states. Advocates are working to remove obstacles to full practice authority for abortion by NPs, CNMs and PAs at the state and national levels. For those interested in providing abortion, obtaining education and training can also be difficult. Educational resources and other learning opportunities have been created, and new ones are emerging. This chapter describes the movement toward abortion care by non-physician advanced-practice clinicians in the USA.

16.2 A Brief History of Nurse Practitioners, Certified Nurse-Midwives and Physician Assistants in Abortion Care in the Twentieth Century

The Jane Collective in Chicago created the nation's first underground, organized abortion support system, an alternative to the largely illegal, unsafe and life-threatening options people resorted to before abortion became legal. Nurses and midwives participated in the Jane Collective, both helping connect those in need of abortions with trained physicians and learning to do abortions themselves [1]. Following the Supreme Court decision on *Roe v. Wade*, many states established criminal abortion laws that restricted abortion to physicians. Only six states (Arizona, Montana, New Hampshire, Oregon, Vermont and West Virginia) [2] did not enact such laws; however their absence has not meant that CNMs, NPs and PAs have been performing abortions. In some states, these clinicians were overtly trained to perform uterine aspiration abortions alongside their physician colleagues, while in others, they may have done abortions, but there is no record of their activity. Data on how many CNMs, NPs and PAs were actually trained or have provided abortion in those states since 1973 are not readily available; however, several studies carried out in Vermont in the 1980s and 1990s did establish that the rates of complications following first-trimester uterine aspiration abortion were comparable between PAs and physicians. [3].

While physician-only abortion laws were ostensibly established to protect women from inadequately trained or illicit abortionists, their intent was not to exclude CNMs, NPs and PAs – which were emergent professions in the USA at that time – from abortion care. However, in ensuing years, antiabortion forces have seized on these laws as an additional policy strategy for limiting access [4]. Nevertheless, in spite of a robust, mounting body of international and domestic evidence that demonstrates the safety, efficacy and acceptability of CNMs, NPs and PAs as providers of abortion, they are not legally able to deliver this service in most states at the time of this writing [5].

In 1975, the Institute of Medicine (now the National Academy of Medicine – see Chapter 4) released the first comprehensive report on the safety and quality of abortion care in the USA. While the report represented an important scientific evaluation of the practice of abortion, it did not recognize nurses and CNMs as providers, even though a CNM expert was on the committee that produced the report [6]. While the report did not state that abortion should only be accomplished by physicians, its only discussion of practice restrictions was focused on states that required a physician panel to certify an abortion was appropriate for a woman who was seeking one; it included no mention of physician-only abortion legislation.

By 1990, concerns about a looming shortage of abortion providers prompted the American College of Obstetricians and Gynecologists (ACOG) and the National Abortion Federation (NAF) to convene a meeting entitled: "Who Will Provide Abortions? Ensuring the Availability of Qualified Practitioners" [7] (see Chapter 4). Representatives from the American College of Nurse-Midwives (ACNM), the American Academy of Physician Assistants (AAPA), and the National Association of Nurse Practitioners in Reproductive Health (NANPRH, now Nurse Practitioners in Women's Health, NPWH) attended. One of the key recommendations from the symposium was that CNMs, NPs and PAs were a qualified, yet untapped sector of the health-care workforce that could help to address the abortion provider shortage. Soon after the gathering, the AAPA and NANPRH issued statements of support for the professions they represented in providing abortion, and the ACNM removed its prohibition on CNMs from performing abortions (Table 16.1). The American College of Obstetricians and Gynecologists also endorsed

the provision of abortion by "other licensed health professionals in collaborative settings."

Six years later, a second convening specifically to address "The Role of Physician Assistants, Nurse Practitioners, and Nurse-Midwives in Providing Abortions: Strategies for Expanding Abortion Access" was held [2]. The aim of that gathering was to further develop legislative and educational strategies to expand opportunities for these advanced-practice clinicians to become part of the abortion workforce. One outcome was the formation of Clinicians for Choice (now Clinicians in Abortion Care), a specialty organization under the umbrella of the National Abortion Federation that focuses on expanding the scope of practice of nurses, CNMs, NPs and PAs to include abortion care.

Although CNMs, NPs and PAs were performing uterine aspiration abortion in some sites around the country, the role started to become more widely recognized in 1999 when a PA litigated her right to provide abortions in Montana and won. [9]. In 2006, an NP in rural Oregon also asserted the legal right to provide uterine aspiration abortion in that state [9]. These developments were paralleled by growing international recognition of the key role of midwives and other licensed professionals in providing safe abortion care. In 2002, the International Confederation of Midwives (ICM) issued an official position statement on "Midwives' Provision of Abortion-Related Services," and subsequently updated their Essential Competencies for Basic Midwifery Practice that included competencies in abortion-related care services (reaffirmed in 2019) [10,11]. A number of other prominent domestic and international professional organizations have followed suit with endorsements of NPs, CNMs and PAs as providers of abortion (Table 16.1).

By 2009, growing interest among CNMs, NPs and PAs in incorporating abortion into clinical practice prompted the development of a guide (*Providing Abortion Care: A Professional Toolkit for Nurse-Midwives, Nurse Practitioners and Physician Assistants*) to help them prepare for and navigate challenges they were likely to encounter in this process [9]. The *Toolkit* featured detailed information and recommendations about how to document relevant clinical skills; investigate state practice regulations and abortion laws; build key professional relationships; and integrate abortion into clinical practice. In 2019, an

Table 16.1 Professional organizations' endorsement of advanced-practice registered nurses (APRNs) as abortion providers

American College of Nurse-Midwives (ACNM)	Midwives as Abortion Providers. 2018. www.midwife.org/default.aspx?bid=59&cat=3&button=Search
American College of Obstetricians and Gynecologists (ACOG)	ACOG: American College of Obstetricians and Gynecologists Committee on Health Care for Underserved Women (2017 reaffirmed). Committee Opinion No. 13: Increasing Access to Abortion 2014. www .acog.org /-/media/Committee-Opinions / Committee-on-Health-Care-for-Underserved-Women /co613 .pdf? dmc=1&ts =20171011T2045552523
American Public Health Association (APHA)	APHA: American Public Health Association (2011). Provision of Abortion Care by Advanced Practice Nurses and Physician Assistants. Policy Statement 20112. www.apha.org/policies-and-advocacy/public-health-policy-statements/policy-database/2014/07/28/16/00/provision-of-abortion-care-by-advanced-practice-nurses-and-physician-assistants
International Confederation of Midwives (ICN)	Midwives' Provision of Abortion-Related Services. 2008, 2014. www.internationalmidwives.org/our-work/policy-and-practice/icm-position-statements/
National Abortion Federation (NAF)	National Abortion Federation and Clinicians for Choice, 2017. Role of CNMs, NPs, and PAs in Abortion Care. 2017. https:// 5aa1b2xfmfh2e2mk03kk8rsx-wpengine .netdna-ssl.com/wp-content /uploads/CNM_NP _PA_org_statements.pdf
National Academies of Sciences, Engineering, and Medicine (NASEM)	National Academies of Sciences, Engineering, and Medicine. 2018. *The Safety and Quality of Abortion Care in the United States.* Washington, DC: The National Academies Press. doi:https://doi .org/10.17226/24950
Nurses for Sexual and Reproductive Health	Advanced Practice Clinicians in Abortion Care Acknowledged as Safe and Effective Providers. 2018. www.nsrh.org/news/6002516
National Association of Nurse Practitioners in Reproductive Health (NANPRH)	National Association of Nurse Practitioners in Reproductive Health (now National Association of Nurse Practitioners in Women's Health, NPWH). (1991). *Resolution on Nurse Practitioners as Abortion Providers*, October 1991. Washington, DC: NPWH, www.npwh.org
World Health Organization (WHO)	WHO (World Health Organization) (2012). *Safe Abortion: Technical and Policy Guidance for Health Systems.* Geneva: WHO. http://apps .who.int/iris/bitstream/handle/10665/70914/9789241548434_eng; jsessionid=68D043152B7571FDB95109E53A09956C?sequence=1

WHO (World Health Organization) (2015). Health worker roles in providing safe abortion care and post-abortion contraception. Geneva, Switzerland: WHO. http://apps.who.int/iris/bitstream/handle/10665/181043/WHO_RHR_15.15_eng.pdf?sequence=1 |

updated web-based version of the *Toolkit* was published that is relevant to all types of licensed providers who want to expand their practice to include abortion [12].

As of publication of this book, CNMs, NPs and PAs are legally able to provide medication abortion in fifteen US states [13] and uterine aspiration abortion in nine, and both types in the District of Columbia (J. Arons, personal communication, July 29, 2019). Several states have ongoing legal cases related to medication abortion, which is now well established as within the scope of practice of CNMs, NPs and PAs in states where they have prescriptive privileges. Telemedicine is another rapidly expanding approach for the delivery of medication abortion in which CNMs, NPs and PAs are extensively involved with great potential to further increase access, especially for rural populations. Finally, CNMs, NPs and PAs are at the forefront of conversations about how to support people's choices and preferences in abortion care, including as part of the growing international and national discussion about self-managed abortion and access to abortifacient medications through the internet. In some countries, Bangladesh and Nepal, for example, nurses are the primary providers of abortion in rural areas, and in most places they are responsible for referrals and advice to pregnant women, particularly regarding the expanding access to medication abortion.

16.3 Background on NP, CNM and PA Education and Scope of Practice

The scope of practice for NPs, CNMs and PAs in abortion care requires understanding of both the state laws enacted following the *Roe* decision and the variations in state legislation regarding the practice authority of each of these professions. Because the regulation of advanced-practice nursing is complex, this section focuses primarily on the education and regulation of advanced-practice registered nurses (APRNs), and only briefly discusses these aspects of PA practice, which are similar, but not identical.

In 2008, the National Council of State Boards of Nursing (NCSBN) recognized that differences in state regulations regarding scope of practice were limiting the portability of APRNs' practices. In response, the organization called for greater uniformity in state laws and regulations regarding advanced-practice nursing, which would in turn facilitate licensure across state lines [14]. While the NCSBN has an established mechanism (referred to as the "Nursing Licensure Compact") that enables registered nurses (RNs) to obtain a multistate license to practice in their state of residence as well as others without needing to apply for separate licenses, this mechanism only exists in three states at the advanced-practice level at this time [15].

In an effort to standardize licensure, accreditation, certification and education of nurses at the advanced-practice level across states, in 2008 the NCSBN in conjunction with a number of other major professional nursing organizations developed *The APRN Consensus Model*, which outlines requirements for practice at the advanced level. This model stipulates that registered nurses must complete an education program that prepares them for a specific role (nurse practitioner, nurse midwife, nurse anesthetist or clinical nurse specialist) and to care for a specific population (family/individual across the life span, adult/gerontology, neonatal, pediatrics, women's health/gender-related or psychiatric/mental health). Nurses choose their advanced educational program based on the role and population in which they plan to practice. In order to enter into practice, graduates must pass a national certification exam for each role they may assume and population they seek to serve [14].

While the NCSBN defines minimum educational requirements, individual state boards of nursing oversee their implementation. In addition, other professional nursing organizations, such as the National Organization of Nurse Practitioner Faculties (NONPF) and the American College of Nurse-Midwives (ACNM), also issue educational and clinical competencies specific to the role they represent and the populations they serve. APRN education programs use these as guides in developing their curricula. All ARPNs have the education to perform basic assessment skills (history taking, physical examination) and clinical management skills, including diagnostic reasoning, on which to build abortion specific skills.

The APRN Consensus Model also recommends a plan for licensure of APRNs as independent practitioners exclusively under the authority of nursing boards and without regulatory requirements for collaboration, direction or supervision from physicians or other health-care professionals. While a number of states have implemented this directive, many still require some level of physician oversight or collaboration for APRNs for a defined period of time or as long as they are licensed in the state [14].

With the NCSBN's mandate to move toward uniformity in state laws, at this time many states have embraced the model; others have not yet made changes to their regulatory language, or have not adopted all portions of the model. This is an ongoing focus of legislative activity at the state level for many APRN interest groups. Notably, the Department of Veterans Affairs (VA), which does not fall under the purview of state boards of nursing or medicine, amended its provider regulations to permit full practice authority to APRNs in three out of the four roles (all but nurse anesthetists) [16]. This allows APRNs in the VA to practice to the full extent of their education, training and certification regardless of state regulations, except with regard to those pertaining to prescription of controlled substances.

The scope of practice regulations for PAs differ from those of nursing. PA scope of practice is based on a formal course of education and is dictated by state laws and regulation; however, to a large extent, it is determined at the practice level in collaboration with collaborating physicians [17].

16.4 Laws and Regulations about Who Can Provide Abortion

While APRNs have succeeded in gaining full practice authority in many states, in the majority of states this does not extend to abortion. As mentioned earlier, most states passed physician-only abortion laws in the 1970s. Therefore, even in states where APRNs have full practice authority, these criminal laws supersede practice regulations, precluding any health-care provider other than a physician from performing an abortion. Only two states – California and Maine -- have passed subsequent legislation to expressly permit NPs, CNMs and PAs to provide abortion at the time of this publication. In several states (Illinois, Washington), attorneys general have recently issued opinions in support of the provision of abortion by NPs, CNMs and PAs; advocates in other states are pursuing similar as well as other legal strategies to expand scope of practice to include abortion. Such efforts can be challenging because of the politicization of abortion as well as professional tensions with organized medicine. Currently, APRNs are able to legally provide medication abortion in approximately 30% of states and uterine aspiration abortion in less than 10% [5].

Unlike the USA, most countries do not rely on local, sometimes contradictory, laws to govern professional practice. If national law permits abortion by APRNs, they may provide it

anywhere, and outside capital cities they are often the main sources of abortion care. This situation exists in nations like Ethiopia (Chapter 29) and Nepal (Chapter 27), where recognition of unsafe abortion as an important cause of maternal mortality led to legalization and inclusion of APRNs in abortion training programs (Chapter 2).

16.5 Safety, Efficacy and Acceptability of NPs, CNMs and PAs as Providers of Abortion

Substantial data from around the world, including the USA, demonstrate that with appropriate training CNMs, NPs and PAs can master the essential skills to provide medication and uterine aspiration abortions safely and effectively [18]. The Health Workforce Pilot Project (HWPP) was a six-year multisite prospective study sponsored by the Advancing New Standards in Reproductive Health (ANSIRH) program at the University of California, San Francisco Bixby Center. [19] The project trained a group of CNMs, NPs and PAs in California to perform uterine aspiration abortions, and evaluated their safety, effectiveness and acceptability to patients. Findings included that the risk of complications associated with the procedure were statistically equivalent whether it was performed by a physician, CNM, NP or PA. In addition, more than 9,000 patients who participated in the study completed a post-abortion survey about their experience, including timeliness of care and level of pain, and no statistical difference by provider type was detected in these outcomes [19].

16.6 Education and Training in Abortion Care for NPs, CNMs and PAs

In addition to the challenges posed by state laws and regulations, NPs, CNMs and PAs who want to provide abortion as part of their clinical practice often encounter obstacles to obtaining education and training. For many, this begins with pre-licensure and pre-certification educational programs, where didactic content and clinical learning opportunities in abortion care are limited or completely absent from the curricula [20,21]. Research detailing the abortion-related didactic and clinical offerings of CNM, NP and PA programs in the USA are limited. One of the few published studies on this subject found that among accredited CNM, NP and PA programs, only slightly more than half included didactic instruction in at least one abortion procedure (surgical aspiration, manual vacuum aspiration [MVA] or medication), and only 21% provided learners with clinical instruction on at least one of the three methods. CNM programs were the most likely to include didactic instruction about abortion in their curricula, but PA programs were more likely to include clinical instruction. Nevertheless, overall, only about one quarter of the responding PA programs offered students this learning opportunity [22]. More research is needed to describe the current state of abortion education in the USA across these professions, as this survey was conducted nearly twenty years ago, prior to the approval and commercial release of mifepristone, which has the potential to expand abortion provision. Some countries (eg, Bangladesh, Ethiopia, Nepal), in conjunction with legalization of abortion, integrated abortion-specific training for APRNs into their health service educational programs (so-called pre-service training). For most others, abortion training remains "in service" (ie, after beginning practice). Ideally, basic abortion skills are learned "pre-service" and are maintained and enhanced "in service" through continuing education programs. Nepal (Chapter 27) provides an example of integrating both into a national abortion training program for health professionals.

The post-graduate abortion training landscape for CNMs, NPs and PAs can also be bleak, as there are not established pathways for acquiring necessary skills and minimal professional support for those interested in becoming an abortion provider. The limited training spots that abortion-providing agencies can offer are often preferentially given to physician learners who face fewer regulatory barriers to implementing these skills. While some abortion-providing health-care agencies offer internal training and support for clinical staff to build the skills and knowledge necessary to provide abortion, for those not employed in such institutions, such opportunities are largely nonexistent.

Overcoming all of the educational, training, institutional, legal and regulatory barriers in order to become an abortion provider requires a high level of motivation and persistence. Nevertheless, there are exemplar institutions, organizations and individuals that have managed to implement education and training programs or acquire abortion training on their own. In this section, we highlight some of these.

16.6.1 Education Programs

Several education programs have been spotlighted for their inclusion of didactic content and/or offering of skills workshops in abortion care [12]. While anecdotal evidence and the experiences of the authors of this chapter suggest that such offerings are not the norm across APRN and PA education programs, they do provide models and suggest that there may be other APRN and PA faculty who include content about abortion in their courses in innovative ways.

16.6.2 Organizational Efforts

In response to deficits in abortion related curricula, in the late 1990s, fledgling chapters of Nursing Students for Choice (NSFC) were established at a number of nursing schools in some parts of the country. Initially, these groups were not well connected; however, over time a national organizational structure was created to provide support and programming, including an annual conference that convenes representatives from student chapters across the country to network and learn skills in abortion care and advocacy for curricula reform. The organization also launched a voluntary clinical externship program for students who did not have opportunities in their education programs, or who wanted to gain additional clinical experience in abortion care. Some chapters also offered their own elective courses on abortion. One model developed by student members of NSFC was the Abortion Care Education (ACE) elective. Based on the experience of implementing this elective, a guide was created so others could replicate and adapt the course for their own campuses. The guide is still available; it includes case studies for unintended pregnancy prevention and care with a strong focus on abortion care are available for nursing educators [23] (Table 16.2).

In 2017, NSFC (which had changed its name to Nursing Students for Sexual and Reproductive Health) merged with the organization Reproductive Health in Nursing (RHN) to become Nurses for Sexual and Reproductive Health (NSRH). NSRH continues to host an

Table 16.2 Abortion education and training resources for nurse practitioners, nurse midwives and physician assistants

Resource	Where to obtain
Abortion Care Education (ACE) Elective	http://nsrh.org/ACE-Elective-Getting-Started
Abortion Provider Toolkit	https://aptoolkit.org
Nurses for Sexual and Reproductive Health (Clinical Externship Program, ACE elective, and other resources)	http://nsrh.org
Early Abortion Training Workbook	https://workbook.pressbooks.com
Midwest Access Project (MAP) Individual Clinical Training	http://midwestaccessproject.org/training-post/
Consortium of Clinical Abortion Training Centers	www.abortiontraining.org
PPNYC Clinical Training and Research Initiative	www.plannedparenthood.org/planned-parenthood-new-york-city/local-education-training/trainings-professionals/clinical-training-and-research-initiative
Reproductive Health Access Project	www.reproductiveaccess.org/abortion/
Clinicians in Abortion Care (CIAC)	https://prochoice.org/health-care-professionals/ciac/
Nursing Education Modules in Unintended Pregnancy Prevention and Care	https://rhnursing.org/area/resources-for-educators/

annual activist conference, a clinical externship program, and to offer other training resources (including the ACE elective guide) for both nursing students and practicing clinicians. The organization's website features information on education and training resources, as well as abortion-related advocacy and activism [24].

Frustrated by the limited training opportunities in abortion care in the USA, some students have gone abroad to further their skills and knowledge. Four advanced-practice nursing students who pursued training outside of their formal education program wrote about their experiences volunteering in a clinic in Mexico City (Chapter 32) where they were able to learn to perform uterine aspiration abortion procedures as well as other key elements of abortion care [25]. It is not known how many US APRN and PA students have traveled abroad to obtain skills in procedural abortion, or in what countries in addition to Mexico such self-arranged trainings occur.

16.6.3 Post-certification Abortion Training

Training in abortion care in the USA is limited for CNMs, NPs and PAs who have completed an education program and are certified (in service training). Some agencies that provide abortion offer educational and skill-building opportunities and mentorship for their employees. In some of the states where physician-only abortion laws were never enacted, models for training CNMs, NPs and PAs to competency in uterine aspiration procedures have been developed. The Vermont Feminist Women's Health Center, which later merged with Planned Parenthood, was a national leader in efforts to train and employ CNM, NP and PA clinicians as abortion providers [26]. Planned Parenthood of NYC was also a frontrunner in training clinicians other than physicians to provide abortion through their Clinical Training and Research Initiative. The program, which was established in 1993 to "close the gap between the need for abortion services and the number of clinicians trained to provide abortions," is still in operation, and aspires to train more CNMs, NPs and PAs in the future (L. Kroll, personal communication, June 14, 2019).

Recently, openings for CNMs, NPs and PAs have been established in several abortion training programs. The Individual Clinical Training Program is an initiative of the Midwest Access Project (MAP) that aims to "train a diverse array of health care professionals who are highly motivated to provide comprehensive reproductive health care in their future practice to underserved patient populations, but who lack access to the clinical training to do so." For individuals accepted into this program, a tailored plan is created to address their learning needs that is also consistent with the scope of practice in the state where they practice. For trainees who work in a state where uterine aspiration abortion is not legally within their scope, training in this procedure is not offered; however, they are given opportunities to learn other skills essential to comprehensive abortion care. While the majority of past MAP trainees have been physicians (including medical students, residents, fellows and practicing physicians), as of 2018 3% were reported to be advanced-practice clinicians [27].

Creating a Clinician Corps (C3), an initiative currently under the auspices of the National Abortion Federation, has spearheaded formation of a Consortium of Clinical Abortion Training Centers "for physicians and advanced practice clinicians that were unable to obtain abortion training during their education or residency and for those who are seeking to refresh or augment their clinical skills." Clinicians in this program are "trained to competency" to be able to deliver care in a variety of settings through a combination of didactics and hands-on learning [28]. Additional information on these training programs, including about eligibility and how to apply, is available on their websites [28] (see Table 16.2).

For CNMs, NPs and PAs interested in providing medication abortion, training is generally easier to access than it is for uterine aspiration procedures. A number of educational resources have been developed, including web-based modules that allow learners to follow a self-paced program suited to their needs. Some organizations, including Clinicians in Abortion Care and the Reproductive Health Access Project, have also sponsored in-person trainings for clinicians to learn about providing medication abortion [29]. Some CNMs, NPs and PAs also seek training in pelvic/early pregnancy ultrasound, as it is not an area of clinical competence upon graduation for all students in these professions.

Because formal post-graduate pathways for CNMs, NPs and PAs to become abortion providers are limited in the USA, those who want to include this service in their clinical practice may find the only way to acquire the knowledge and skills they need is to develop their own education and training plan. *The Early Abortion Training Workbook*, an "interactive curriculum to train new reproductive health care providers to competence," includes a tool for assessing, developing training plans and guiding learners as they build their skills and knowledge in early abortion care [30] (see Table 16.2). A vital first step in this process is evaluating the learner's existing skills and knowledge to determine their learning needs. Then, depending on what relevant clinical knowledge and skills they already possess (ie, performing pelvic examinations, pregnancy options counseling, pregnancy test interpretation, pelvic ultrasound, paracervical anesthesia, conscious sedation, medication abortion and endometrial biopsy using MVA), an individualized training program can be created. The *Workbook* is appropriate for CNM, NP and PA learners, as well as physicians.

Based on a study of providers who participated in the previously mentioned HWPP project, Freedman and Levi offer insights about how CNMs, NPs and PAs develop confidence and competence in integrating uterine aspiration abortion into their practice. Their findings may be useful for preceptors and faculty trainers to better understand the process of developing new technical skills among CNM, NP and PA learners [31]. In addition, the *Abortion Provider Toolkit* includes information about documenting abortion-related education and skill acquisition through a professional portfolio [12]. Clinicians are advised to keep records proactively in case of any regulatory challenge or investigation regarding their competence or scope of practice in this contentious area of care.

16.7 Conclusion

The report by the National Academies of Sciences, Engineering, and Medicine states that prohibiting NPs, CNMs and PAs from performing abortions can cause delays for patients and hinder the effectiveness of care [4]. Delays can lead women to seek abortions at later gestations, which may increase the potential for complications, use more costly emergency rooms for follow-up care and further burden patients with travel and logistical concerns. Given the evidence that CNMs, NPs and PAs provide safe and effective abortion care that is acceptable to patients, and that these clinicians are more likely to practice in rural areas [32], it is clear that there is a missed opportunity to tap a pool of qualified potential abortion providers in the USA.

References

1. Kaplan L. *The Story of Jane: The Legendary Underground Feminist Abortion Service.* New York: Random House; 1995.

2. National Abortion Federation. *The Role of Nurse Practitioners, Physician Assistants, and Nurse-Midwives in Providing Abortion: Strategies for Expanding Abortion Access.* Washington, DC: National Abortion Federation; 1997.

3. Freedman MA, Jillson DA, Coffin RR, et al. (1986). Comparison of complications rates in first trimester abortions performed by physician assistants and physicians. *Am J Pub Health.* **76**:550–554.

4. National Academies of Sciences, Engineering, and Medicine. *The Safety and Quality of Abortion Care in the United States.* Washington, DC: The National Academies Press; 2018.

5. The Policy Surveillance Program, a Law Atlas Project. State abortion laws. http://lawatlas.org/page/abortion-law-project. Accessed July 27, 2019.

6. Institute of Medicine (IOM). *Legalized Abortion and the Public Health.* Washington, DC: National Academy Press; 1975.

7. National Abortion Federation. *Who Will Provide Abortions? Ensuring Availability of Qualified Practitioners (Recommendations from a National Symposium).* Washington, DC: National Abortion Federation; 1990.

8. National Abortion Federation. Role of CNMs, NPs, and PAs in Abortion Care. https://5aa1b2xfmfh2e2mk03kk8rsx-wpengine.netdna-ssl.com/wp-content/uploads/CNM_NP_PA_org_statements.pdf. Accessed July 30, 2019.

9. Taylor D, Safriet B, Dempsey G, Kruse B, Jackson C. *Providing Abortion Care: A Professional Toolkit for Nurse-Midwives, Nurse Practitioners and Physician Assistants.* http://apctoolkit.org/wp-content/themes/apctoolkit/index.html. Accessed July 30, 2019.

10. International Confederation of Midwives. Midwives' provision of abortion-related services. Position statement. www.internationalmidwives.org/assets/files/statement-files/2019/06/midwives-provision-of-abortion-related-services-eng-letterhead.pdf. Accessed July 7, 2019.

11. International Confederation of Midwives. *Essential Competencies for Midwifery Practice.* Koninginnegracht, The Netherlands: International Confederation of Midwives; 2019.

12. Taylor D, Safriet B, Kruse B, Dempsey G, Summers L. Welcome to the *Abortion Provider Toolkit.* UCSF Bixby Center for Global Reproductive Health. 2018. http://aptoolkit.org/. Accessed July 7, 2019.

13. Guttmacher Institute. *State Policies on Abortion Rights.* Washington, DC: Guttmacher Center for Population Research Innovation and Dissemination. www.guttmacher.org/united-states/abortion/state-policies-abortion. Accessed June 15, 2019.

14. National Council of State Boards of Nursing. *APRN Consensus Model.* www.ncsbn.org/aprn-consensus.htm. Accessed July 30, 2019.

15. National Council of State Boards of Nursing. APRN Compact. www.ncsbn.org/aprn-compact.htm. Accessed July 30, 2019.

16. Sofer D. VA grants most APRNs full practice authority. *Am. J Nurs.* 2017;**117**(3):14.

17. American Academy of Physician Assistants (AAPA). PA Scope of Practice. Issue brief. 2017. www.aapa.org/wp-content/uploads/2017/01/Issue-brief_Scope-of-Practice_0117-1.pdf. Accessed July 30, 2019.

18. Barnard S, Kim C, Park MH, Ngo TD. Doctors or mid-level providers of abortion. *Cochrane Database Syst Rev.* 2015;(7):CD011242.

19. Weitz TA, Taylor D, Desai S, et al. Safety of aspiration abortion performed by nurse practitioners, certified nurse midwives, and physician assistants under a California legal waiver. *Am J Public Health.* 2013;**103**:454–461.

20. Cappiello J, Coplon L, Carpenter, H. A systematic review of sexual and reproductive health care content in nursing curricula. *J Obstet Gynecol Neonatal Nurs.* 2017;**46**:e157–e167.

21. Simmonds K, Foster AM, Zurek M. From the outside in: a unique model for stimulating curricula reform in nursing education. *J Nurs Educ.* 2009;**48**(10):583–587.

22. Foster AM, Polis C, Allee MK, Simmonds K, Zurek M, Brown A. Abortion education in nurse practitioner, physician assistant and certified nurse-midwifery programs: a national survey. *Contraception.* 2006;**73**(4):408–414.

23. Nurses for Sexual and Reproductive Health (NSRH). Welcome to the ACE Elective! http://nsrh.org/Abortion-Care-Education-(ACE). Accessed July 30, 2019.

24. Nurses for Sexual and Reproductive Health (NSRH). http://nsrh.org/. Accessed July 30, 2019.

25. Taylor A, Hathaway A, Luneau M, McKenna F, Cappiello, J. Four narratives on abortion

training in Mexico City. *Womens Healthcare*. 2016;4 (4):78–81.

26. Freedman MA, Jillson, DA, Coffin RR, Novick, LF. Comparison of complication rates in first trimester abortions performed by physician assistants and physicians. *Am J Public Health*. 1986;**76**.5:550–554.

27. Midwest Access Project (MAP). https:// midwestaccessproject.org/ what-we-do/individual- clinical-training/. Accessed July 30, 2019.

28. National Abortion Federation (NAF). https://prochoice.org/. Accessed July 30, 2019.

29. Reproductive Health Access Project (RHAP). www .reproductiveaccess.org/. Accessed July 30, 2019.

30. *The Early Abortion Training Workbook*. San Francisco: Advancing New Standards on Reproductive Health (ANSIRH). www.ansirh.org/ publications/training/early- abortion-training-workbook. Accessed July 30, 2019.

31. Freedman L, Levi A. How clinicians develop confidence in their competence in performing aspiration abortion. *Qual Health Res*. 2014;**24**:78–89.

32. Barnes H, Richards MR, McHugh MD, Martsolf G. Rural and nonrural primary care physician practices increasingly rely on nurse practitioners. *Health Aff (Millwood)*. 2018;**37** (6):908–914.

Chapter

17

A Guide for Creating a Program in Sexual and Reproductive Health-Care Education

Angela Dempsey and Katharine O'Connell White

17.1 Introduction

Building a new program to advance clinical services and educate health-care trainees in sexual and reproductive health care is a multifaceted endeavor and should be tailored to individual sites. However, there are common threads that connect such programs. This chapter provides a stepwise framework for developing a program inclusive of developing clinical services, designing a rotation with strong learning objectives and curriculum, addressing partial participation in abortion care by trainees and managing partnerships with other training sites. The pragmatic framework presented in this guide also addresses how to develop institutional support and ensure long-term sustainability of the program beyond the start-up phase. Though many terms we've used apply to academic medicine, this framework could be utilized in other settings.

17.2 Developing Clinical Services

17.2.1 Conduct a Needs Assessment

Program directors are frequently faced with the challenge of beginning or improving clinical services. A needs assessment helps determine which service(s) are most feasible and impactful for patients or resident education.

Which of the services listed in Table 17.1 is already provided? Consider whether there is an unmet need that supports either initiating a new service or improving an existing service. Such need may be supported by clinical data, conversations with other providers or staff, patient satisfaction survey results or comparison to other sites.

Whichever services you plan to add or expand, thoughtful conversations with key leaders, such as operations managers, clinic/practice managers,

Table 17.1 Examples of potential services

Contraception	Miscarriage Care
• Contraceptive care integrated into gynecology care • Contraceptive care for medically complicated patients • Routine and challenging implant and IUD insertions and removals • Immediate postpartum LARC • Contraception consultation services	• Counseling about management options • Medical management with mifepristone and misoprostol • Aspiration in an ambulatory setting • Management of women with medical complications
Abortion Care	Abnormal Pregnancy
• Counseling about management options • Medication abortion with mifepristone and misoprostol • Procedural abortion in an ambulatory setting • Procedural abortion in an operating room • Hospital based services for second-trimester or complicated abortions	• Diagnosis and management of pregnancy of unknown location • Ectopic pregnancy diagnosis and management • Diagnosis, management and follow-up of molar pregnancy

LARC: long-acting reversible contraception; IUD, intrauterine device departmental or division chiefs, nursing and other staff leaders and others, can give you information about volume, space and staff considerations. Conversations should address:

- Space planning: Are there vacant or underutilized procedural spaces at your site (eg, in vitro fertilization [IVF], colonoscopy, ophthalmology) that might be available for procedures for pregnancy loss and/or abortion?
- Regulatory environment: Does your site have restrictions that impact provision of miscarriage and induced abortion care?
- Medication abortion provision: Is mifepristone on formulary? Is it restricted to outpatient use or also available for inpatient use? Which providers are registered? If mifepristone is not on formulary, what is the process for submitting a new formulary agent for approval?
- Block time availability: How does operating room (OR) block time or non-block time work at your site? How might this impact your service provision?

17.2.2 Plan for New Service Implementation

One you have selected a service that you would like to implement or improve, summarize the information from your needs assessment in a way that you can share with other stakeholders, including a justification for your project. Next, create a logistical plan that addresses needs for space, equipment, personnel, trainees, patient flow, financial considerations and strategic partnerships.

- Plan your space, including the proposed clinical space, with considerations of how often you will need to use it, and whether physical upgrades or a new space is needed for optimal service provision.
- List major equipment (eg, ultrasound or suction machine) and minor equipment (eg, tenacula, ring forceps, dilators, metal specula, needle extenders) that need to be purchased. Include equipment that will need to be regularly purchased (eg, cervical os finders or manual vacuum aspiration [MVA] equipment).
- Identify existing clinical staff to support the new service and any need to hire new

personnel. Suggest staff training and designate who will be responsible for ordering major, minor, and disposable equipment.
- Determine which trainees would ideally participate in the service (eg, on a family planning rotation, member of the obstetrics and gynecology [ob-gyn] team).
- Create a plan for patient flow. Identify what types of patient encounters you will be able to provide through your new service and your patient capacity per block/session. Project the anticipated increase in capacity over the first year of service. Explain how patients will be scheduled and how referrals will be handled.
- Plot financial considerations including how you will bill, whether insurance covers the proposed service or if a cash payment price is needed, and how utilizing patient financial assistance through National Abortion Federation (NAF) membership might help. Based on reimbursement for your new service, estimate how many patients you need to see at a minimum to support your time, utilization of clinical space and use of clinical staff.
- Identify strategic partners in your new service implementation or improvement and determine how to best enroll them in your plan. Partners may include operating room management/nursing, anesthesia personnel, labor and delivery management/nursing, pharmacy, emergency department management/nursing, ambulatory practice management/nursing, pathology department, mortuary department, central processing and operations staff who are in charge of ordering single-use equipment (IUDs and implants, laminaria/Dilapan, MVA equipment).

A month-by-month timeline for implementation can help keep the project on track. Don't forget to measure the successes or impacts of your program at the end of year one following new service implementation by tracking volume of patients, patient satisfaction, revenue generation, trainee satisfaction, and so on. Think about how you can prospectively collect data to utilize in evaluation of your program.

17.2.3 Introduce the New Service

Once you have identified the need and created a project plan to implement the new service, determine which stakeholders would benefit from hearing the details directly from you:

- Operating room staff
- Anesthesia personnel
- Labor and delivery staff
- Clinic staff
- Physicians
- Trainees
- Referral sources
- Emergency department
- Services such as pathology, pharmacy and central processing

Electronic communication or in-person meetings will be appropriate for different stakeholder groups. For in-person meetings, aim to reach as many people as possible, through staff or faculty meetings. Bring multiple groups together when possible by inviting broad stakeholder groups to an existing meeting (eg, invite nursing staff and faculty from other departments to a Grand Rounds presentation).

When preparing your communications, regardless of whether these will be verbal or written and to which audiences, be strategic! Consider sharing the service justification from your needs assessment. Specific patient stories are powerful for describing the need for your services. Decide on two or three clear talking points that are the most important to communicate to your audience and recap them at the end of your presentation. Prepare responses to anticipated objections that your audience might raise. It is important to create an environment where staff, colleagues and trainees can comfortably share concerns with you. You may consider the following: limiting the audience at certain presentations, using polling software for anonymous comments and questions, utilizing a comment box and inviting follow-up questions or comments by email or phone.

Once you have completed the internal rollout of your new service, it's time to expand your communication beyond the institution. New clinical services benefit from external marketing to community practices and patients. In many institutions, external marketing needs to be conducted in conjunction with departmental and institutional gatekeepers, who can grant you permission to market your services externally through physical materials such as brochures and business cards as well as via a web presence.

Once you have permission to create an external marketing plan, use the human resources in your institution (eg, departmental business manager, hospital marketing department, service line director, informational technology staff). Consider the myriad possible marketing strategies: physical brochures, business cards, department or hospital websites, or an independent website (eg, www.abortionclinics.com in the USA).

In your overall marketing plan, think about both patients and providers who need to hear about your service. For both audiences, consider what approaches and materials are most useful and where they should be located. How to obtain an appointment may be the most important piece of information; ensure your contact information is clear and accurate.

If external marketing is not supported by your department or institution, there are other strategies that you might employ to facilitate patients reaching your service. These approaches may involve internal marketing to key departments (eg, Grand Rounds, resident education time), to the general hospital or university community (eg, intranet, email newsletters) and education of institutional schedulers to route patients or providers who call in with questions to the appropriate person.

17.3 Designing a Rotation

A reproductive health education program ideally includes a family planning rotation that (1) meets training accreditation requirements, (2) allows trainees to accomplish intentionally crafted learning objectives to prepare them to gain competence, (3) capitalizes on the strengths of existing faculty and clinical services and (4) addresses unique site-specific challenges.

17.3.1 Build the Rotation Schedule

Most rotation schedules need to be designed around unique challenges (eg, a distant freestanding partner clinic) and strengths of a site. This framework will help you build a rotation schedule that fits your needs.

1. List all the sites that offer potential educational opportunities for trainees (eg, abortion clinic, miscarriage clinic, contraception clinic, freestanding partner clinic, operating room, procedures clinic, ultrasound).

Table 17.2 Sample rotation schedule form

		Mon	Tues	Wed	Thurs	Fri	Sat	Sun
AM	Activity							
	Preceptor							
PM	Activity							
	Preceptor							

2. Propose an ideal weekly schedule for trainees using a table format (Table 17.2).
3. Consider whether scheduled or self-directed rotation didactics offer the best fit.
4. Invite key stakeholders such as residency program leadership, trainees, participating faculty and/or clinic leadership to discuss the proposed rotation schedule.
5. Guiding questions for the stakeholder meeting and any needed next steps may include the following:
   a. Are there preceptors for each activity?
   b. Is there clinical space to accommodate each activity?
   c. Does the clinical volume support the number of learners planned for each activity?
   d. Are additional affiliation agreements needed for external training sites?
   e. Can the proposed schedule stand weekly or are additional versions needed?

17.3.2 Generate Learning Objectives for Trainees

Setting learning objectives for the education program helps trainees clearly understand the value and intent of the offered educational experiences, as well as how these experiences fit into their overall training and future practice. Thoughtful and comprehensive learning objectives also help residents understand what gaps may occur in their education should they decide to partially participate in some opportunities.

Generate learning objectives for each of the various domains in which learners should gain concrete clinical skills, knowledge or communication skills. Common domains for family planning-focused training include the following:

- Provision of contraception, abortion and miscarriage care

- Evidence-based and patient-centered counseling about contraception, abortion and miscarriage care
- Advocating for patients' access to sexual and reproductive health services

Learning objectives may also be driven by assessment tools, such as Accreditation Council for Graduate Medical Education (ACGME) milestones (Figure 17.1) [1].

For programs that integrate experiences at both an academic center and freestanding partner clinic, learning objectives may be shared by both sites or individualized by site. Make sure that objectives are inclusive of many skills gained through the rotation, even for learners who choose to partially participate in the clinical care. For example, all learners – even those who do not do uterine aspiration abortion during the rotation – benefit from many skills such as preoperative assessment, ultrasound for gestational dating, management of conscious sedation and pregnancy options counseling. Thus, it is important to include these in learning objectives. In addition, the ability to reflect on one's beliefs about abortion and professional responsibilities to patients is important. You might include a learning objective around this skill, such as, "At the end of this rotation, each trainee will be able to articulate their personal boundaries around provision of abortion care to future patients and colleagues."

Once a formal list of learning objectives is crafted, determine your plan to inform the trainees of the objectives and track their progress toward meeting them. Typically, educators review the objectives during an orientation to the program and/or rotation. Tracking progress toward meeting the objectives may be as informal as sitting with the trainee at rotation midpoint and endpoint to review progress and chart a strategy for accomplishing unmet objectives, or as formal as an electronic evaluation system that captures data from each trainee.

Family Planning — Patient Care				
Level 1	Level 2	Level 3	Level 4	Level 5
Verbalizes basic knowledge about common contraceptive options	Demonstrates a basic understanding of the effectiveness risks benefits complications and contraindications of contraception including emergency contraception and pregnancy termination	Counsels on the effectiveness risks benefits and contraindications of available forms of contraception Counsels on the effectiveness risks benefits and contraindications for male and female sterilization Performs intra-uterine and implantable contraceptive placement Demonstrates ability to perform basic first-trimester uterine evacuation (medical and surgical)	Formulates comprehensive management plans for patients with medical diseases complicating their use of contraceptive methods Manages complications of contraceptive methods and pregnancy termination Determines the need for consultation referral or transfer of patients with complex complications Demonstrates ability to perform basic second-trimester uterine evacuation (medical and surgical)	Applies innovative and complex approaches to family planning and implements treatment plans based on emerging evidence

Comments: Not yet rotated ▢

Figure 17.1 ACGME Family Planning Milestone. © 2013 Accreditation Council for Graduate Medical Education and American College of Obstetrics and Gynecology; Reproduced with permission from the Accreditation Council on Graduate Medical Education

17.3.3 Build the Curriculum

The curricular materials provided to trainees during a rotation should deepen their knowledge base about family planning topics, augment their ability to provide accurate, evidence-based care directly to patients and reinforce the hands-on education they receive while working with patients. An effective curriculum is tailored to the training level of the learner, organized to complement the clinical activities of the rotation, fills knowledge gaps that are predictably not gained through clinical experiences and is aligned to support the stated learning objectives of the rotation. For example, when a resident combines a clinic session in which they provided several uterine aspiration procedures with reading a chapter about uterine aspiration in the first trimester, their newly acquired knowledge and skills are solidified more deeply. Or when exposure to second-trimester uterine aspiration is limited, curricular material about surgical technique of second-trimester procedures and management of potential complications provides important knowledge for future practice that cannot be gained through clinical experience. Other important considerations for those designing curriculum include whether to include simulation and whether the curriculum will be self-directed, led by an educator or a combination of both.

17.3.4 Incorporate a Values Clarification Exercise

Values clarification exercises or professionalism workshops help learners, staff, and faculty engage in the self-reflection necessary to articulate their thoughts about abortion and raise self-awareness of the roots of their beliefs. For many, this may be the first time that they have been encouraged to explore these values and think critically about how their individual values framework may impact patient care as well as their choices around the provision of clinical services. Resources, such as the National Abortion Federation's *The Abortion Option*, exist to help directors incorporate this type of activity into their rotation [2]. Important considerations when incorporating a values clarification into a rotation include determining whether a local faculty member or external party would be best suited to lead the session based on your site's climate and strategizing to optimize learner participation and their perception of safety in discussing a difficult topic.

17.4 Addressing Partial Participation in Abortion Care

Although abortion training is an important, required aspect of training for providers of sexual and reproductive health care, programs must respect individuals' moral or religious objections. That said, conscientious refusal has limits, and does not mean that a learner should be allowed to opt out of all abortion training. Partial participation allows the flexibility to respect trainee boundaries while maximizing education [3]. The following includes resources and ideas for developing an effective approach to help trainees navigate decisions about participation in abortion training.

17.4.1 Determine Participation

Each program should host a direct discussion in which trainees clarify their participation level. Ideally, this conversation would:

- Be led by a person who is knowledgeable about the program but also perceived as approachable by trainees
- Be scheduled at a time when the trainee and teacher are not sleep-deprived or rushed
- Occur in a space that provides privacy and optimizes the comfort level of the trainee

This dialogue can build rapport between teacher and trainee, establish common ground around patient well-being and reinforce a culture of mutual respect regardless of views toward abortion. Consider including the following elements in each discussion:

- Program expectations or policies around trainee participation
- Learning objectives that may be more difficult to meet with partial participation
- Open-ended questions to ascertain the trainee's goals and objectives for the training and the presence of any objections or unease with participating in abortion care
- Clarification of the specific boundaries the trainee wants to observe (eg, abortion indications, gestational age limits)
- Alternative activities as appropriate to optimize the educational value of the training

Because trainees may approach their decision about participation very early in their careers, it may be based only on their feelings or perceptions from outside of medicine. Consider key things you would like your trainees to consider when deciding on participation level. Examples of useful resources to provide in advance of the face-to-face discussion include the following:

- Institutional or national policies on conscientious objection
- American College of Obstetricians and Gynecologists (ACOG) Committee Opinions [4–6]
- Relevant program or accreditation guidelines on abortion education

Developing a policy helps training programs codify their approach to partial participation. Policies ensure a standard approach with each trainee and provide support should conflict arise. To formalize a policy, collaborate with departmental education leaders such as the chairperson and residency program director to achieve consensus on expectations for training and process for handling partial participation. Such a policy may, but need not, specify activities that the trainee will or will not perform. In addition, the policy can specify materials to be reviewed by trainees as well as the role of the trainee in ensuring coverage and achieving learning objectives through alternative mechanisms.

17.4.2 Respond to Partial Participation

An initial step once a trainee has elected partial participation is to examine the rotation schedule to determine whether you can honor their boundaries and meet the learning objectives within the existing schedule or whether it will be necessary to create alternative clinical experiences, didactics, projects and so on. Consider engaging the trainee in this problem solving to ensure they acquire the knowledge and skill they need by rotation's end given their chosen participation level. As you develop your plan for partial participators, take care not to inadvertently create incentives to limit participation (eg, an alternative surgical assignment). In line with professional standards following graduation, the partially participating trainee should work with peers to ensure coverage of patient care when they are unable to provide it. Consider readdressing the trainee's participation level during the rotation to explore whether they remain comfortable with previously set boundaries and to ensure they feel those boundaries are being respected.

It is important to articulate for the trainee the myriad skills, such as counseling, ultrasound and post-procedure care, that can be developed at the site, even in the setting of limited abortion provision. Trainees may also deepen their understanding of patient experience when seeking abortion that will inform their care of patients throughout their career.

17.5 Managing Partnerships with Freestanding Clinics

Programs that need to partner with a freestanding clinic to provide abortion training and meet program objectives may consider the following parameters to establish and optimize the partnership.

A central challenge when partnering with a freestanding clinic is integrating learners from your program into a workflow that may prioritize efficiency. When establishing the parameters of the partnership, articulating the following details help both program and clinic plan strategically and optimize sustainability of the relationship:

- How do learners affect clinic workflow?
- How does clinic workflow impact achievement of program learning objectives?
- Can learner balance procedural training with skill development in ultrasound, counseling and post-procedure care without disrupting efficiency?
- Is there a minimum expectation of case volume or mix when trainees are present?
- Which provider(s) will supervise the trainee experience and care on site?
- Will the clinic evaluate trainees?
- What activities are available to optimize learning for trainees who have an objection to abortion provision?
- May trainees participate in scholarship or quality improvement opportunities?
- What governs use of the institution's name in affiliation with the partner site?
- Who in the clinic can work with institutional representatives to discuss financial sustainability after any start-up funding expires?

Freestanding clinic partners may encounter regular protester activity that impacts trainees. Consider whether any additional safety measures are necessary with the inclusion of trainees as well as your strategy to both prepare trainees for protesters before attending clinic and debrief with them afterward. The debrief session may present an opportunity to highlight for trainees the

ramifications of stigmatization of abortion on their patients. For dedicated staff of a freestanding clinic, it may be a new experience to work with trainees who have varying comfort levels with abortion care. Staff development and a mechanism for them to provide feedback provides needed support to optimize everyone's experience.

Graduate medical education (GME) programs often require an executed affiliation agreement for trainees to work and learn outside of the academic center. The residency program director or coordinator, the designated institutional officer (DIO) or GME administrator can provide an institutional template for these agreements and guidance about the required signatures.

Setting a policy for coverage of clinical services at the partner site demonstrates to the partner how you value the relationship, ensures that patients receive care and legitimizes the educational value of the experience to the trainees. Such a policy may address plans for planned leave of the supervising physician, procedures to be followed during resident sick leave or vacation and language to preclude shifting of trainees from the partner site to other services without advanced notice and reason. To highlight the rationale for such a policy, consider outlining the multiple educational objectives of training at the site in the text of the policy.

17.6 Gaining and Sustaining Institutional Support

Securing support from leaders and stakeholders in your institution and enrolling them in your program's success optimizes program launch and long-term sustainability. Such leaders include, but are not limited, to chief executive officers, chief medical officers, department chairs, division chiefs, medical school deans, DIOs, GME officers and residency program directors.

Efforts to ensure the survival of your program should begin during the early phases of development of your program. Identification of the priorities of your institutional leaders allows use of strategic language in emails, conversations and so on that helps all to see how your program aligns with these priorities. Leaders may have concerns such as the public reputation of the hospital, patient satisfaction, recruiting quality faculty and residents and balancing their budget. Identify how your program can support these objectives –

grateful patients and good patient care for hospital administrators, enthusiastic learners and institutional reputation for academic leaders and the like. Try to identify potential objections that these leaders may have with a sexual and reproductive health training program. Counter these objections with data, published literature, patient stories and patient letters. Have key program objectives available in writing to share during interactions.

For programs including abortion care, think about the strategic ways to describe your program/services to others in the institution and community. Terms such as *abortion*, *pregnancy termination*, *family planning* and *pregnancy loss* may resonate differently with your colleagues, trainees, institutional leaders and patients. When naming your clinic, service or program, consider the advantages and disadvantages of a generic name (such as Women's Health) versus a specific name (such as Women's Options Center). When discussing abortion care and services, think through what fears, concerns or past experiences might be triggered for the stakeholders most influential to the long-term success of your program. Awareness of these concerns may shape your language and approach when discussing the program.

Direct contact with institutional leaders helps you establish your reputation with them and build relationships. A relationship is important when you need to address controversial situations. Opportunities to interact with leaders occur through committee participation, administrative roles or regularly held meetings. Don't be afraid to ask your chairperson to advocate for you to participate in these opportunities. It is important to engage early with staff who will be vital to new service delivery (eg, leadership in nursing and anesthesia) so that they do not become obstacles later. Finally, when decisions are being made that might impact your program, ask for a seat at the table. For leadership hires and clinical space changes, ask to be included in decision making. This involvement ensures that your program needs and sustainability are being considered.

17.7 Program Sustainability

Program sustainability is a function not only of revenue generation but also the degree to which you can embed the program and services into the fabric of the department, demonstrate value to and for the trainees, introduce innovation in education and clinical service and enroll leaders in the mission of the program. In addition, avoiding burnout yourself is a key factor in program sustainability.

17.7.1 Map Financial Sustainability

Multiple elements factor into your program's ability to financially support itself following the period of grant funding. You may want your clinical services to be integrated with other departmental services, until your increased volume warrants a separate cost center. Financial managers are helpful in understanding the metrics that the department tracks, which, in the USA, include relative value units (RVU), actual reimbursement, payer mix and others, and how these metrics align with typical services you will provide. Clarify whether there are targets required to justify each clinical session – number of patients, a certain number of RVUs or an amount of revenue generated. Table 17.3 identifies common procedures that generate revenue in family planning care and their associated billing code and RVU. Reimbursement varies by site, payer and other institution-specific factors.

17.7.2 Hire a Program Coordinator

A strong program coordinator is one of the important elements of ensuring your success. When interviewing candidates, have a clear understanding of the tasks for which they are responsible and what skill sets – medical, administrative, research – you need them to possess. Seek assistance from department administrators when navigating the human resources processes. It can be advantageous to hire someone who is already a part of your institution, as they already have useful knowledge when navigating institutional bureaucracy and can utilize existing networks. Additionally, a coordinator who is a licensed nurse or clinician could potentially generate revenue for patient counseling, follow-up phone calls and so on.

17.7.3 Embed Clinical Services into the Department

Part of creating a sustainable program involves integrating the new services and education you offer into the daily workings of your department. Think about ways to make yourself and your

Table 17.3 Current US Procedural Terminology (CPT) codes, Evaluation and Management (E&M) Codes and Relative Value Units (RVUs) for common family planning procedures

Procedure	CPT or E&M	Work RVU
IUD insertion	58300	1.01
IUD removal	58301	1.27
Implant insertion	11981	1.48
Implant removal	11982	1.78
Implant removal and reinsertion	11983	3.30
Tubal ligation pre-op visit	99205/99215	3.17/2.11
Laparoscopic tubal ligation	58600-5, 58615, 58670–1	3.94-5.91
Laparoscopic salpingectomy	58700	12.95
Procedure	CPT	Work RVU
Insertion of cervical dilators	59200	0.79
D&C for spontaneous abortion	59812	4.44
D&C for missed abortion, 1st trimester	59820	4.84
D&C for missed abortion, 2nd trimester	59821	5.09
Diagnostic D&C	58120	3.59
Therapeutic abortion, 1st trimester (D&C)	59840	3.01
Therapeutic abortion, 2nd trimester (D&E)	59841	5.65
Paracervical block	64435	1.45
Ultrasound guidance for procedures (not only TOP but difficult IUD removal/insertion)	76998-26	1.20
Abdominal ultrasound, pregnant	76815	0.65
Vaginal ultrasound, pregnant	76817	0.75
Vaginal ultrasound, not pregnant	76830	0.69

D&C, dilation and curettage; D&E, dilation and evacuation; IUD, intrauterine device; TOP, termination of pregnancy

program indispensable to the overall department. Have a concrete understanding of the benefits that you and your program bring, which may include contributions to:

- Clinical resources such as evidence-based protocols; streamlined abortion, contraception care and miscarriage care; management of pregnancy of unknown location, non-tubal ectopic and molar pregnancies; and management of patients with genetic anomalies or maternal comorbidities
- Academic offerings such as Grand Rounds, quality improvement reviews and morbidity and mortality rounds

- Education for trainees and medical students including didactic curricula, research mentorship, clinical opportunities and student interest groups

17.7.4 Track Patient Volume

It is critical for new directors to track patient volume to justify the program's financial and education value. These data will measure the financial impact of the services, justify sustained support for the program, help with tracking trainees' experience and contribute to grant applications and reports. In addition, data about patient care could be used for quality improvement or research projects (with institutional review board approval.)

Passive tracking from billing or electronic medical record data may be the easiest way to track volume. The information gathered in this way may be limited to location of service, billing provider, service provider and billing data.

Active tracking through a database you create is more labor intensive but allows you to collect more information about patients, and allows you to track volume at multiple sites:

- Referral source
- Provider name
- Procedure category and indication
- Patient demographics, medical history and clinical care course

The database should be accessible to multiple people at different sites, utilizing available technology (e.g. Google Sheets) and secure storage if you are collecting any patient identifiers to maintain confidentiality.

17.7.5 Track Learner Experience

Data regarding the experience of your learners can demonstrate the impact of your program, guide program improvements, and support long-term sustainability. Consider the evaluations currently used by your department and whether you can create an evaluation that includes customized elements.

You may want to consider capturing:

☐ Resident satisfaction with didactic and clinical training

☐ Number of certain procedures

☐ Procedures of importance to accrediting organizations (eg, ultrasounds)

☐ Resident perception of degree of competence with certain procedures

☐ Degree to which the rotation allowed residents to meet the specified learning objectives

☐ Suggestions for improvement to specific areas of the rotation

☐ Information about resident experience at each clinical site

☐ Narrative comments on strengths/weaknesses/unique aspects of the training

☐ Contribution to counseling, psychosocial and advocacy skills

☐ Understanding patients' challenges in navigating the health-care system

17.8 Conclusion

Ensuring access to comprehensive reproductive health services for patients now and into the future requires widespread availability of education programs. Building a successful sexual and reproductive health-care education program requires attention to many domains including clinical services, rotation design and curriculum, participation policies, training partnerships and long-term sustainability. When building a program, using a comprehensive, thoughtful framework like the one presented here creates a sustainable foundation upon which future growth can more easily occur.

References

1. The Obstetrics and Gynecology Milestone Project. *J Grad Med Educ.* 2014;6:129–143.

2. National Abortion Federation. *The Abortion Option: A Values Clarification Guide for Health Care Professionals.* Washington, DC: National Abortion Federation, 2005.

3. Steinauer JE, Hawkins M, Turk JK, Darney P, Preskill F, Landy U. Opting out of abortion training: benefits of partial participation in a dedicated family planning rotation for ob-gyn residents. *Contraception.* 2013;87:88–92.

4. American College of Obstetricians and Gynecologists. ACOG Committee Opinion No. 385 November 2007: the limits of conscientious refusal in reproductive medicine. *Obstet Gynecol.* 2007;110:1203–1208.

5. Committee on Health Care for Underserved Women. ACOG Committee Opinion No. 612: abortion training and education. *Obstet Gynecol.* 2014;124: 1055–1059.

6. Committee on Health Care for Underserved Women. ACOG Committee Opinion No. 613: increasing access to abortion. *Obstet Gynecol.* 2014;124: 1060–1065.

Chapter

18

Creating and Implementing a Curriculum for Reproductive and Sexual Health Training Programs

Laura MacIsaac and Rachel Masch

18.1 Purpose

A curriculum in reproductive and sexual health serves as the foundation on which the learner builds and integrates knowledge in the family planning field. Curricula built from diverse sources of information encourage a comprehensive experience by "challenging [learners] to elaborate, explain, justify and/or compare and contrast information [and to] encourage them to apply information to clinical ... problems" [1]. In the USA, accreditation organizations at all levels of medical education – undergraduate, graduate and continuing medical education – require written curricula with clearly defined educational objectives, methods and evaluations to address core competencies in health-care delivery. Residency and fellowship training programs use milestones as the backbone for structuring objectives, curricula and assessment of learners at various levels. Globally, many countries require in-service training exams, licensing exams and maintenance of certification exams that expect mastery of medical knowledge acquired through educational curricula. In addition, a robust reproductive and sexual health curriculum can ensure that the next generation of medical providers obtains the necessary knowledge and skills to address the needs of the populations they serve. Medical educators must develop materials, clinical experiences and evaluation tools that hold the learners, faculty, and educational institutions accountable to these societal needs.

A conceptual framework for curriculum development, such as Kern's six-step model, incorporates the following: (i) problem identification and general needs assessment, (ii) targeted needs assessment, (iii) goals and objectives, (iv) educational strategies, (v) implementation and (vi) evaluation and feedback [2]. More specifically, to help clarify the purpose and scope of a program, start with a checklist [3] that identifies:

○ The target audience, with particular attention to their level of training
○ Goals and objectives of the rotation
○ The content to be covered and over what period of time
○ How the didactic experience will be integrated into clinical training
○ How the curriculum materials will be reviewed and with/by whom
○ How to verify an adequate level of mastery of the subject matter
○ How the curriculum is kept current/up to date
○ The relevant milestones and how they have been met (see Chapter 19)

18.2 Needs Assessment and Target Audience

18.2.1 Needs Assessment

The first step in building a sexual and reproductive health curriculum is to do a thoughtful needs assessment. This analysis must identify gaps in the current educational experience, taking into account the needs of all stakeholders – the patients, providers, the teaching institution, the health-care delivery system and, most broadly, society. A good needs assessment describes how an educational intervention can contribute to solving the health-care problem at hand. Components of the assessment provide information on the target audience of learners, the outcomes to be achieved and the resources available. Consider the following when building a needs assessment:

● The number of learners
● The number of faculty

- How the time will be split among all of the different learning methods available
- The available resources
- Whether there is reliable access to inter/intranet and other technological tools

A targeted needs assessment more clearly defines the learners, their level of baseline fluency with the material (cognitive, psychomotor skills and other behavioral competencies) and the time frame in which the learning experience will be completed.

18.2.2 Target Audience/Adult Learning

Ideally, a curriculum should be flexible enough to meet the needs of diverse learners, based on how it is organized and utilized. Understand your target audience: learners in family planning may be at different stages of their professional growth, but all have a wide variety of past experiences that dictate their approach to learning new materials. There is a large body of research about how adults learn, and when building a curriculum for these learners, it is important to remember that adults learn if [4]:

○ They want to learn
○ The learning is relevant to their current situation
○ They are told the "why" and not just the "what"
○ They can use past experiences to solve current problems.

In addition, durable learning in adults requires them to challenge what they think they know and apply critical thinking and reflection to openly confront long-held cultural beliefs and prior knowledge. Lastly, adults learn best by doing, so presenting them with cases, patients and situations that are relevant to their clinical experiences will help cement didactic concepts and elevate critical thinking [5].

The target learning community may be approaching a reproductive and sexual health curriculum from very different areas of health care, as well as from varying tiers of education. These may include:

- Student, resident, fellow (in nursing or medicine or social science)
- Health educators/counselors
- Nurses
- Advanced-practice clinicians (APCs)
- Physicians from various disciplines

The level of training, prerequisite skills and prior knowledge and experiences of the learner will dictate which materials/chapters from the comprehensive curriculum will be assigned and evaluated. It is important to remember that the various career stages may not correspond to familiarity or previous exposure to the subject matter; an experienced provider from a non-women's health specialty who is using the curriculum to obtain evidence-based information for her patients may use more of the basic materials to meet her objectives. The curriculum can include a wide range of topics and depth, and the instructor and learner can decide which parts are most relevant for their purposes and goals. The organizational structure should encourage flexibility, so that different learners from different levels of training as well as across different areas of health care will be able to extract appropriate components and build a curricular program to suit their needs.

18.3 Educational Strategies: Goals, Objectives and Content

18.3.1 Goals and Objectives

Once the needs of target learners and desired outcomes have been gathered and organized, clear goals and objectives can be written and reviewed together to ensure that both learner and faculty have aligned aims. Specific outcomes for the learner fall into one of three categories: cognitive (knowledge), affective (professionalism, values clarification) or psychomotor (skills). When resources (including time) are limited, prioritization of objectives facilitates rational allocation of those resources.

An agile and dynamic curriculum can adapt to fit the needs of learners of different levels and from different areas of the health-care system. It can also be used by one learner or a cohort of students. A horizontal structure allows a learner to select from a broad range of topics within the overall syllabus. Adding "verticality" to this structure, however, allows the material to be organized by depth of complexity – from beginner to master. Thus, the first tier of a certain topic or section can be assigned to beginners (eg, students) and include basic chapters and review articles, whereas the next tier of materials is more complex and challenging, and may include literature reviews, practice bulletins, national or international guidelines and original research. The highest level in a subject area includes modules that support "train the trainer" expectations.

18.3.1.1 Content Framework: Building Your Library

A comprehensive syllabus of current concepts in reproductive and sexual health enables trainees to enhance their fund of knowledge and use evidence-based decision making to reinforce their clinical training and to better counsel patients. The outline in Figure 18.1 is a suggested list of the major topics and subtopics to be included in a reproductive and sexual health syllabus. Depending on each site's or learner's needs, these modules can be addressed in their entirety or taught individually. Each of these topics can be

linked to additional online materials for an enhanced learning experience. In the USA, the Accreditation Council for Graduate Medical Education (ACGME) uses milestones to track a learner's progress in obstetrics and gynecology (ob-gyn) residency programs [6]. Milestones are the most common method to organize learning objectives and assign learning. (See Chapter 19.)

A modular format, by major topic heading, breaks the syllabus up into manageable blocks on which to base a learning schedule. The schedule can vary depending on the overall duration of the learning experience, on the level of the trainee and on the desired objectives and milestones to be mastered. One module, or a combination of them, may be assigned each week, which allows the

---

1. Gender equality

   - Safe sex, safe abortion, global statistics, abortion mortality, countries as case studies, economics, policy (cite local law), access to effective contraception and public health, reducing unintended pregnancies and sexually transmitted infections (STIs)

2. Counseling & Consent

   - Psychosocial; ambivalence; challenging social situations; shared decision and informed consent; how to effectively counsel on complications (recommend a video)

3. Pain control for medical and surgical abortions

4. Surgical abortion in the first trimester

5. Surgical abortion in the second trimester

6. Complicated/challenging abortions

7. Medication abortion in the first trimester

8. Induction abortion in the second trimester

9. Early Pregnancy Loss (EPL)

10. Pregnancy of Unknown Location (PUL)

11. Short-acting contraception

12. Long-acting contraception

13. LBGQTIA+ (Lesbian Gay Bisexual Transgender Queer/Questioning Intersex Asexual +)

Figure 18.1 Example Table of Contents for Reproductive and Sexual Health Syllabus

learner to focus their didactic activities on the materials within those specific sections. Or, if the learner is there for only a short time, picking the topic(s) that is/are of most interest can achieve their personal objectives. Administering a pre-test and post-test to learners for each module helps them identify gaps, focuses their learning and helps with retention of information [7].

18.4 Implementation

18.4.1 Prerequisites

"Implementation is critical to the success of any curriculum. It is the step that converts a mental exercise to reality" [2].

Fulfill the following prerequisites before starting implementation:

- Procure resources:
    - Faculty development in creative and effective teaching skills (online courses can minimize cost and time away)
    - Dedicated time for the learner to interact with curriculum and the faculty to teach
    - Opportunities for the learner to demonstrate knowledge
    - Materials such as paper, binders, copiers and/or computers, simulation supplies
- Identify and address the barriers to implementation
- Pilot the curriculum before introducing it to all targeted learners
    - Allows assessment of usability and gives opportunities to make adjustments
- Assign the curriculum to the target audience on a schedule and by module
- Assign roles and a time frame
    - Who will teach/evaluate what content, when and by which methods
- Refine the curriculum over successive cycles (next section).

18.4.2 Teaching Methods

Using multiple and diverse methods to introduce, teach to mastery, and then integrate medical knowledge and skills will facilitate the learner's ability to achieve and maintain higher-order and complex objectives. Cognitive, psychomotor or attitudinal/behavioral objectives are best taught

by a separate set of teaching methods for each. The most effective approaches for each are outlined below:

- Cognitive skills:
    - Assigned readings in a syllabus
    - In-person or video lectures
        - Based on adult learning theory, successful lectures are those that are interactive, e.g. using audience response systems or active audience participation with case-based scenarios [8]
    - Online resources: webinars, interactive case-based scenarios
    - Small group discussions
- Psychomotor skills:
    - Simulation (see Chapter 22)
    - Supervised clinical experiences
    - Standardized patients
    - Role-playing
- Attitudinal/professional skills:
    - Role-modeling
    - Audio or video reviews of standardized patient interactions
    - Values clarification programs

Educational technology affords the opportunity to expand access to many learners. Online curricula can be blended with face-to-face learning and reading. Technological advances in medical education are expanding rapidly. If the resources are available, animation and virtual reality in a simulation environment can efficiently introduce the psychomotor skills needed for surgical training prior to experience with patients. Video gaming has been used for both psychomotor skills acquisition as well as complex decision making [5] but requires more extensive resources.

When curricula are accessible via cloud computing, learners with access to computers and the internet are able to review interactive materials at many different times and locations. For those without this access, a binder with the required written content, organized by learning objective and competency, provides the written aspects of the curriculum. Lectures with slides can be printed and placed in binder. Assure that all necessary copyright permissions have been obtained.

Healthy, high-functioning health-care teams are essential to optimize patient safety and provider wellness. Team-based care relies on expert interpersonal communication, psychological safety and mutual respect of all team members [9]. If the learner does not have alternative opportunities to master these skills, they can be taught during the reproductive and sexual health rotation with workshops on professionalism, team-based care and values-clarification.

Incorporating different teaching modalities into the experience can ensure that the learner remains interested and engaged and has successfully assimilated the required material. Mastery of educational content learned by different modalities is more effective as well as durable.

18.5 Evaluation and Modification

18.5.1 Evaluation of the Learner

At each stage and module, and at the end of an educational program, learners are evaluated for progress on their milestones and success toward fulfilling all goals and objectives. Evaluations start by clearly articulating the observable and measurable skills and knowledge base that are expected to be mastered at the end of each section of the curriculum (a formative assessment) and then again at the completion of the course as a whole (a summative assessment). Formative assessments throughout the rotation/course enable the learner to identify their areas of strength and weakness, and address specific gaps in their knowledge, while also alerting the educator to the areas that need more focus. With periodic formative assessments, feedback can be integrated into each learner's progress throughout the experience. By tracking the progress of each learner at regular intervals, constructive action is able to be taken, if necessary, while the student is still immersed in the training experience. Summative assessments are an objective way to ensure that the overall course objectives have been met. They can also afford both the educator and the student an opportunity to evaluate the experience and give feedback on what areas of the curriculum were strong and which need modification.

There are several types of formative assessments. For cognitive objectives, the learner can complete a pre-test prior to beginning the rotation. This serves to give both the learner and the educator a benchmark of the trainee's fund of knowledge. From there, the syllabus is reviewed and a schedule determined that correlates with the length of the rotation. The learner should know in advance what sections of the syllabus they will be held accountable for and by when, and then each module of the curriculum has an assessment – whether it is a quiz, a two-way question/answer exchange, a case/patient-based scenario or an interactive computer program. These formative assessments allow for periodic assessment of fluency in the cognitive objectives, proper navigation of the curriculum in all its aspects, and should match the objectives and milestones that have been previously discussed. After the completion of the rotation, a comprehensive post-test that addresses all of the sections can be given to ensure adequate retention and recall of the material. Summative post-tests should mirror portions of other exams that may be required during residency, fellowship or licensing evaluations. Evaluation of clinical skills is discussed in Chapter 19.

18.5.2 Evaluation of the Program

The development of a successful curriculum never really ends; it evolves based on evaluation results, new learners and updated information. It is important to have a strategy that continually revises and reforms the curriculum based on how well it is meeting the instructional purposes and needs of its target audience. Keep the syllabus dynamic. New resources can be added, and older or less relevant ones removed to keep the curriculum streamlined and not overwhelming to the learner. The following are suggestions for keeping the curriculum relevant, manageable and meeting the users' needs:

- Keeping in mind copyright laws and ensuring that you have permission to use the content, search for new sources relevant to the topic:
  - by module, and
  - by content modality (written, video, interactive, simulation)
- Assess the need to add or delete major topics/sections
- Assess the navigation of material from a user's perspective
- Purge older/irrelevant references from each domain
- Revise assessment tools

○ One strategy to keep the syllabus relevant to the audience: request that each learner adds and deletes at least one question to the curriculum assessment tool and/or to each module's quiz [10]

Evaluation of the program can be used not only to drive the ongoing improvement of a curriculum, but also to gain support and resources, and, in educational research endeavors, to answer questions about the effectiveness of a specific section of the curriculum or the relative merits of different educational approaches. An added benefit to a regular (eg., annual) evaluation of an educational program is that it promotes trust and investment in the program leadership. A critical component of this annual program evaluation is a thorough review of the curriculum and all of its components. In the USA, the ACGME requires every residency and fellowship program to perform an annual program evaluation (APE) at least once per year and to make recommendations to improve each program in the domains of educational leadership, faculty, curriculum, teaching methods and assessment tools. The evaluation of an educational experience provides a quantitative, systematic approach for collecting data to analyze the effectiveness and efficiency of that training, and can also be utilized for resource allocation at the departmental leadership level.

To summarize, curriculum creation and implementation should include the following steps:

- Assessment of needs: patient, provider, institution, society
- Identification and description of the target audience (learners)
- Formulation of clear goals, objectives and milestones to be achieved
- Determination of content to create a syllabus
- Creation of a learning schedule agreed upon by trainer and learner
- Implementation using a diverse range of learning modalities (books, videos, interactive sessions, flipped classrooms, case-based simulation programs)
- Evaluation of both the learner and the program at regular intervals (at least annually)
- Modify and incorporate feedback from the end user, the learners.

A well-built and dynamic curriculum in sexual and reproductive health creates the essential framework through which learners can achieve mastery and competence in the knowledge and skills required to provide outstanding family planning care.

References

1. Hauer KE, Boscardin C, Brenner JM, van Schaik SM, Papp KK. Twelve tips for assessing medical knowledge with open-ended questions: designing constructed response examinations in medical education. *Med Teach*. 2020;**42**(8):880–885. doi:10.1080/0142159X.2019.1629404.

2. Kern D. Overview: a six-step approach to curriculum development. In P Thomas, DE Kern, MT Hughes, BY Chen (Eds.), *Curriculum Development for Medical Education: A Six-Step Approach*, 3rd ed. Baltimore, MD: Johns Hopkins University Press; 2016:5–9.

3. Interstate Renewable Energy Council. Basic guidelines for training curriculum: key components of a curriculum. https://irecusa.org/workforce-education/training-resources/best-practices-the-series/best-practices-2-curriculum-program-development/key-components-of-a-curriculum/. Accessed July 11, 2019.

4. Taylor David CM, Hamdy Hossan. Adult learning theories: implications for learning and teaching in medical education: AMEE Guide No. 83. *Med Teach*. 2013;**35**(11):e1561–1572. https://doi.org/10.3109/0142159X.2013.828153

5. Thomas P, Abras C. Step 4: educational strategies. In P Thomas, DE Kern, MT Hughes, BY Chen (Eds.), *Curriculum Development for Medical Education: A Six-Step Approach*, 3rd ed. Baltimore, MD: Johns Hopkins University Press; 2016:57–83.

6. Council of Resident Education in Obstetrics and Gynecology – American College of Obstetricians and Gynecologists (CREOG-ACOG). *Educational Objectives: Core Curriculum in Obstetrics and Gynecology*, 11th ed. Washington, DC: American College of Obstetricians and Gynecologists; 2016.

7. Sweet LR, Palazzi DL. Application of Kern's six-step approach to curriculum development by global health residents. *Educ Health (Abingdon)*. 2015 May–Aug;**28**(2):138–141. doi:10.4103/1357-6283.170124

8. Hermsen JL, Mokadam NA, Verrier ED. Flipping the classroom: how to optimize

learning in the didactic setting. *Thorac Surg Clin.* 2019;**29**(3):279–284. doi:https://doi.org/10.1016/j.thorsurg.2019.04.002

9. Yang SC. The alternative surgical curriculum. *Thorac Surg Clin.* **29**(3):291–301. doi:10.1016/j.thorsurg.2019.04.003

10. Kurtz JB, Lourie MA, Holman EE, Grob KL, Monrad SU. MCQs: creating assessments as an active learning strategy: what are students' perceptions? A mixed methods study. *Med Educ Online.* 2019;**24**:1. https://doi.org/10.1080/10872981.2019.1630239

19

Assessing Competence in Family Planning Skills through Milestones

Sabrina Holmquist

One of the cornerstones of any training program is defining and measuring competence: what knowledge, skills and attitudes must a graduate of the training program demonstrate in order to be considered competent, or ready for independent practice? How can incremental progress toward competence be measured and recorded? In this chapter, we will explore the conceptual framework of competency-based medical education and the evolution of competencies to milestones in formal graduate medical education. We will describe how the milestones for the Fellowship in Complex Family Planning were developed and implemented, and finally we will explore how milestones can be used to assess and document learner competence outside of a traditional medical training model, using the framework of mastery learning.

19.1 Competency-Based Education and Training in Medicine

Both physician and nursing education programs employ a competency-based education and training (CBET) model, in which learners are expected to demonstrate *clinical competency* in a defined set of objectives prior to being entrusted to provide independent patient care. Clinical competency is defined in the nursing literature as "the overarching set of knowledge, skills and attitudes required to practice safely and effectively without direct supervision" (the UK-based Nursing & Midwifery Council), and by the Accreditation Council for Graduate Medical Education (ACGME) as the "knowledge, skills and attitudes necessary for entry into unsupervised practice." The goal of a CBET model, according to the World Health Organization, is "a health professional who can practice medicine at a defined level of proficiency, in accord with local conditions, to meet local needs" [1]. Renamed competency-based medical education

(CBME) by the ACGME in 1999, CBME is defined as "an outcomes-based approach to the design, implementation, assessment and evaluation of a medical education program using an organizing framework of competencies " [2]. Principles and characteristics of CBME are listed in Table 19.1.

Medical education regulatory bodies in North America began developing conceptual frameworks embracing CBME principles in the 1990s, beginning with the Royal College of Physicians and Surgeons of Canada. The Royal College, which oversees medical education for all Canadian-trained physicians, developed the CanMEDS model in 1996 (Figure 19.1), whose main purpose is "to define the necessary competencies for all areas of medical practice and provide a comprehensive foundation for medical education and practice in Canada" [4]. This framework, which has undergone two revisions, most recently in 2015, has been adopted by dozens of countries worldwide, and is currently "the most widely accepted and applied physician competency framework in the world" [5].

In 1999, the ACGME, in collaboration with the American Board of Medical Specialties (ABMS) introduced the conceptual framework of the six domains of clinical competence (Figure 19.2). The Outcome Project, as this initiative was dubbed in 2001, sought to "focus education on the competency domains, enhance assessment of resident performance and increase utilization of educational outcomes for improving residents' education" [6]. This general competencies framework was adopted by all US graduate and continuing medical accrediting, certifying and licensing organizations, thus shaping the content, quality and standards of medical education for all practicing US physicians. However, while the Outcome Project represented an improvement over previous accreditation systems,

Table 19.1 Principles and characteristics of competency-based educational modules [3]

Principles	Characteristics
1. Competencies are role derived (eg, physician, physician assistant, nurse practitioner), specified in behavioral terms and made public.	1. Learning is individualized.
2. Assessment criteria are competency based and specify what constitutes mastery level of achievement.	2. Feedback to the learner is critical.
3. Assessment requires performance as the prime evidence but also takes knowledge into account.	3. Emphasis is more on the exit criteria than on the admission criteria.
4. Individual learners progress at rates dependent on demonstrated competency.	4. Modules requires a systematic program (approach).
5. The instructional program facilitates development and evaluation of the specific competencies.	5. Training is modularized
	6. Both the learner and the program have accountability.

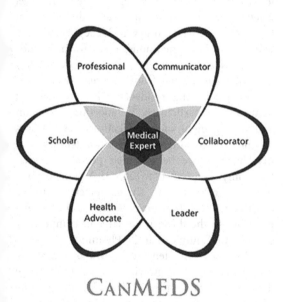

Figure 19.1 CanMEDS framework

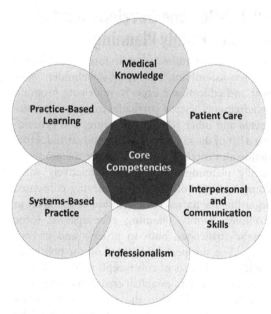

Figure 19.2 ACGME six core competencies

implementation proved thorny. Lack of a shared mental model of competency both within and between disciplines, as well as a paucity of standardized assessment instruments and curricula, led to wide variation in both what was taught and how competence was assessed. In an effort to operationalize the competencies in a meaningful way, and provide a developmental framework on which to build residency and fellowship programs, the ACGME introduced the Next Accreditation System in 2007, which first introduced the concept of milestones in graduate medical education [7].

19.2 Milestones and Graduate Medical Education

Milestones are the latest iteration of the ACGME's ongoing effort to implement a continuous accreditation process for graduate medical education programs. Based on the Dreyfus model of skill acquisition [8], "milestones are competency-based developmental outcomes (eg, knowledge, skills, attitudes, and performance) that can be demonstrated progressively by residents and fellows from the beginning of their education through graduation to the unsupervised practice of their specialties" [9]. Practically speaking, milestones provide a narrative description of the performance levels along a developmental continuum that learners are expected to demonstrate for skills, knowledge, and behaviors in the six competency domains. Milestones have been developed by specialty groups across the continuum of graduate medical education, and were implemented for obstetrics and gynecology (ob-gyn) residency training beginning in 2013. Milestones have since been developed and implemented for the four fellowships in ob-gyn certified by the American Board of Medical Specialties (ABMS); in 2015, work was begun on milestone development for the Complex Family Planning fellowship.

19.3 Milestone Development for Complex Family Planning

The process of authoring milestones for any field involves assembling a group of stakeholders, content and educational experts; reviewing program requirements, shared curricula, competency statements and other relevant literature; and generating a list of the knowledge, skills and attitudes that define an expert in the field. While the academic family planning community is relatively small compared with other fields, achieving consensus regarding the narrative description of an expert in Complex Family Planning encompassed some unique challenges, both in process and in outcome. As a subspecialty focused on the politically controversial areas of contraception and abortion care, it is crucial to establish credibility as medical experts not just within the medical community but increasingly in the media, the courts, the legislature and the court of public opinion. By defining *expert* in a way that is statistically rigorous, free of bias and incorporates the expertise of a quorum of experts in the field, Complex Family Planning gains legitimacy within the larger community of practice, evaluation and research in fellowship education, and "produc[es] highly competent physicians to meet the health and health care needs of the public" [9]. This rigorous process must also define scope of practice widely enough to encompass the complexities of providing comprehensive reproductive health care and abortion for medically complicated persons without excluding the general reproductive health-

care practitioner from providing routine contraception and abortion care for straightforward, medically uncomplicated persons. The ultimate goal of the Complex Family Planning milestones is to define and measure learner progress toward becoming a Complex Family Planning expert, without limiting contraception and abortion provision to those who are fellowship trained and thus further reducing the number of abortion providers in the USA.

All ACGME-accredited milestones follow a similar format, shown in Table 19.2.

The Complex Family Planning milestone template deviates slightly from the ACGME residency milestone template in that level 1 represents a deficiency rather than a floor; entry-level fellowship milestones begin at level 2 whereas entry-level resident milestones begin at level 1. Level 2 fellowship milestones are drawn directly from the relevant level 4 ob-gyn residency milestones, which describe a practitioner ready for independent practice, and theoretically the competency level of an incoming fellow. In recognition that not all graduating residents will have reached competency, particularly in abortion provision and management of complications, level 1 was retained to document progress for fellows who may have started behind their peers. Milestone taxonomy is described in Table 19.3; general competencies refer to the six competency models described in the Outcome Project, and subcompetencies to the thirteen domains of competency defined for Complex Family Planning.

These subcompetency domains, as well as the milestone sets and individual milestones, were developed from the *Fellowship in Family Planning Guide to Learning* (GTL), a document that provides a comprehensive educational curriculum, including program aims and competency-based goals and objectives, in accordance with the ACGME Common Program Requirements for post-graduate fellowships. The GTL is a comprehensive, granular description of the skills and knowledge required of a fellowship graduate; it provides an endpoint, but does not describe the trajectory of a learner. The milestones provide that trajectory, describing the specific knowledge, skills and attitudes expected as learners progress from incoming fellows to fully qualified Complex Family Planning experts.

The Complex Family Planning milestones were written by a single author, piloted for a

Table 19.2 Milestone template for ACGME and Complex Family Planning fellowship

	Milestone Description: Template				
	Level 1	Level 2	Level 3	Level 4	Level 5
ACGME residency framework	Expectations for a beginning resident	Milestone performance above entry level, but lower than mid-residency expectations	Milestone performance at mid-residency level	Ready for independent practice in the specialty	Aspirational level; exceeds expectations
Complex Family Planning framework	**Critical deficiencies**[*] – The fellow demonstrates milestones at a lower than expected level for a graduating resident[*].	The fellow demonstrates milestones expected for a **graduating resident/** incoming fellow or **early learner.**	The fellow is making progress toward achieving the requisite milestones; **mid-learner.**	The fellow has achieved fellowship milestones **sufficient for graduation/ independent practice,** including expert-level proficiency in the practice and teaching of family planning.	The fellow has progressed beyond fellowship proficiency and has achieved **aspirational** levels, including original and substantive contribution to the body of scientific and clinical knowledge and practice.

[*] While a "critical deficiencies" level has been omitted for most other specialties, it was retained for the Complex Family Planning milestones in order to capture residents whose family planning residency training was deficient, and document progress for fellows who may have started behind their peers.

Table 19.3 Milestone taxonomy

General competency

Sub-competency

Set of milestones

M1: Anatomy and Physiology of Reproduction: Medical Knowledge

Level 1	Level 2	Level 3	Level 4	Level 5
Incomplete working knowledge of pelvic anatomy. Incomplete understanding of the physiology of the normal menstrual cycle.	Demonstrates knowledge of the anatomy and function of pelvic structures, cervical canal and uterine cavity, including vascular and neurologic supply. Demonstrates in-depth knowledge of the physiology of the normal menstrual cycle. Demonstrates basic knowledge of the physiology of conception *and how various contraceptive methods interrupt these processes*.	Demonstrates in-depth knowledge of menstrual cycle variations due to normal as well as pathologic causes, and is able to use a focused diagnostic approach to generate a comprehensive management plan. Specific milestone	Demonstrates the ability to formulate evidence-based management plans for women with complex co-morbid conditions. Able to provide expert consultation regarding contraception in women with complex conditions affecting their menstrual cycle. Provides instruction and/or mentorship to learners in the areas of reproductive anatomy and/or physiology.	Contributed to research and/or clinical care guidelines in the areas of the physiology of conception, reproductive endocrinology as it relates to pregnancy and/or contraception and new applications of contraceptive technology on the physiology of reproduction.

period of nine months and then vetted within the larger academic fellowship community using a modified Delphi method. Originally described by the RAND corporation in the 1950s, the Delphi method (or Delphi technique) is a widely accepted method of achieving consensus among a group of experts in a particular content area concerning real-world knowledge [10]. The method consists of conducting a series of surveys over two to four iterations to collect data from a panel of experts, with the goal of achieving group consensus utilizing an anonymous feedback process to which statistical methods can be applied. The Delphi method was chosen for a number of reasons. For example, it collates expert opinion anonymously, minimizing the dominant individual effect (in which participants with the most seniority or the loudest voices dominate a conversation). It also provides a controlled feedback process, minimizing the noise created when participants in an open discussion focus on individual concerns or side conversations. Finally, the Delphi method facilitates the use of statistical analysis to decrease bias from dominant voices, coercion or group pressure for conformity – everyone's vote, reported anonymously, counts the same. The Delphi method has been used to develop consensus milestones and assessment tools in a number of other fields, including milestones in Pulmonary/Critical Care Medicine for fellows, Neurology and Emergency Medicine for residents and Emergency Medicine for medical students.

Three rounds of surveys were conducted using the Delphi method: round 1 solicited both quantitative and qualitative responses concerning the number and content of the individual milestone subcompetencies. Responses were used to create a structured round 2 survey identifying areas of consensus (defined as >80% of respondents *not* suggesting revisions) and summarizing suggested revisions, on which participants voted. Areas lacking consensus after the second round were included in the final survey. All Delphi surveys were developed by the primary milestones author, and distributed using web-based survey software. Twenty-five fellowship directors (83%) from all regions of the country participated in some portion of this 20-month study; completion rates for the three rounds were 50% (9/18), 63% (12/19) and 86% (12/14), respectively. Of the 222 total subcompetencies across 15 original milestone areas, 119 (54%) achieved consensus in the first round, and 91% in the second round, including 19 subcompetencies in new or merged milestone areas. A 100% consensus across all subcompetencies was achieved after round 3; however, 13 additional questions regarding subcompetency order and content remained without consensus. These final areas were discussed and consensus obtained at an in-person fellowship director's meeting in the spring of 2018, at which point the final 13 Complex Family Planning milestones were finalized and introduced to all fellowship programs in July 2018.

19.4 Assessing Milestones: Best Practices

Milestones provide a framework on which to measure learner progress, but they do not provide the tools by which progress is measured. Indeed, in their *Milestones Guidebook* (2016), the ACGME specifically notes, "The entire Milestones document (set) . . . was never intended to serve as a regular assessment tool. . . . Instead, the Milestones should inform the use and development of assessment tools aligned with the curricular goals and tasks" [11]. When assessing milestone progress, there are three main factors to consider: the assessee (the learner), the assessor (the preceptor) and the assessment tool. We will consider each of these elements separately, and then discuss systems that bring them together.

19.5 The Learner

In order to be full participants, learners needs to be familiar with what is expected of them, the roadmap to get there and how their progress will be measured along the way. When implementing milestones, there are a number of suggested best practices to assure that learners are actively engaged in their own learning:

- Milestones should be shared with learners at the beginning of their fellowship or rotation, so they can develop a shared understanding of the learning goals and requirements for competence.

- Learners should be encouraged to develop an individualized learning plan (ILP), guided by the milestones and informed by an initial self-assessment, with feedback from their preceptor. This learning plan should be reviewed with their fellowship director or main preceptor at least twice annually.

- Learners should be equipped with the tools and opportunity to seek out direct observation and feedback from all clinical preceptors, as well as complete self-assessments at predetermined check-in intervals, not less than every six months. These assessments can be compared to other measures of performance and used to adjust the ILP.

- Learners should be empowered to provide feedback on the milestones themselves, and actively participate in milestone piloting and revision.

As described in the CBME model, learners are active participants in and have equal accountability for their educational program. Involving learners at all levels of milestone development and assessment can strengthen both the program and the quality and engagement of its graduates.

19.6 The Assessor

Any assessment program is only as good as its assessors; variation in learner ratings for a given assessment is invariably related to the assessor rather than the tool. Consequently, orienting all precepting faculty to the structure, content and purpose of the milestones is essential. Core faculty will need a global understanding of the milestones and assessment system, whereas clinical or research preceptors may only need to understand the subcompetencies applying to their setting and

Table 19.4 Milestones for the Fellowship in Complex Family Planning

Milestone Number	Competency Area	Sub-competency	Example of Level 2 Milestone (expected of incoming fellow)
M1	M	Anatomy and physiology of reproduction	Demonstrates basic knowledge of the physiology of conception and how various contraception methods interrupt these processes
M2	MK	Contraception	Demonstrates basic knowledge of combined hormonal contraceptives including pharmacology, mechanism of action, efficacy and side effects
M3	PC	Contraception	Counsels on the effectiveness, risks, benefits, and contraindications of all forms of available contraception
M4	MK/PC	Medical management of induced abortion or pregnancy loss in the first trimester	Demonstrates knowledge of all medical methods of first trimester medical uterine evacuation
M5	PC	Medical management of induced abortion or pregnancy loss in the second trimester	Counsels about and performs medical uterine evacuation in the second trimester, including appropriate selection and dosing of prostaglandin analogs
M6	PC	Surgical management of induced abortion or pregnancy loss in the first trimester	Demonstrates the ability to independently perform basic first trimester surgical uterine evacuation
M7	PC	Surgical management of induced abortion or pregnancy loss in the second trimester	Demonstrates the ability to perform basic second trimester surgical uterine evacuation, with supervision/assistance
M8	PC	Diagnosis and management of extra-uterine and pregnancy of unknown location (PUL)	Utilizes non-surgical and surgical methods to manage patients with tubal ectopic pregnancy
M9	ICS	Patient-centered communication and counseling	Demonstrates the ability to provide unbiased, evidence-based, nondirective pregnancy options counseling
M10	ICS	Communication with health-care teams	Communicates effectively with physicians and other health care professionals regarding patient care
M11	P	Professional ethics and accountability	Successfully navigates conflicts between patient preferences that are discordant with personal beliefs (Level 3)
M12	SBP	Public policy and advocacy	Demonstrates an awareness of the need for patient advocacy as it relates to reproductive health care and family planning
M13	PBLI	Research design, statistics and publication	Develop a hypothesis-based research project involving clinical subjects, bench research, analysis of an existing dataset or a combination of these, with mentorship (Level 3)

MK, Medical Knowledge; PC, Patient Care; ICS, Interpersonal and Communication Skills; P, Professionalism; SBP, Systems-Based Practice; PBLI, Practice-Based Learning and Improvement the assessment tools they will encounter. For example, a preceptor in a high-volume clinical setting may only need to focus on procedural and communication milestones, whereas a research mentor will need to understand and assess scholarly milestones. Best practices in training and supporting preceptors include:

- Orient faculty to the milestones at the beginning of the academic year, and provide ongoing faculty development in the areas of feedback, effective precepting, documenting teaching activity for promotion (where applicable) and working with challenging learners.
- Encourage preceptors to directly observe learners in a variety of settings, and provide both formative (for the purpose of learning, often given during or immediately after direct observation) and summative (for the purpose of assessment, often given remote from direct observation) feedback. Narrative feedback (in the form of comments rather than completion of checkboxes) is especially valuable.
- Provide preceptors with feedback and assessment tools that are short, easy to complete and targeted to their practice setting. Web- or app-based feedback tools that are accessible on a mobile phone, can be initiated by the learner, take less than five minutes to complete and aggregate data electronically are especially useful.
- Provide preceptors with feedback regarding their assessment completion, timeliness and quality. Providing assessors with feedback on their feedback will result in more useful learner assessments, and better feedback directly to the learners. Provide tangible evidence that their assessment efforts are vital to the program.

19.7 The Tools

Milestone assessment tools should closely mirror the activities that are being assessed, and should reflect the skills and attributes described in the milestones. Table 19.5 summarizes common assessment methods for each of the six core competencies.

Where possible, existing assessment tools with proven utility should be used or modified rather than creating tools de novo. Assessment utility, or how well an assessment works, relies on a number of assessment characteristics [12]:

Table 19.5 Sample assessment methods for the general competencies organized by ACGME six core competencies

Competency	Assessment method
Patient care, including surgical/procedural skills	Direct observation Procedure evaluation forms Quality performance measures Simulation Case logs
Medical knowledge	Summative exam (written or oral) Assessment of clinical reasoning: SNAPPS Didactic preparation and participation
Professionalism	Multi-source feedback Direct observation
Interpersonal and communication skills	Direct observation Multi-source feedback Simulation/standardized patients Observed teaching and assessment of teaching skills
Practice-Based Learning and Improvement	Quality improvement (QI) measures: application of evidence-based medicine to clinical practice Presentation of the literature/journal club Research activities (if applicable)
Systems-Based Practice	QI measures Multi-source feedback

- Validity: how well does the assessment measure what it's supposed to measure?
- Reliability: how accurate, or reproducible is the assessment tool? If two different assessors use the tool to assess the same learner, will they come up with the same assessment?
- Educational impact: does what you're assessing really matter?
- Acceptability: Is the tool in a format and of a length that is acceptable to your assessors?
- Feasibility: is the tool accessible, cost-efficient (in terms of money and time), and incorporable into the teaching setting?

Ideally, a truly useful assessment tool will demonstrate all five characteristics. This can sometimes be a balancing act – an exhaustive surgical check-list or a resource-intensive simulation that demonstrates exceptional inter-rater reliability but takes so long or so many resources to complete that no one does it is not feasible or acceptable, and consequently is not worth using. The goal of an assessment tool is not perfection, but it should be an easy-to-complete tool that provides timely, valid and useful feedback to the learner and the program director, and measures progress along the milestones with the eventual goal of documenting competency reliably.

19.8 Putting It All Together: Milestone Check-Ins, Demonstration of Competence and Remediation

Once you have written, refined and rolled out your milestones, oriented your learners and your preceptors and identified and deployed your assessment instruments, it's time to put your system into practice! Initially, you will need to determine the following:

1. How often will you conduct learner assessments?
2. How will you collect and aggregate the data?
3. How often will you review the data, and with whom?
4. How will you make decisions regarding promotion and eventual graduation?
5. How will you determine the need for and design a remediation plan?

19.8.1 Collecting Learner Assessments

The frequency of learner assessments depends on the type of competency or milestone being assessed, the location of the activity (clinical care vs research for example) and the assessor. Patient care milestones that focus on clinical or surgical skills are best assessed immediately after the clinical session or case, by an assessor who observed the care first-hand and can offer immediate feedback. Assessors should be encouraged to share formative feedback verbally with the learner in the moment; this can also be captured using a web- or app-based evaluation form that can be completed on a smart phone. Many residency and fellowship training programs employ health-care education management software packages (eg, MedHub^{TM}, New Innovations^{TM}, myTIPreport^{TM3}) which provide

procedure-specific assessment forms that can be completed in a matter of minutes with the preceptor and learner together. The primary advantage of these electronic systems is the data can be captured in the moment and immediately available in aggregate to the fellowship program director and the learner. Forms can also be tailored to the clinical setting or the specific procedure being performed, and performance indicators can be tied directly to the milestones. Downsides of these system include high subscription costs, training faculty to use the system and potential data overload (though too *many* assessments is rarely an issue!). Written assessment forms are a cheaper, potentially more accessible option but rely on the assessor or the learner to collect and turn the forms in to a coordinator who then has to enter the data manually.

Longitudinal milestones, such as research or public policy and advocacy, may be more amenable to periodic summative assessment. The ACGME has established clear guidelines regarding the minimum frequency of learner assessment: Learners must be assessed at the end of every core rotation, or at minimum every three months, and must have data from multiple evaluators. Healthcare education management software can aggregate a variety of assessment types from multiple assessors, map results to milestones and provide longitudinal progress reports on the individual fellow, individual milestone or program level. These tools can prove invaluable to the fellowship director and committees responsible for documenting fellow progress to competence.

19.8.2 Milestone Review: Promotion, Graduation and Remediation

The ACGME requires the program director to meet with the learner at least semi-annually to review milestones progress, revisit their individual learning plan, and identify areas of strength and possible enrichment, as well as areas for development. If deficiencies are noted in the learner's performance or they fail to progress, a plan detailing the area of concern, remediation plan, performance goals and timeframe for achievement must be documented, and an interim check-in scheduled. The program director must generate an annual summative evaluation as well as a final evaluation documenting competence across all of the milestone areas and learner readiness to enter independent practice. The following best practices in milestone documentation and review are suggested:

- Initial milestones assessment should occur in the first few months of training, to establish baseline performance and determine whether the learner has any deficiencies that need to be addressed in an expedited manner. For a fellow, For example, they a family planning fellow may have had no exposure to second-trimester procedures in residency.
- The individual learning plan should note areas of particular deficiency or initial expertise and be used to guide rotation order, length and experience to match a particular learner's needs.
- Milestone review at eighteen months, or six months prior to anticipated program completion, should document an adequate trajectory to competence. If the learner has any deficiencies that may result in their not achieving competence at the completion of their training, these should be addressed with a clear and realistic plan including performance goals and periodic check-ins that will allow them to reach competence by the completion of their program, or clearly demonstrate where they have fallen short. This will prevent the unpleasant discovery that the learner is not competent for independent practice at graduation, when there is no time left for remediation.

In ACGME-accredited programs, the program director is aided in this considerable responsibility by the clinical competency committee (CCC), which must consist of at least three people with substantive knowledge of the fellow's performance in a variety of settings, and include at least one core faculty member. The CCC must convene at a minimum every six months to review all learner assessments, milestone progress and advise the fellowship director regarding learner progress and promotion to the next level. This meeting must occur prior to the director's semi-annual meeting with the resident or fellow, at which time recommendations for remediation or short-interval review are communicated. The CCC provides independent review of the learner's progress, and documentation from this committee is invaluable in supporting readiness for independent practice, certifying competence and in the rare cases where learners must be placed on probation or dismissed from their training program.

19.8.3 Using Milestones Outside of a Formal Graduate Medical Education Program

While milestones were developed to measure progress and competence in formal graduate medical education programs, the concept can easily be applied to medical education or procedural training occurring outside of traditional GME programs. The ACGME Outcomes Project (2001) and the Next Accreditation System (NAS, 2007) have attempted to superimpose an outcomes-based assessment model onto the traditional education system, which relies on longitudinal patient experiences structured by time and location. In the traditional physician training model, learners progress through clinical clerkships, residency, fellowship and finally continuing medical education activities (measured in hours spent), with the assumption that learners will be exposed to a sufficient number of cases to achieve competency. This system does not reliably result in clinical competence, however. Numerous studies across a plurality of medical fields have demonstrated both skill and knowledge deficits due to ineffective clinical training [13]; some learners are able to demonstrate competence at the conclusion of their training period, whereas others require more time. This may be particularly true for abortion care, which is often insufficiently covered in residency training programs, and is entirely absent in fields other than ob-gyn and a limited number of family practice residency programs [14]. For providers who wish to perform abortions but did not receive training to competence during their medical training and choose not or are unable to complete a Complex Family Planning fellowship, milestones can be used to design, measure and document competency in abortion provision outside of the traditional medical training establishment, employing a mastery learning model.

Mastery learning, in which learners work to achieve specific educational competencies over a variable period of time, has been shown to yield more uniform competence among learners as compared to a time-defined model. As described by McGaghie in a 2015 publication, "Mastery learning means that trainees acquire essential knowledge, skills, and affective and professionalism attributes measured rigorously and compared with fixed achievement standards, without limiting the time needed to reach the outcome.

Mastery learning results are uniform with little or no variation among learners. By contrast, educational time can vary among learners" [15].

Mastery learning has [at least] the following seven complementary features [16]:

1. Baseline, or diagnostic testing;
2. Clear learning objectives, sequenced as units usually in increasing difficulty;
3. Engagement in educational activities (eg, deliberate skills practice, calculations, data interpretation, reading) focused on reaching the objectives;
4. A set minimum passing standard (eg, test score) for each educational unit;
5. Formative testing to gauge unit completion at a preset minimum passing standard for mastery;
6. Advancement to the next educational unit given measured achievement at or above the mastery standard; and
7. Continued practice or study on an educational unit until the mastery standard is reached.

When coupled with a competency-based education model, whose endpoint is demonstrated competency rather than time served, mastery learning yields a uniformly qualified group of learners, ready for independent practice. Operationally, competency-based education provides the framework for the educational system, and mastery learning serves as a model for how a learner progresses through it.

Designing a CBME program to teach abortion care outside of the traditional GME system using a Mastery Learning conceptual framework would involve the following steps:

1. Identification of the competencies required for independent abortion provision in a diversity of settings, depending on the needs of the community
2. Determination of the specific medical knowledge and clinical skills required for the full spectrum of abortion provision and complications management, broken down into performance levels, or milestones

3. Progressive arrangement of the above milestones, both within a skill set or module (eg, first-trimester uterine aspiration) and between modules of care (eg, medication abortion, followed by first-trimester uterine aspiration, followed by provision of IV sedation)
4. Identification of curricular materials that map to each milestone, and the skills, time, training and materials needed by training providers to facilitate learner progress to mastery
5. Development of milestone assessment tools to document the progressive development of learner competence, skill mastery and readiness for independent practice
6. Data collection and program evaluation, to assure goals are being met and allow for continuous quality improvement of the educational program

ILPs would be constructed based on the learner's baseline skills and desired level of competence. For example, a physician may be competent to provide uterine aspiration abortion to twelve weeks' gestation, but wish to increase to sixteen weeks. Their learning plan would look very different from that of a nurse practitioner who wants to start providing medication abortion in their community. The number and scope of milestones and the time needed to reach mastery would vary for each learner, but the definition of competence or mastery, based on standardized milestones for each clinical skill, would remain the same. Training programs could then adjust their assessment program to match their learner's needs, employing best practices and validated tools defined by the ACGME but shortening check-in intervals and changing the number and type of assessors as indicated. The development of robust mastery-based learning programs in abortion provision for providers outside of GME training has the potential to increase the number of abortion providers more rapidly and with significant less expense and fewer resources than traditional GME training programs.

References

1. McGaghie WC, Miller GE, Sajid AW, Telder TV. *Competency-Based Curriculum Development in Medical Education*. Geneva: World Health Organization; 1978.

2. Frank JR, Snell LS, Cate OT, et al. Competency based medical education: theory to practice. *Med Teach*. 2010;32 (8):638–645.

3. Elam S. *Performance-Based Teacher Education: What Is the State of the Art?* Washington, DC: American Association of Colleges for Teacher Education; 1971.

4. Royal College of Physicians and Surgeons of Canada. About CanMEDS. www

.royalcollege.ca/rcsite/
canmeds/about-canmeds-e

5. Frank JR, Snell L, Sherbino J.
    (Eds.). *Can Meds
    2015 Physician Competency
    Framework*. Ottawa: Royal
    College of Physicians and
    Surgeons of Canada; 2015.

6. Swing SR. The ACGME
    Outcome Project: retrospective
    and prospective. *Med Teach*.
    2007;29:648–654.

7. Holmboe ES, Yamazaki K,
    Edgar L, et al. Reflections on
    the first 2 years of milestone
    implementation. *J Grad Med
    Educ*. 2015;7(3): 506–512.

8. Dreyfus S, Dreyfus H. *A Five-
    Stage Model of the Mental
    Activities Involved in Directed
    Skill Acquisition*. Berkeley:
    University of California
    Operations Research Center;
    1980. Monograph. www.dtic
    .mil/dtic/index.html

9. Accreditation Council for
    Graduate Medical Education.
    Milestones. www.acgme.org/

acgmeweb/tabid/430/
Programand?
InstitutionalAccreditation/
NextAccreditationSystem/
Milestones.aspx

10. Hsu Ca-C, Sandford BA. The
    Delphi technique: making
    sense of consensus. *Pract Assess
    Res Eval*. 2007;12(10). http://
    pareonline.net/getvn.asp?v=
    12&n=10

11. Holmboe ES, Edgar L, Hamstra
    S. *The Milestones Guidebook
    Version 2016*. Chicago:
    ACGME; 2016.

12. Norcini J, Anderson B, Bollela
    V, et al. Criteria for good
    assessment: consensus
    statement and
    recommendations from the
    Ottawa 2010 Conference. *Med
    Teach*. 2011;33:206–214.

13. Issenberg SB, McGaghie WC.
    *Looking to the Future.
    International Best Practices for
    Evaluation in the Health
    Professions*. London: Radcliffe
    Publishing; 2013:341–359.

14. Steinauer JE, Turk JK,
    Pomerantz T, Simonson K,
    Learman LA, Landy U.
    Abortion training in US
    obstetrics and gynecology
    residency programs. *Am
    J Obstet Gynecol*. 2018 Jul;
    219(1):86.e1–86.e6.

15. McGaghie WC. Mastery
    learning: it is time for
    medical education to
    join the 21st century.
    Acad Med. 2015;90:
    1438–1441.

16. McGaghie WC, Siddall VJ,
    Mazmanian PE, Myers J,
    American College of Chest
    Physicians Health and Science
    Policy Committee. Lessons for
    continuing medical education
    from simulation research in
    undergraduate and graduate
    medical education:
    effectiveness of continuing
    medical education: American
    College of Chest Physicians
    Evidence-Based Educational
    Guidelines. *Chest*. 2009;
    135(3 Suppl):62S–68S.

Chapter

20

Educating and Mentoring Medical Students in Family Planning

Carla Lupi

20.1 Background

The emergence of family planning in recent years as an element of the required curricula at some US medical schools is cause for celebration. This increase is owed to pressures and support from different fronts, including student activists calling out the neglect of this critical area of women's health; committed faculty joining the ranks of educational leaders in women's health; and medical education reformers advocating for the need to align curricula to address major public health needs. While most working in the field over these years can agree that progress has been made, the extent of the progress is not clearly known, as systematic and periodically collected data on family planning as a topic in US undergraduate medical education (UME) are lacking. That said, the limited available evidence consistently reveals large gaps [1]. In a recent survey of fourth-year students from thirty-seven US medical schools, 72% rated as inadequate their clerkship and preclinical education in knowledge of abortion. Forty-five percent found their learning of contraceptive technology and counseling significantly lacking [2]. An assessment of knowledge among fourth-year students at a Canadian medical school uncovered a degree of misinformation that could significantly and negatively impact patient care [3].

While family planning educators can easily view these lapses as the consequence of missing content, the larger medical education community has recognized over the past two decades that even when content is included in a curriculum, students do not walk across the graduation stage with many of the core skills and knowledge included in that curriculum [4]. This stark fact points to deficiencies in the traditional curricular approaches of medical education and has led to a recent movement toward curricula organized as systems of competency or outcomes-based education. This approach includes working across the

entirety of a medical school program to provide developmentally appropriate opportunities for knowledge acquisition and application, for repeated skills practice with feedback, for intentional development of professional identity and for participation in advocacy toward improved health outcomes for patients and communities. Systems-based approach also requires moving beyond assessment done simply to pass courses and clerkships [5] to assessment that aggregates and holistically synthesizes assessment data to make repeated judgments of evolving trainee competence [6].

While adoption of outcomes-based systems has begun, obstacles exist and most institutions are far from realizing full-scale implementation. Therefore, at a larger level, the challenges of the family planning educator community within UME going forward are twofold. First, educators must continue to overcome factors that have historically marginalized family planning and abortion in medical curricula. These factors include overt resistance from institutions and faculty who are uncomfortable with or morally opposed to family planning services, the need to tailor learning to the range of students' ethical positions and a continued devaluing of women's and reproductive health in health professions education. Second, family planning educators must partner with other medical educators to achieve a successful system of outcomes-based education.

Family planning educators and medical students can find themselves in a variety of roles with respect to building family planning curricula and reforming undergraduate medical education: advocating for inclusion, mentoring students, teaching, designing instructional elements, designing assessments of learning and/or designing and overseeing larger scale curricular reform. Regardless of the specific role, faculty members or students may be interested in careers in academic medicine that focus on medical education.

This chapter addresses individuals in each of these situations, calling out frameworks and resources currently available to draw from.

20.2 Advocating for Curricular Inclusion

Successfully advocating for curricular inclusion of family planning care requires having clear arguments and a strategy based on understanding curricular management and quality improvement at the institution. Careful preparation is one component of minimizing resistance to inclusion. Following a widely accepted framework for curricular design [7], they should be able to outline the public health need for family planning care and then determine what in fact is and is not in the curriculum. As the Liaison Committee on Medical Education (LCME) has recently mandated the establishment [8] of continually updated databases, or "curriculum maps," that allow searching of the entire curriculum by various identifiers, faculty and students should be able to obtain this information from the offices of education deans. An important caveat here is that these databases are often limited to where and how a content area or skillset is taught. Information on when or how, if at all, assessment occurs, is less often easily available but equally if not more valuable. For example, a curriculum map may show that contraception is taught in a problem-based learning session and that contraceptive counseling is taught in a clerkship but have no information about assessment. Without assessment of contraceptive counseling in the clinical and/or in simulation, for example, the success of the teaching is not known.

With this information in hand, the next step is to determine gaps – the difference between what should be and what is actually in the curriculum. When considering what should be, a generally accepted starting point is the acknowledged goal in undergraduate medical education of developing the "general undifferentiated medical student" who is prepared to enter a residency and ultimately practice in any specialty of their choice. The vast majority of these "undifferentiated" students will care for reproductive-aged women and men who, if heterosexually active, will spend most of their reproductive-aged years needing pregnancy prevention. While attending to contraception is largely in the domain of primary care, doctors providing specialty and subspecialty care will still encounter patients for whom the risks of pregnancy are well above average and for whom contraceptive care requires additional judgment and expertise. Given the continuing high rates of unintended pregnancy in the USA, and the frequent use of pregnancy testing in outpatient, inpatient and emergency room (ER) settings, almost all physicians will encounter patients to whom they will have to convey news of an unintended pregnancy. Therefore, the likelihood that most medical students will need some if not all of the following "core knowledge and skills" during residency and in practice is high:

1. Knowledge and skills required for contraceptive counseling, including the ability to screen for intimate partner violence and reproductive coercion

2. The ability to access and apply updated information on all available contraceptive methods

3. The skill of routine screening regarding intentions for pregnancy to determine the need for contraception (or pre-conception care)

4. The skill of conveying the news of a positive pregnancy test and initiating non-directive pregnancy options counseling

5. The ability to examine one's own emotions, values and attitudes regarding patients and their circumstances, and mitigate potential threats to person-centered and timely care and to patient autonomy during contraceptive counseling, non-directive pregnancy options counseling and abortion counseling

6. The early skills of identifying resources and advocating for patients with limited resources and/or obtaining care in under-resourced systems

With the gaps identified, educators must move on to considering where to make the case and exactly how to frame their case for filling the gaps.

In recent years, accreditors have begun to mandate a move away from curricular management driven by departments and course directors to a more centralized model of committees and subcommittees with student and broad faculty representation. These structures can and do facilitate change; advocates are beginning to leverage them to do so [9].

Beyond calling out the needs of the "undifferentiated medical student," what other arguments will resonate with those in curricular management roles and on committees? One is the potential for the learning of proposed curricular content to contribute to the school's educational program outcomes – a list of the learning outcomes expected of all graduates. The LCME requires that schools use these outcomes to guide all curricular change and to monitor curricular success. While the expression of these outcomes varies substantially between schools, they are often organized around one of the two sets of competency domains used in US medical education. The five skills defined above fit easily within either set of domains.

Two sets of overlapping competency domains are used in US medical education, the six domains of the Accreditation Council for Graduate Medical Education (ACGME) and the eight domains of Physician Competency Reference Set (PCRS) adopted by the Association of American Medical Colleges (AAMC) in 2014. Contraceptive counseling, delivering the news of a positive pregnancy test and screening for intimate partner violence and reproductive coercion situate within the domains of patient care and interpersonal and communication skills. Accessing updated and valid information is a skill within practice-based learning and improvement while advocating in limited and under-resourced circumstances falls within systems-based practice. Therefore, the inclusion of family planning in an undergraduate medical curriculum provides additional opportunities to learn skills that are transferable. For example, conveying the news of a positive pregnancy test to a woman who does not want a pregnancy at that time requires an approach and responsiveness that apply when delivering other "bad" news. Identification of one's own values around reproductive circumstances and decisions and using that information to mitigate compromise of patient autonomy is also required for physicians who may face requests around futile care, discontinuance of pacemakers or refusal of treatment. The knowledge, skills and attitudes here come under the domains of professionalism in both the PCRS and the ACGME frameworks.

Another argument relevant to the larger curriculum derives from the newer imperative of social accountability of medical education to prepare graduates to address major public health challenges, health disparities and health-care inequities through caring for individual patients, working at the health-care systems level and advocating for larger change [10]. In fact, some version of social accountability forms the value-added proposition for the establishment of most of the new medical schools that have emerged in the past fifteen years. External foundations are funding projects within schools to strengthen curricula with respect to social accountability and are supporting the development of metrics to track and compare the social accountability of medical schools. The social accountability argument for including family planning in US undergraduate medical education is robust for several reasons. First, the provision of contraception is a clearly effective means of reducing unintended pregnancy and its consequences while the provision of the most effective contraceptive methods in the USA is largely under the control of physician practice. Second, unintended pregnancy and abortion involve glaring health disparities and health-care inequities. Third, the core skills defined above are developmentally appropriate for undergraduate medical education. Deferring their learning to a much more variable system of graduate medical education training is simply not efficient.

Another justification for curricular inclusion, while dwarfed by all of those above, is that knowledge of contraception and abortion is expected on some high-stakes examinations.

20.3 Teaching Medical Students and Designing Instructional Materials

Faculty may find themselves largely in the role of teachers and instructional designers, having been asked by a clerkship or course director to deliver an hour or more of mandatory instruction.

20.3.1 Crafting or Determining Learning Objectives

Course and clerkship directors who enlist faculty in teaching may provide clear learning objectives or simply some topics. Teachers who receive only topics should take the first step of a serious educator and define learning objectives. Writing good learning objectives requires defining what learners should be able to do as a result of the instruction. Teachers can begin with revisiting the core skills and knowledge outlined above and identify which may fit with the topics that were assigned. Well-crafted learning objectives may also be found in instructional materials that have been developed by others (organizations are listed in Section 20.3.3).

Faculty who must write their own objectives yet lack experience should consider obtaining help. Learning objectives look deceptively simple on the surface, but writing good ones is a skill that most educators hone with significant practice. Possible resources include a senior educator faculty member within a department, a faculty member of an institutional teaching academy or a faculty developer available through the office or department of medical education or academic affairs. (Medical schools are required to provide resources and support to faculty in the development and delivery of curricula.)

20.3.2 Ensuring That Proposed Objectives Build on Prior Learning in the Curriculum

Faculty teaching at one point in the curriculum should develop a clear understanding of what has already been covered and assessed. This knowledge will inform planning to avoid unnecessary redundancy, to identify opportunities for purposeful redundancy (learning of knowledge and skills that should be repeated to enhance retention) and to effectively build on prior learning. Students appreciate faculty who are aware of their prior curriculum, who identify when and why they are repeating material and who summon prior material to facilitate their learning of new material.

Connecting with faculty who have taught relevant material earlier in the curriculum is also an opportunity to review their material and build relationships that may support expanded development of the curriculum at a later date. It will also likely help access information on student performance on relevant test questions or simulation examinations. For example, if a faculty member who is designing a session to teach contraceptive counseling dialogues with those who teach reproductive pharmacology, reproductive system cancers and/or thromboembolic disease, they might work to ensure the delivery of consistent and clinically relevant content and highlight places to reinforce overlapping content. The clinical skills director who likely oversees assessment from simulation may have information on whether the template for history and physical includes

attention to pregnancy intentions or risk of unintended pregnancy and on how students performed on those elements. Faculty teaching contraceptive counseling, non-directive pregnancy options counseling or both should know the prior curriculum on intimate partner violence, especially opportunities for simulated practice of screening. If students have had ample learning of knowledge and skills required for addressing intimate partner violence, then revisiting these and building on them to include screening for reproductive coercion could be a logical next step.

In connecting with the directors of courses that cover communication skills or evidence-based medicine, clerkship and clinical faculty may realize that students are learning frameworks that can easily and effectively be applied to family planning. Repeated use of the same framework is an important strategy to achieve the important goal of retained learning, that is learning students will carry across the graduation stage. For example, the framework for "breaking bad news" may apply to delivering the news of a positive pregnancy test to a patient who has not yet expressed her intentions around pregnancy. Working in a different competency domain, family planning educators can collaborate with faculty who teach evidence-based medicine (EBM) by calling out the key primary literature and guidelines that inform family planning care and by engaging learners in critical appraisal of family planning literature using the templates introduced in the earlier EBM curriculum.

Because ethical issues may arise even when a teaching session does not explicitly include objectives dealing with ethical reasoning, teachers working at any point in the curriculum should have familiarity with the frameworks for ethical reasoning and professional identity formation[1]

---

[1] Professional identity formation (PIF) is a newer component of recommended education across major professions. PIF is the process by which learners adopt and/or reconcile their personal values with those of the profession. The process occurs, whether explicitly addressed in the curriculum or left entirely to the learner's experience of the curriculum. The outcomes of this process determine the learner's ultimate readiness to engage in fulfilling their social contract within the profession. The recent Carnegie Foundation report on medical education identifies attention to PIF as one of the four major areas of needed reform [5].

used in that curriculum. Family planning educators should ask those knowledgeable about the previous curricula in ethics and professional identity formation questions such as the following:

a. Are reproductive health examples used?
b. What bioethical principles are covered with these examples?
c. What frameworks do students learn for ethical reasoning?
d. Have they learned the processes for evaluating their emotions, values and attitudes surrounding care of patients who present moral and/or emotional challenges for them?

Finally, family planning educators should know how the curriculum at their institution fosters student learning of approaches to advocacy and collaboration with other health professionals and communities, especially when learning occurs in under-resourced settings, states posing substantial non-financial barriers to access or states with restricted government funding for family planning and abortion. Knowledge of this prior curriculum is particularly important for educators in the clinical setting. While all students do not necessarily need to apply advocacy skills in the care of patients needing family planning care, their learning of these skills overall will be enhanced as they see them applied to family planning.

Faculty teaching in the didactic space, whether they be ethicists, pharmacologists, policy experts or physiologists, are typically very interested to learn about how clinical teachers help students see the relevance of what they teach and how clinicians build on what they teach. They will often be highly receptive to input on how to increase the relevance of what they teach to opportunities you may provide for clinical learning.

20.3.3 Deciding on Instructional Methods and Delivering Content

Once learning objectives are defined, the next decision concerns instructional method. The most important consideration is selecting the instructional method that aligns with the learning objectives. For example, lecturing may provide background knowledge for a skill, but it cannot replace opportunities to practice that skill, whether it's appropriately using information resources or screening for intimate partner violence. Skills development requires active-learning strategies. (Other major considerations are the size of instructional groups, the faculty member's skills and experience and perhaps the availability of online platforms and professional instructional designers.)

Faculty members relatively new to these decisions should consider consulting the faculty developer available through the institution or department of medical education. These individuals can help in every stage of the design of instructional sessions and can provide teaching observations and the coaching necessary to furthering skills. All faculty, and especially faculty new to teaching should see this coaching as key to developing skills with active-learning formats, such as facilitating small group discussions, conducting interactive large group teams-based learning sessions, running online discussion boards and overseeing simulated practice with standardized patients. Without guidance and coaching, faculty often stumble on first attempts (because it's not easy), and as a result, students conclude that the active-learning method is not effective when in fact the faculty was simply not prepared to use it effectively.

Another strategy for those new to teaching in active learning formats is to use materials developed and tested by another educator whenever available and focus initial efforts on delivering in the format rather than creating the material. A handful of websites offer access to previously used and refined instructional materials for family planning and abortion, including Innovating Education in Reproductive Health, MedEd Portal, the Association of Professors of Gynecology and Obstetrics and Reproductive Health Education in Family Medicine.

For those who may be creating PowerPoints and have not received training in the basics of effective slide design, consultation with the institution's instructional designer or faculty developer again can be highly useful. More than aesthetics are at play. Research from cognitive psychology clearly shows that good slide design enhances learning, whereas poor slide design undermines learning [11]. Another benefit of working with a faculty developer and/or instructional designer is that they are also knowledgeable about resources across the institution, including simulation and other faculty with skills and knowledge that might be of help.

Faculty developing their own materials, planning to make their role as an educator important to their academic promotion and success and/or hoping to make their product widely available to those at other institutions should ask the faculty developer about appropriate steps in the initial design and delivery process to structure their work as a scholarly project that may ultimately be suitable for peer-reviewed publication.

20.4 Including Instruction and Experiences That May Not Be "Necessary" at the UME Level

While using a manual vacuum aspirator for uterine evacuation and inserting an intrauterine device (IUD) or implant are not among the "core skills" defined above, students respond favorably to these opportunities to practice with simulated materials. While they do not need to engage in this practice with the goal of becoming competent, participating in these activities may contribute to their ability to counsel patients about these procedures and enhance their memory of the related information.

Arguments can also be made to ensure that all students interact with patients seeking abortion, even if they do not participate in their care or will ever provide abortions. First, abortion is common. In the USA, it is more common than appendectomies and cardiac catheterizations, for example, and many other procedures [12,13]. Second, just as exposure to patients with life-altering stroke or kidney disease makes real the seriousness of preventing and controlling hypertension, exposure to patients seeking abortion does the same for contraception. Third, students who may have negative stereotypes or overly simplified notions of women's reasons for seeking abortion will have the opportunity to see the complexity and nuance of women's realities and perhaps begin to develop an empathy that will serve them in caring for similar patients, and a greater respect for those who provide abortion care. Finally, some students will go on to become leaders of medical organizations and health-care systems, and as a result of their exposure might be more favorably influenced in these leadership roles to see the critical roles of comprehensive contraceptive provision and compassionate abortion care for women and their families, and the contribution of family planning curricula to strengthening foundational skills in person-centered care.

The students most likely to "opt out" or not to "opt in" to rotating in a clinic providing abortions are the ones for whom this exposure could have the most meaningful impact. Therefore, any feasible strategy to foster their openness to "opting in" or "not opting out" should be explored. One strategy is clear and standardized communication should come from the clerkship director or other faculty member to all students about the value of the opportunity for all students, regardless of future specialty plans. Another strategy is ensuring the student's ability to control what they observe and/or participate in. For example [14], some will be willing to listen in on a counseling session and perhaps stay with a patient in recovery, but not observe ultrasounds or any part of a procedure. They may be willing to ask a patient at a post-procedure visit about her emotional reactions. It may also be helpful to ensure that each student is paired upon arrival to the clinical site with a nurse or other provider who knows what the student has agreed to, and to whom they can communicate at any moment a change in their comfort with what they have chosen to do.

20.5 Assessing Medical Student Learning: Didactic, Clinical and Programmatic

Clinical learning is a complex process, and assessing clinical performance is considered one of the larger, if not the largest, challenge in medical education today. Graduating students who are not competent constitutes a breach of our obligation to the public and to graduate medical education. As mentioned earlier, recent studies have confirmed that a significant proportion of medical school graduates are unable to perform core skills that are covered in the curriculum. If methods for assessing these skills are falling short, then methods for assessing the core skills of family planning in UME, which in fact build on these skills, will also be lacking.

In response to these gaps, medical schools are beginning to implement newer approaches to assessment designed to promote both consistent learning over time and long-term retention of knowledge and skills. These approaches include shifts in methods, adoption of the framework of entrustable professional activities, "just-in-time" assessments such as the mini-Clinical Evaluation Exercise (mini-CEX), the use of assessment for learning, the use of promotional and graduation objective structured clinical examinations (OSCEs) and, most important, the design of programmatic assessment. Family planning educators who are serious about graduates attaining the core family planning skills and carrying those into residency will benefit from understanding the overall system of assessment at their school and considering the opportunities for improving the assessment of family planning knowledge and skills using the best of the available system.

20.5.1 Using Simulation

For uniform assessment of skills, most schools now use OSCEs at different points in the curriculum. More than 100 schools in the USA, as of 2016, required passage of a third or fourth year OSCE for graduation [15]. OSCEs typically consist of eight to twelve scenarios with standardized patients and/or simulation mannequins that assess clinical behaviors, including communication skills, examination and procedural skills and/or teamwork. Contraceptive counseling and non-directive pregnancy options counseling are well suited to this method. Including at least one of them in a promotional and/or graduation examination signals to students the importance of these skills to their readiness for residency (MedEd Portal contains simulation encounters for assessment of both skillsets) [16,17]. Family planning educators should also ask to see all simulation encounters involving a reproductive-aged woman to determine whether the appropriate screening for contraceptive need and/or possibility of unintended pregnancy is included, and if so, whether performance on these items is a requirement for passage.

Simulated encounters can also be adapted assess ethical reasoning and evidence-based medicine skills. For example, in a contraceptive counseling scenario, examinees can have access to the World Health Organization or country-based medical eligibility criteria, which in the USA is available through the Centers for Disease Control and Prevention. After the encounter, they can be asked to write an explanation of how they used the resource.

20.5.2 Using Just-in-Time Assessments

These are structured assessments of specific clinical encounters or skills performed in the clinical setting. Typically, faculty (or residents) observe the encounter and then complete a short form of ten or fewer questions about competency domains, specific behaviors and/or the need for supervision or help in completing the encounter or skill. Ideally, this assessment is communicated as feedback to the learner immediately to promote learning (ie, assessment for learning). The majority of validity data for this method comes from graduate medical education. A systematic review of one version (the mini-CEX), its utility, including validity, in both UME and GME is pending [18].

This approach is also being piloted by several medical schools for assessing student performance of entrustable professional activities (EPAs). If students have at least a few opportunities to practice contraceptive counseling during clinical rotations (which meets the definition of an EPA), then the platform of just-in-time assessment could provide them feedback to promote their continual learning and data for use by faculty to judge their final level of competence.

20.5.3 Programmatic Assessment

Originating in the Netherlands, programmatic assessment is a relatively new approach in North American medical education, and for several reasons is now widely considered the most promising alternative to the inadequate approach of simply passing examinations specific to required courses and clerkships. Programmatic assessment is "a centrally planned, coordinated approach [that] entails collecting multiple pieces of information to generate holistic views of learners and their progression" [6]. It provides learners continual and meaningful feedback to promote their learning to foster their own self-directed learning and facilitates well-grounded judgements for readiness for promotion and graduation. Reports of the implementation, outcomes and validity of programmatic assessment have been emerging with greater frequency in recently in published literature.

Family planning educators interested in assessment should learn about their institutions' structures and/or plans for programmatic assessment through the office or department of medical education. They might consider what assessment data across a curriculum could contribute to a family planning or reproductive health "portfolio," and inquire about the feasibility of having this data "tagged" for periodic review. Such data might include OSCE encounters, just-in-time assessments, essay examinations in ethics and reflective writing on encounters with patients that evoke difficult emotions, attitudes and/or ethical challenges.

20.6 Mentoring Medical Students

As is the case with mentoring in general, mentoring students in family planning and abortion can take different forms and serve different goals. In family planning, these goals include role-modeling as an abortion provider, facilitating residency application and supporting the student's growth as an educator, scholar, researcher and/or activist/advocate. Below are just a few examples of the forms this mentorship may take.

In family planning, the role-modeling is particularly important for replacing any negative stereotypes of abortion providers with the reality of compassionate, dedicated and scholarly physicians. Mentors also serve as advisors for chapters of student advocacy organizations such as Medical Students for Choice, and in this role can guide students in facilitating extracurricular educational sessions and workshops. These sessions can provide opportunities for helping students develop formal teaching skills, such as those for teaching psychomotor skills that can be applied during a papaya workshop or a session on IUD and implant insertion. For those going into obstetrics and gynecology or family medicine, or considering post-residency fellowship training in family planning, mentors can provide students pointers on how to discuss their interest in family

planning during the residency application process and facilitate contact with supportive faculty at programs of interest.

Collaborating with students in the development of teaching materials and assessment tools offers some of the most rewarding and unique opportunities to mentor. Students may identify gaps in the curriculum and/or lend their voices to those acknowledged by a faculty member. A faculty member can prepare them to effectively advocate to a curriculum committee, guide them through the process of developing instructional materials, involve them in designing an elective or include them on a teaching team. If done with a scholarly approach, these efforts may result in materials suitable for peer-reviewed publication or presentation, thus providing another avenue for supporting the mentee's growth.

Faculty members have also worked with students to develop patient navigator programs for women facing barriers – for example, in obtaining long-acting reversible methods or abortions – and to advocate at the legislative level.

20.7 Conclusion

Recent decades have seen substantial – albeit incomplete – improvement in the incorporation of family planning into undergraduate medical education. With the movement of health professions education overall into an outcomes-based framework, family planning educators who bring content that is powerfully aligned with the imperative of social accountability are in a unique position to benefit from and contribute to the reform movement in medical education. The way forward begins with well-reasoned advocacy for curricular integration, thoughtfully designed curricula, and assessment of this education as offered here.

References

1. Steinauer J, LaRochelle F, Rowh M, Backus L, Sandahl Y, Foster A. First impressions: what are preclinical medical students in the US and Canada learning about sexual and reproductive health? *Contraception*. 2009; 80(1):74–80.

2. Veazey K, Nieuwoudt C, Gavito C, Tocce K. Student

perceptions of reproductive health education in US medical schools: a qualitative analysis of students taking family planning electives. *Med Educ Online*. 2015;20:28973.

3. Cessford TA, Norman WV. Making a case for abortion curriculum reform: a knowledge-assessment survey of undergraduate medical

students. *J Obstet Gynaecol Can*. 2011;33(6):580.

4. Angus SV, Vu TR, Willett LL, Call S, Halvorsen AJ, Chaudhry S. Internal medicine residency program directors' views of the core entrustable professional activities for entering residency: an opportunity to enhance communication of competency along the continuum. *Acad Med*. 2017;92(6):785–791.

5. Cooke M, Irby DM, O'Brien BC. *Educating Physicians: A Call for Reform of Medical School and Residency*. Vol. 16. New York: John Wiley & Sons; 2010.

6. Hauer KE, O'Sullivan PS, Fitzhenry K, Boscardin C. Translating theory into practice: implementing a program of assessment. *Acad Med*. 2018;93(3):444–450.

7. Thomas PA, Kern DE, Hughes MT, Chen BY. (Eds.). *Curriculum Development for Medical Education: A Six-Step Approach*, 3rd ed. Baltimore, MD: Johns Hopkins University Press; 2016.

8. Liaison Committee on Medical Education, Association of American Medical Colleges, American Medical Association. *Functions and Structure of a Medical School: Standards for Accreditation of Medical Education Programs Leading to the MD Degree*; 2019. http://lcme.org/publications/. Accessed September 21, 2019.

9. Stumbar SE, Brown DR, Lupi CS. Developing and implementing curricular objectives for sexual health in undergraduate medical education: a practical approach. *Acad Med*. 2020;95(1):77–82.

10. Boelen C, Pearson D, Kaufman A, et al. Producing a socially accountable medical school: AMEE Guide No. 109. *Med Teach*. 2016;38(11):1078–1091.

11. Mayer RE. Applying the science of learning: evidence-based principles for the design of multimedia instruction. *Am Psychol*. 2008;63(8):760–769.

12. Hall MJ, Schwartzman A, Zhang J, Liu X. Ambulatory surgery data from hospitals and ambulatory surgery centers: United States 2010. *Natl Health Stat Report*. 2017;(103):1–15.

13. Finger KR, Stocks C, Weiss AJ, Steiner CA. *Most frequent operating room procedures performed in U.S. hospitals, 2003–2012*. 2014. Healthcare Cost and Utilization Project. Statistical Brief #186.

14. Martinez R, Minor D, Lupi C. Abortion care education: What exactly do students want to see and do, and what do they do? Paper presented at the SGEA Regional Conference, Orlando, FL; 2019.

15. Association of American Medical Colleges. *SP/OSCE Final Examinations at US Medical Schools*; 2019. www.aamc.org/data-reports/curriculum-reports/interactive-data/sp/osce-final-examinations-us-medical-schools. Accessed September 21, 2019.

16. Lupi C, Mechaber A. Objective structured clinical examination: contraceptive counseling for long acting reversible methods. *MedEdPORTAL*. 2011;7:9021. https://doi.org/10.15766/mep_2374–8265.9021

17. Lupi CS, Ward-Peterson M, Castro CA. Non-directive pregnancy options counseling: online instructional module, objective structured clinical exam, and rater and standardized patient training materials. *MedEdPORTAL*. 2017;13:10566. https://doi.org/10.15766/mep_2374–8265.10566

18. Mortaz Hejri S, Jalili M, Shirazi M, Masoomi R, Nedjat S, Norcini J. The utility of mini-Clinical Evaluation Exercise (mini-CEX) in undergraduate and postgraduate medical education: protocol for a systematic review. *Syst Rev*. 2017;6(1):146.

21

The Role of Students in Advocating for Training in Sexual and Reproductive Health Care

Lois V. Backus and Rebecca Henderson

21.1 Introduction

Medical students are uniquely placed in the medical education system to advocate for improvements in their education. Stigmatized aspects of sexual and reproductive health care, such as abortion, are areas where this constituency can be powerful advocates if organized to use their collective power to influence educational change. Formal education on abortion is limited in medical schools [1], and organized efforts by medical students and others to promote the integration of all aspects of sexual and reproductive health care, including abortion, within medical education have been shown to be effective strategies resulting in greater access to comprehensive education on family planning topics [2].

Medical education in the USA is highly competitive and consists of four years of formal schooling at the graduate level following a baccalaureate degree. The awarding of the medical doctor (MD) degree is followed by three or more years of highly structured clinical training in the medical specialty that each physician chooses. In some areas of the world, foundational medical training is incorporated into post-secondary education and can be six years or longer followed by a number of years as a training doctor. In all cases, medical education provides a lengthy time period during which students may become engaged in advocacy work on behalf of their future patients. Medical student engagement with family planning advocacy, both focused on educational change and on better access to care for patients, can help to normalize abortion and contraception within medical practice by ensuring routine discussion of these controversial topics in the educational milieu.

Within medical schools, medical students interested in learning about all aspects of family planning in their medical education have successfully achieved changes in curricula at the institutional level through collective efforts [2]. In addition, a number of organizations now support the efforts of these interested medical students, including Medical Students for Choice (MSFC), which was founded more than 20 years ago and now supports medical students at more than 220 medical schools worldwide. The American Medical Student Association (AMSA), the medical student division of the American Medical Women's Association (AMWA) and other student organizations collaborate with MSFC at individual medical schools. Organizations focused on ensuring access for training physicians as they move through their training years have also developed, such as the Ryan Residency Program, which helps obstetrics and gynecology (ob-gyn) residency programs integrate abortion training, and the Fellowship in Family Planning, which enables motivated trained physicians to obtain additional expertise in family planning practice. This chapter uses MSFC as a model for successfully engaging medical students in the effort to incorporate all aspects of sexual and reproductive health care into medical education.

21.2 Abortion in Medical School Curricula

In the USA, the legalization of abortion in the early 1970s did much to increase access to safe procedures, but did little to improve the lack of education about abortion in medical school curricula. It was not until 1993, the year that the first abortion-providing doctor was killed in the USA by an antiabortion extremist, that medical students became aware of the lack of any formal education about abortion in their education [3] and formal efforts to organize medical students began.

Medical education is typically divided between clinical and non-clinical, or classroom-based instruction. In the USA generally, the first two years are non-clinical, followed by two years that are clinically focused, with students rotating through various "clerkships" throughout the hospital. Although ob-gyn is one of the major "clerkships" during US medical students' clinical training, training in abortion and other aspects of sexual and reproductive health are often limited [1]. Classroom education focused on women's health care within the non-clinical curricula frequently provides little, if any, information about abortion [4].

The published studies of medical curricula on abortion clearly show deficits in formal education on abortion, both in the non-clinical and in the clinical curricula of many medical schools. Only 19% of the third-year ob-gyn clerkship directors surveyed reported a lecture specifically about abortion in the non-clinical, or preclinical curriculum. While 45% of third-year ob-gyn clerkships offered some clinical exposure to abortion, participation rates were very low [1]. A review of the preclinical curriculum in medical schools published four years later found that 67% of the medical schools responding had some abortion content in their non-clinical curricula [4]. However, Steinauer, et al. also found that two thirds of medical students reported spending less than thirty minutes of class time on all aspects of abortion, and one third received no education on the topic at all. Simultaneously, they reported that the first medication approved in the USA to treat erectile dysfunction, sildenafil, received more than three times as much required classroom time than abortion and birth control combined [4].

Regardless of legal status, abortion remains common throughout the world. It is more common in developing regions than in regions with greater access to contraception. Despite its frequency, however, abortion content is minimal or non-existent in most medical school curricula. Little literature describes the implementation of abortion-specific curricula for medical schools internationally; however, medical training programs vary worldwide. For example, in Turkey, where abortion is illegal, only 56% of medical students had heard of medication abortion [5]. A cross-sectional study of knowledge of abortion and reproductive health in India found that 84%

of senior medical students had no clinical practice in abortion during medical training [6].

Outside the USA, MSFC works with medical students in twenty-four other countries, including nine countries in Africa that have laws restricting legal abortion, and in the Republic of Ireland, where abortion was illegal until very recently. Formalized education on abortion did not exist in those countries prior to MSFC members' efforts to promote its inclusion. A tactical focus on the effects of unsafe abortion have helped students in their quest for formalized education on abortion [7]. A student from Burundi said this about his education:

> In the course of my training in OBGYN, four adolescent girls died and six suffered hemorrhage due to unsafe abortion. Other women told me that they had been forced to stop contraceptive methods by their husbands or mothers-in-law. I need sufficient education to help every woman with her choices.

Training opportunities outside the formal educational institution can be helpful as well, because medical students are often reluctant to address controversial issues within their schools. Physicians and other sexual and reproductive health (SRH) providers in communities with medical schools can be an important resource for these extracurricular opportunities for medical students. For instance, MSFC has more than 100 SRH sites that offer educational opportunities for medical students within their facilities. Faculty supporters, mentors and local community providers can also be helpful to students seeking legitimacy within their educational institutions. In one case in the USA, a group of medical students advocating for conversations among their fellow students regarding the use of condoms was threatened with formal censure by five school administrators who alleged that their open promotion of condom usage was inappropriate. The group's faculty advisor, an internist, interceded on the group's behalf and achieved a resolution of the administrators' concerns while the group worked to obtain the support of their student body.

Another medical student described the value of the creation of an organized abortion-supportive community as being particularly important for those studying in areas where abortion was not considered to be a normal part of women's health-care services:

(n=224)

	Average # of educational events organized by chapter	% of chapters Involved in curriculam reform	% of chapters with a faculty advisor
ALL CHAPTERS	**5.5**	**45.4%**	**47.1%**
All US Chapters	4.9	47.8%	57.5%
US Northeast	5.9	64.9%	67.6%
US Southeast	4.2	25.7%	40.0%
US Midwest	5.1	67.6%	64.9%
US West	4	24.0%	56.0%
Canada	4.13	53.3%	26.7%
Africa	13.2	14.3%	42.9%
All other International Chapters	5.7	45.5%	9.1%

Data are from MSFC's survey of student leaders in Spring 2019

Figure 21.1 MSFC chapter activities, spring semester 2019

Since I got involved with MSFC I feel like my actions are meaningful and the organization is clearly transforming the lives of numerous medical students and the whole population at large. MSFC is very different from other organizations in that it helps you to set objectives and provides you with the means necessary to achieve them. (MSFC Member Communication)

Currently, MSFC data show that only 47% of chapters have a faculty advisor supporting their work (Figure 21.1). Of the current US-based chapters with faculty advisors, 64% are faculty members who are trained through the Ryan Program or Fellowship in Family Planning. Medical students, even acting without faculty support, can provide valuable educational opportunities within their institutions, but faculty support offers benefits in addition to directly supporting the students' advocacy efforts.

21.3 Recent Changes in Medical Training and Policy

The inclusion of abortion in medical curricula has been facilitated in the USA by major professional organizations that set curricula and guide the standard of educational practice. While the Accreditation Council for Graduate Medical Education (ACGME) mandates that all US residency programs in obstetrics and gynecology provide comprehensive women's health-care training, including training in abortion [8], policy toward undergraduate education is less clear. In November 2014, the American College of Obstetricians and Gynecologists (ACOG) released a committee opinion on abortion training and education, urging "continued efforts to destigmatize and integration abortion training into medical education as a critical element of women's healthcare" [9]. The Association of Professors of Gynecology and Obstetrics (APGO) includes the development of a thorough understanding of abortion in their educational objectives of ob-gyn undergraduate medical education [10].

Moving national and international medical organizations forward on abortion policy has taken many years of coordinated effort. For instance, in 1995 MSFC's first national advocacy project in the USA was a petition to the ACGME that supported including abortion as a required part of ob-gyn residency training. This first national medical student effort supported efforts within larger medical organizations to persuade the ACGME to include an explicit requirement for abortion training in all US obstetrics and gynecology residency programs. More recently, medical students and alumni of MSFC have advocated for abortion-positive policies within their state medical societies[1] and joined in advocacy efforts within pediatrics, internal medicine and family medicine specialty organizations.

Internationally, a rapidly changing environment around safe abortion practice worldwide led the World Health Organization (WHO) to update and revise their guidelines in 2012 [11].

21.4 Supporting Effective Medical Student Activism

Engaging communities of medical students that advocate together for family planning education within medical education curricula helps combat the stigma that often surrounds abortion and other sexual and reproductive health-care topics. In addition to localized impacts, the presence of communities of peers and mentors is critical to sustaining efforts across regions, through all levels of medical education, and into the realm of medical practice. A clear focus on community building is at the heart of the model that MSFC uses to advocate for the integration of family planning content in non-clinical medical education, clinical medical education, residency training and medical services.

Classic community organizing strategies have been shown to be effective for developing and sustaining these communities of medical students, resulting in positive change in medical education even in countries where abortion is illegal. In fact, in countries where abortion is highly restricted or illegal, the dangers of unsafe abortion may increase medical students' sense of urgency for improved training and education on abortion. Furthermore, medical students who join organized efforts such as MSFC value their inclusion in the larger community of engaged students and leaders. Collaboration with this worldwide community helps more isolated students to feel a part of a global movement implementing change worldwide.

> With MSFC I get to extend my own network and to see my impact grow exponentially. It is through MSFC that I met some of the most promising opinion-makers involved in social change around the globe. Through shared experience and joint programs, we were able to put our talents toward a greater cause. MSFC give me the motivation and the capacity to do more. (MSFC Member Communication)

From the application process through graduation, medical school is an intensive environment for learning. Students in this intensive environment are greatly sustained by friendships and collaborative work with other students sharing their values. Such interactions not only serve to feed student's social and emotional needs, but reinforce shared values. Student members frequently describe this process in terms of the importance of finding "[their] people," enabling them to stay in medical school, to succeed in collaborative efforts, and to promote shared goals.

Faculty mentors are also an important source of support for medical students. As the Fellowship in Family Planning has grown, more qualified physician mentors have become available to medical students, particularly in large training institutions. Access to mentors continues to be difficult for many medical students interested in reproductive health, however, as relatively few physicians worldwide are either qualified or willing to provide leadership and mentoring on abortion.

The community organizing framework used by MSFC and other organizations is particularly effective with medical students because it empowers local students to choose the focus and the tactics that they use to make change on their campus. The creation of a national and worldwide community of learners facilitates the sharing of experiences of advocacy and change, and students can use this knowledge to build change on their own campuses. Medical students generally feel that they are without power within medical institutions, but the community organizing approach allows students to use their community as a foundation to influence change. Where one lone voice may not be heard, fifty can have a powerful impact.

Within medical schools, students use the bonds created within their activist communities to address issues related to family planning that are often considered highly controversial, and to help mobilize students who would not otherwise engage with these topics. Whether it is a request to update medically inaccurate content in the curriculum or a proposal for a comprehensive series of curriculum additions, a single student

---

[1] See https://msfc.org/michigan-msfc-members-demand-abortion-training-opportunities-residents/

may be easily ignored or labeled "difficult," but a request from an organized, prepared group of students is more likely to be received respectfully.

21.4.1 Curricula Change

Changing the curricula in medical school can be a complex process that takes place over several years. In the USA, changes to the formal curricula often involve institution-wide curriculum committees through which changes to the curriculum are carefully vetted. MSFC provides students with a step-by-step guide, freely available on their website[2] that informs medical students of various tactics that can be utilized in a successful effort to change the curriculum.

Recently, an MSFC chapter in Uganda conducted a successful campaign resulting in the addition of new curriculum elements in all areas of sexual and reproductive health in all five years of the medical curriculum [7]. At any given time, one quarter to one third of MSFC chapters are engaged in formal efforts to reform their schools' curriculum (see Figure 21.1).

21.4.2 Extracurricular Education within Institutions

While engaging in formal curriculum change efforts can result in larger, lasting educational change, a focus on providing extracurricular opportunities for SRH training can ensure consistent learning opportunities for medical students at all levels of their education that fill in gaps in the formal curriculum. Educational events organized by groups of medical students add much to medical education and can ensure that aspects of medical practice, such as abortion, are included in the broader educational package that medical students can access in their institutions even if that medical care is not available through the hospital system. In a typical semester, for instance, MSFC chapters organize more than five of these extracurricular education events (see Figure 21.1).

MSFC and other organizations also provide medical students with a broad array of educational resources that can be used to facilitate these extracurricular activities or for individualized

learning.[3] Among MSFC chapters, these extracurricular educational events provide their campus communities with thousands of workshops, lectures and panel discussions on SRH topics each year.

21.4.3 Clinical Training Opportunities for Medical Students

Since clinical training opportunities are limited in most medical schools [1], extracurricular and external clinical training opportunities for medical students to enhance the limited opportunities available within their non-clinical and clinical curriculum can also be an effective way to introduce medical students to sexual and reproductive health care in a clinical setting. Providers of SRH services can be important resources to medical students in their local communities. For instance, the Health Development Initiative in Rwanda supports medical students at the University of Rwanda who are seeking clinical experiences in SRH. MSFC provides funding and a worldwide network of training sites that support student learning in this way. These opportunities to observe, listen and learn in a medical facility providing abortion, contraception and other sexual health services exposes students to patient needs and clinical issues in an important way [12].

21.5 Strategies That Work

As an organization, MSFC employs three main strategies in order to build and sustain communities of medical student activists at individual schools, and to foster a worldwide network of activists at all stages in medical training:

1. **Connectivity:** The first key element of MSFC's community building strategy ensures that the larger MSFC community is accessible to any interested medical student, and connects interested students to each other. MSFC maintains an internet-based network that allows for rapid communication with staff members who offer support, guidance and reinforcement to medical students. Medical students new to the community are also connected with other medical students who have established chapters in their region to

---

[2] See https://msfc.org/medical-students/curriculum-reform/

[3] See https://msfc.org/medical-students/event-resources/

facilitate peer-to-peer guidance and mentorship.

2. **Support:** MSFC fosters growing communities of students by providing effective resources that support medical student activity. MSFC produces and maintains educational resources to support activist efforts based on best practices and past successes. These materials include detailed guides for advocating for curriculum change and for hosting educational events on topics that are often not covered in the formal medical curriculum. These resources enable medical student chapters to host activities that are likely to be successful in educating peers and implementing change at home institutions.

3. **Flexibility:** Finally, a key aspect of MSFC's community building activities includes an active commitment to remaining flexible and responsive to changes in formal and informal policy environments. Abortion in medical education is subject to rapid change due to societal, political, legal and policy factors, and MSFC responds quickly to those changes, developing and testing new strategies for overcoming new challenges and effectively addressing new opportunities. Further, as social and policy landscapes may differ radically by region or institution, MSFC's

strategies must accommodate each new setting in order to best support student chapters.

21.5.1 The Spread of Medical Student Activism

Medical student interest in abortion and other aspects of sexual health has remained high throughout the past two decades. MSFC, as an example, has seen steady growth in student interest at medical schools since its inception, beginning with a few chapters in 1993 and growing to 224 chapters in 25 countries in 2019. Although much of that growth has been organic, it has been sustained by the organizational focus on connecting with students that reach out to the organization, supporting them financially, and being flexible, allowing for local student decision making regarding the change they choose to work toward. These three principles seem particularly important for students working in environments without faculty support.

For MSFC, initial growth in the number of medical schools with active chapters resulted primarily from outreach strategies targeting members of the AMWA, AMSA and other medical student cohorts that potentially could be interested in abortion advocacy. Those strategies resulted in a strong US network of roughly

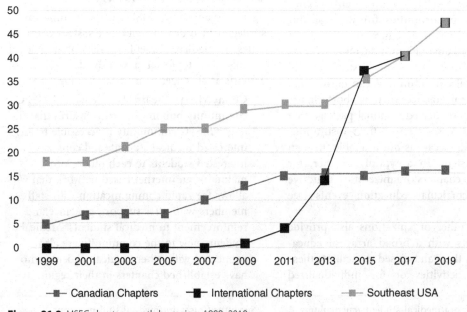

Figure 21.2 MSFC chapter growth by region, 1999–2019

90 chapters after several years. Growth that took place after 1999 resulted primarily from communication strategies, including direct outreach between medical students and internet-based strategies that developed throughout the first decade of the new millennium. Since 2001, growth followed in specific geographic areas of interest chosen by the organization. For instance, in the early 2000s, MSFC chose to focus on growth in the US Southeast. From fewer than 20 schools with active chapters, growth occurred steadily, and MSFC chapters now exist in almost 50 schools there, including at the only medical school in Mississippi. In the USA, of the 166 chapters at the time of publication, 72 are in medical schools with Ryan Programs or Fellowships in Family Planning.

Canadian medical schools also became a special area of focus in the early 2000s, and MSFC now supports chapters at every medical school in Canada except the francophone schools. A French language version of the website was launched in 2019 to facilitate those students' participation.

International expansion beyond Canada began with interest from medical students in Ireland, Israel and at the American University in Beirut in 2009. Students at the University of Rwanda became engaged with this work in 2012, ushering in a strong wave of expansion throughout Africa. In 2019, MSFC is sustaining chapters in ten African countries, six countries in Europe, three countries in Latin America and two countries in Asia.

21.5.2 Characteristics of Medical Student Activism Internationally

Promoting organized activism among medical students varies little from country to country. Differences in the educational environment, however, can be significant, especially with respect to legal and cultural norms surrounding aspects of sexual and reproductive health. One example of these differences involves medical student activism in the Republic of Ireland [13]. In Ireland, a strongly Catholic country, abortion was illegal, and its illegal status was added to the country's constitution in 1983. Although small changes to the constitution allowed citizens to travel to obtain abortion, allowed doctors to provide referral information and permitted abortions to save a

woman's life, the lack of experienced abortion providers led to patient deaths. MSFC began supporting chapters in Ireland in 2009 in an environment dominated by cultural oppression surrounding abortion and a complete lack of any education or training options on abortion.

In addition to traditional chapter support, MSFC developed a partnership with abortion providers in the UK willing to provide training opportunities for students from medical schools in Ireland. Recently, the MSFC chapters joined with a broad national coalition of organizations seeking to overturn the eighth amendment to the Irish constitution that outlaws abortion. The amendment was overturned by popular vote in 2018, and MSFC's members in Ireland will be the first generation of abortion providers in Ireland.

In Bulgaria, medical students have ample access to learning opportunities about abortion, but very little regarding contraception. There, the MSFC chapters focus on promoting education about the full range of contraceptive options as well as other aspects of sexual health such as LGBTQ health issues.

Regardless of the legal and cultural issues, student activism is able to identify and focus on the learning issues that seem most urgent or pertinent to their particular environment. Whether the support comes from an advocacy organization such as MSFC, from local faculty or from a local advocacy organization, outside support is crucial to sustain interest and change-related activities beyond the relatively short timeline of each student's time in medical school.

21.6 Measuring Outcomes

Measuring the success of medical student driven strategies against a group's chosen goals is an essential part of the organized effort to make long-standing change. For instance, MSFC regularly collects data from members who participate in the organization's programs in order to measure (1) the effectiveness of the specific program against predetermined outcomes; (2) the overall impact of the program on participants' knowledge, attitudes and intention to provide abortion; (3) the characteristics of medical students choosing to participate; and (4) the comparative contribution of the particular program toward the organization's broader goals. In order to accomplish this, MSFC has systems in place that measure outcomes related to group activity as well as outcomes affecting individuals.

Measures for group activity include measures of curriculum change, group activity level and impact and institutional environment. These measures are analyzed over a number of years to measure factors at the chapter level that (1) enable chapters to assess positive or negative trends related to potential chapter strengths and weaknesses; (2) identify changes in the policy environment at individual institutions that affect student activities; and (3) enable the assessment of broader changes in educational environment around abortion and other SRH topics. For example, from 2011 to 2018, medical student demand worldwide for abortion training presentations and equipment as well as training resources for male vasectomies have more than doubled in all regions (Figure 21.3). This may reflect both greater awareness of the need for vasectomies, abortion access issues in the USA and efforts to liberalize abortion laws in much of Africa. MSFC has responded by increasing the number of resources available to meet the demand.

Outcomes related to program impact on individual students are measured through the use of program evaluation surveys that are administered before and after participation in a specific program. Responses are analyzed to assess changes in participants' reported intention to provide abortion in their future practice as well as knowledge and attitude changes. Multi-year analysis of the changes in participants' intention to provide abortion in their future practice allows MSFC to ensure that each program is effectively moving medical student participants toward abortion provision. It also enables the organization to do comparative analyses of the various training programs in order to better target organizational resources on those programs achieving the strongest outcomes.

21.7 Specialty Choice as a Factor in Abortion Provision

An additional important factor that impacts the ability of students who intend to provide abortion is medical specialty choice. Formalized abortion training is available in the USA to medical trainees in the majority of ob-gyn residency programs and in some family medicine residency programs. Therefore, while students attending MSFC events may intend to provide abortions, if their career choices lead them into other specialties, their ability to get this training and incorporate abortion into clinical practice may be limited. In 2015, MSFC alumni were surveyed in order to better understand outcomes in terms of specialty choice and abortion provision. More than half of

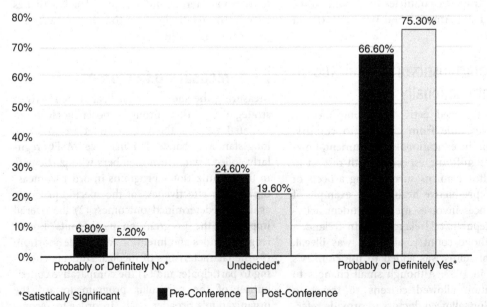

Figure 21.3 Change in intention to provide abortion among participants in MSFC's Conference on Family Planning, 2011–2018

MSFC alumni respondents reported that they specialized in either family medicine or ob-gyn. Steinauer et al found that developing a commitment to abortion provision *while in medical school* was the strongest predictor of abortion provision among practicing ob-gyns [14].

Students often become engaged in activities such as MSFC early in their medical education, before they have made decisions regarding specialty choice. Formalized activities promoting sexual and reproductive health education may therefore influence specialty choice, encouraging engaged students to pursue training that will incorporate abortion.

Among those students choosing specialties that do not incorporate direct abortion delivery, engagement in advocacy activities such as MSFC seems to lead to continued advocacy for these services within their practice. One MSFC alumna reported being the only anesthesiologist in her institution willing to support abortion procedures. Others report becoming engaged in community efforts promoting access to safe abortion services.

The bonds created through the building of communities of students also support individual students as they make decisions about their careers following graduation from medical school. Programs that have increased the availability of abortion training within residency training such as the Ryan Residency Program in ob-gyn and the RHEDI (Reproductive Health Education in Family Medicine) program have given interested medical students in the USA an organized place to seek the training they desire while pursuing the specialty they chose. Beyond residency, the Fellowship in Family Planning has provided hundreds of young physicians with an opportunity for a fellowship in family planning practice. This relatively new career pathway has helped to mainstream abortion education in the USA and could be a useful model elsewhere.

Growing numbers of medical student applicants requesting abortion training during their residency interviews have helped solidify abortion training in a growing number of residency programs. The yearly presence of a group of highly qualified applicants who feel both committed to choosing a residency program that will allow them to gain abortion training, and empowered to ask about this training during residency interviews, is pushing programs to include access to abortion training in order to attract more competitive applicants.

Where a single applicant might be easily ignored, these large numbers of residency applicants asking about abortion training have encouraged programs to consider adding this training to their curriculum.

21.8 Conclusion

Although formal content on sexual and reproductive health, and specifically family planning and abortion, remains rare in many medical schools around the world, the sustained effort to engage medical students in this effort has helped drive the integration of abortion training opportunities in formal medical curricula and foster interest in the incorporation of abortion into medical career plans. A supportive community for students helps to connect students with similar values, and prevents students from feeling isolated, stigmatized, or marginalized. More structured support for students, which can be provided by organizations like MSFC, such as clinical education materials and training in advocacy, also can help to empower students and help them to feel that they are able to respectfully and professionally drive institutional change. MSFC's network shows that peer-to-peer mentorship as well as helping to connect students to senior faculty mentors helps students gain exposure to abortion early in training. Organized and supported groups of medical students can enhance advocacy efforts in sexual and reproductive health as well as mobilizing medical providers early in their education in order to fill gaps in the abortion workforce and create a long-standing network of supportive abortion providers worldwide.

Furthermore, the leadership skills acquired by MSFC group leaders has helped create a large group of committed and effective physician activists who are advocating for patients' access to family planning through their roles as physicians, medical faculty, researchers, and administrators. Former MSFC members are now in medical leadership roles in 50% of the Planned Parenthood affiliates in the USA, and serve as department heads in a host of primary care specialties for large medical institutions throughout the USA and at family planning programs in more than thirty medical centers. Former members of MSFC are now providing abortion care in forty-two US states and five Canadian provinces, as well as in the UK and several countries in Africa. They are leaders in the reproductive health and reproductive justice movements, as well as in professional medical societies worldwide.

References

1. Espey E, Ogburn T, Chavez A, Qualls C, Leyba M. Abortion education in medical schools: a national survey. *Am J Obstet Gynecol.* 2005;**192**(2):640–643.

2. Evans ML, Backus LV. Medical students for choice: creating tomorrow's abortion providers. [Editorial] *Contraception.* 2011;**83**(5):391–393.

3. Joffe C. The crisis in abortion provision and pro-choice medical activism in the 1990s. In ER Solinger (Ed.), *Abortion Wars: A Half Century of Struggle, 1950-2000.* Berkeley: University of California Press; 1998:320–334.

4. Steinauer J. First impressions: what are preclinical medical students in the US and Canada learning about sexual and reproductive health? *Contraception.* 2009;**80**(1):74–80.

5. Mihciokur S, Akin A, Dogan BG, Ozvaris SB. The unmet need for safe abortion in Turkey: a role for medical abortion and training of medical students. *Reprod Health Matters.* 2014;**22**(Suppl 44):26–35.

6. Hogmark S, Klingberg-Allvin M, Gemzell-Danielsson K, Ohlsson H, Essén B. Medical students' knowledge, attitudes and perceptions towards contraceptive use and counselling: a cross-sectional survey in Maharashtra, India. *BMJ Open.* 2013;**3**(12):e003739.

7. Mulyamboga P. Curriculum reform at an international university in Uganda. 2019. https://msfc.org/curriculum-reform-in-uganda/

8. Accreditation Council for Graduate Medical Education. *ACGME program Requirements for Graduate Medical Education in Obstetrics and Gynecology.* Chicago: ACGME; 2014. www.acgme.org/acgmeweb/

9. The American College of Obstetricians and Gynecologists Committee on Health Care for Underserved Women. Abortion training and education. Committee Opinion Number 612. November 2014.

10. Association of Professors of Gynecology and Obstetrics. *APGO Medical Student Educational Objectives,* 10th ed.

Crofton, MD: APGO; 2014. https://obgyn.msu.edu/images/communities/resources/APGO%20Med%20Student%20Obj%2010%20Ed%20.pdf

11. World Health Organization. *Safe Abortion: Technical and Policy Guidance for Health Systems,* 2nd ed. Geneva: WHO; 2012.

12. Pace L, Sandahl Y, Backus L, Silveira M, Steinauer J. Medical Students for Choice's reproductive health externships: impact on medical students' knowledge, attitudes and intention to provide abortions. *Contraception,* 2008; **78**(1):31–35.

13. O'Shea M. Education in abortion care in Ireland: Medical Students for Choice (MSFC) taking a lead. *TSMJ.* 2017;35–41.

14. Steinauer J, Landy U, Filippone H, Lube D, Darney PD, Jackson RA. Predictors of abortion provision among practicing obstetrician-gynecologists: a national survey. *Am J ObstetGynecol.* 2008; **198**(1):39.e1-e6.

Chapter

22

The Role of Simulation in Sexual and Reproductive Health-Care Training

Lisa M. Goldthwaite

22.1 Introduction

Those in medicine may be familiar with the Halstedian apprenticeship model of "see one, do one, teach one" for surgical training. While there is still validity to graded responsibility and apprenticeship, this simple model is outdated. There has instead been a shift toward incorporating simulation-based procedural skills training into medical education. This evolution is practical and necessary for many reasons. Restricted resident work hours, variation in surgical volume, increasing variety of surgical techniques, heightened pressure for mitigating medical errors and pressure for efficient operating times all contribute to a need for an expansion of surgical educational tools outside of the operating room. Using simulation in surgical training is also in line with the motor skill learning theory, where mastery is recognized to occur in three stages [1]. The first stage is cognition, in which the learner seeks to understand a new task. The second stage is integration, where the learner translates knowledge into motor behavior. The third and final stage is automation, which occurs when the learner develops speed and precision with the motor task. All three of these stages of motor skill learning can be supported through surgical simulation.

In the field of family planning specifically, there are several powerful roles for procedural simulation training. First and foremost, as described above, simulation training can serve as a tool for basic skill acquisition. It can also provide opportunities for improving counseling and communication and emergency response team training. Finally, simulation training can foster an environment for discussion, advocacy and sparking interest in the field of sexual and reproductive health.

22.2 Surgical Education

It is recognized that participatory learning (discussion, hands-on practice and teaching others) leads to higher retention rates for learners compared to passive learning (lectures, reading, audio-visual and demonstration) (Figure 22.1) [2]. In all fields of surgical training, moving from a didactic teaching approach to a participatory approach benefits trainees. In surgical training, simulation is an excellent means for participatory learning in a low-stress, low-stakes environment.

Simulation tools come in many forms and can broadly be divided into low- and high-fidelity simulators. Low-fidelity simulators include bench models and laparoscopic box trainers, for example. High-fidelity simulators include virtual reality tools, animal models and cadavers. In general, low-fidelity simulation is less expensive and helpful for beginning learners, or for learning a specific, finite skill set. They are generally portable and reproducible in a variety of environments, including low-resource settings. They can be used in groups or taken home for individual practice. High-fidelity models are often much more expensive, but are better for advanced skill acquisition and trainee evaluation. The basic skills required to perform abortions and contraceptive procedures are well suited for low-fidelity simulation models, and several have been developed and implemented widely in various settings.

22.2.1 Uterine Aspiration Abortion

For surgical uterine aspiration abortion training, a uterine model is necessary. While many commercially available uterine models exist, a simple and commonly used model is the papaya. The papaya model can be used to teach bimanual exams, tenaculum placement, paracervical blocks,

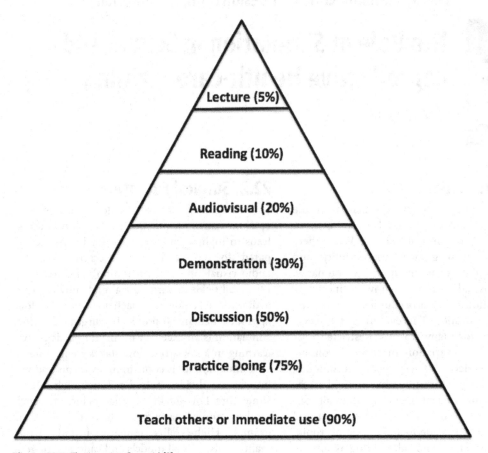

Figure 22.1 The Learning Pyramid [2]

cervical dilation, uterine evacuation and placement of intrauterine contraceptive devices (IUDs). This fruit is similar in size and shape to a uterus, with a stem end that mimics the cervix (Figure 22.2). Papayas can be found in a variety of sizes and are therefore able to represent the size spectrum of first- and second-trimester gravid uteri. By peeling off or puncturing the stem end, one can dilate the "cervix" and enter the simulated "endometrial cavity." Uterine aspiration of seeds simulates the evacuation of products of conception. When the cavity is empty, the learner can even sometimes appreciate a gritty texture with the curette, mimicking the uterine cri.

This model is ideal for beginning learners, including medical students, junior resident physicians or any clinician working to integrate first-trimester uterine aspiration abortion care into their practice. Many residency programs (obstetrics and gynecology and family medicine) and global family planning organizations use some version of a papaya workshop for their training programs. Comprehensive workshop curricula are available online [3].

The papaya model has been evaluated in both medical student and resident physician training environments. Steinauer and colleagues evaluated a medical student curriculum utilizing the papaya model to train students on a number of uterine procedures, including uterine aspiration abortion [4]. Among those students surveyed, 90% rated the simulation workshop as highly valuable. In addition, there was a significant increase in correctly answering knowledge-based questions at the end of the workshop, which persisted to the end of the rotation (p<.0001). Paul and Nobel assessed a similar papaya workshop implemented for family medicine resident physicians [5]. Among trainees surveyed, 92% rated the value of the simulation training as "high" and 73% reported that it would change the way they would manage patients. In addition, trainees reported a 55% decrease in perceived difficulty of the procedure and a 275% increase in procedural confidence.

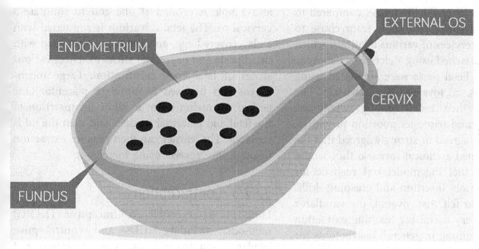

Figure 22.2 The papaya as a uterine model [3]

In addition to the papaya, other fruits can be used to simulate the uterus for first-trimester abortion. The dragonfruit (also known as pitaya) is another excellent low-fidelity fruit model that has been described [6]. It is often inexpensive and, like the papaya, mimics the size, shape and internal "grittiness" of the aspirated uterus. Unlike the papaya, it is usually red on the inside, which can be an added benefit of the model in mimicking blood.

22.2.2 Dilation and Evacuation

The steps of the dilation and evacuation (D&E) procedure for second-trimester abortion require a more advanced model than a papaya or dragonfruit. While many of the steps are similar to those of a first-trimester uterine aspiration abortion, forceps to remove fetal parts are required for D&E. Many models have been developed for D&E training. In general, a uterine model with a cervix large enough to accommodate forceps is necessary. Commercially available uterine models such as the ZOE and NOELLE (Gaumard Scientific, Miami, FL) are frequently available at training hospitals for obstetric and gynecologic simulations, but they are not well suited to D&E training, given their uterine and cervical sizes and rigidity. The Mama-U Postpartum Uterus Trainer (Laerdal Global Health, Stavanger, Norway) is a reasonable size for a D&E model; however, the thin mesh is at risk of damage through the use of D&E forceps and must be handled with care. Simple, low-fidelity models have been described

using plastic water bottles, rice containers, wine totes, stuff sacks, melons and other forms that can mimic the uterine cavity. Items commonly used to simulate fetal parts within various uterine models include cat toys and Ping-Pong balls. Both can be loose inside the uterine model or fastened to the inside of the model with Velcro. Baldwin and colleagues studied the fidelity of three such examples of D&E models [7]. All three models were previously used in various teaching settings, but none had been evaluated by researchers in the field of family planning. Model 1 used cat toys attached with Velcro in a large plastic container, with a cervix constructed of foam. Model 2 was a water bottle with a stuffed form inside that had detachable parts attached with Velcro to the body of the form, along with a removable cover and placenta, also attached with Velcro. Model 3 was a water bottle containing pieces of baguette bread. Models 2 and 3 used the rigid opening of the bottle to simulate the cervix. Fifty-five second-trimester abortion providers participated in the study, rating the realism of the various components of each model. Overall, Model 2 had the most parts that were considered realistic, including the placenta. The foam cervix of Model 1 was rated as realistic. All parts of Model 3 were rated as not realistic. When asked whether they would like to use each model for teaching, 80% responded yes for Model 2, but only 28% responded yes for Model 1 and 9% responded yes for Model 3.

York and colleagues sought to improve on these types of models by designing a low tech, but somewhat higher-fidelity model compared to those described above [8]. Their team chose to create silicone cervices of various dilations, which could then be attached using Velcro to a neoprene uterine model. Fetal parts were simulated using Ping-Pong balls, cat toys and Nerf dart tags. The prototype was then tested among twenty-one experienced second-trimester abortion providers. All participants agreed or strongly agreed that the model represented a clinical scenario they would encounter and that the model was realistic for teaching extraction, insertion and grasping skills. Participants also felt that, overall, the simulator was useful or very useful for teaching extraction skills and for training in general. Instructions for this and other simulation models can be found on the Innovating Education in Reproductive Health website [9].

York and her team then went on to design and evaluate a D&E simulation-training curriculum for obstetrics and gynecology (ob-gyn) resident physicians using this newly developed D&E model [10]. The curriculum is available online [11]. The resident physicians first underwent a 2-hour training session in the simulation-training environment. Then, residents on a family planning rotation underwent additional simulation training using mastery learning techniques. Residents were only allowed to start performing D&E procedures on patients after reaching minimum passing standards on an evaluation checklist. Once they were operating, a skilled supervising surgeon evaluated their performance and provided feedback intra- and post-operatively. Among the 10 resident physicians included in the full analysis, the time to reach a minimal passing score on the simulator ranged from 40 minutes to 3.5 hours. All performed at least three observed operative cases, and seven performed at least six cases. Objective Structured Assessment of Technical Skills (OSATS) ratings improved from case one (19.7) to case three (23.5; $p = .001$) and to case six (26.8; $p = .005$). Overall, they found that simulation training with mastery learning techniques transferred to a high level of performance in the operating room using a checklist, and the OSATS assessments showed improvement in performance over subsequent cases following the training curriculum.

Another low-fidelity model that may be more available in a low-resource setting uses a melon as a uterine model [11]. The melon is hollowed out

and a hole is created at one end to simulate a cervical os. The fetal calvarium is simulated with a clay-covered egg, and limbs are simulated with dried pasta and pepperoni sticks to reflect various stages of fetal bone calcification. Large mushrooms can be used to simulate placenta. One end of the melon is cut to allow for insertion of the fetal and placental models, and then the lid is replaced. The learner can then practice extraction through the "cervix" using forceps.

22.2.3 Contraception

Long-acting reversible contraceptive (LARC) methods, including IUDs and contraceptive implants, require procedures for insertion and removal. These procedures are well suited for simulation training.

22.2.3.1 Intrauterine Device

Regardless of the type of IUD being used, the steps of insertion are generally quite similar. Learners can benefit from understanding the steps of insertion on a model and can also benefit from understanding the specific characteristics of each commercially available insertion device. A number of low- and high-fidelity models for IUD insertion are commercially available and widely used. The papaya as a uterine model (described above) can be used to teach IUD insertion. As with uterine aspiration abortion, the papaya accommodates insertion of instruments and IUDs into the cavity, and allows for an appreciation of reaching the fundus. Another common model is a simple uterine disk model, available from most IUD manufacturers. They consist of a flat, round disk with a transparent uterine cavity and a cervical opening. These are ideal for understanding and practicing the mechanism of deployment for each specific IUD. Another commonly used low-fidelity model is a desktop pelvic model, such as the Gaumard S502 Family Planning Educator (Gaumard Scientific, Miami, FL) or the Sister-U Multi-Uterus Trainer (Laerdal Global Health, Stavanger, Norway). While still low fidelity, these models have more extensive anatomy to help incorporate learning on each step of IUD insertion, beyond simply deploying the device. They both offer visualization into the uterine cavity to watch the IUD insertion or confirm post-insertion position. They are durable, small and portable. A more anatomically complex pelvic model, such as the ZOE Gynecologic Skills Trainer (Gaumard Scientific, Miami, FL), can be used to practice many pelvic procedures, include IUD insertion. This model contains a vulva, vagina, cervix and uterus. It does not allow for visualization into the uterine cavity. It is more anatomically realistic, which may allow for a better simulation of the procedure as a whole. It is also more expensive and less portable. Finally, high-fidelity virtual reality simulators are also available for IUD insertion, such as the PelvicSim (VirtaMed, Zurich, Switzerland). These pelvic models include built-in sensors that provide haptic feedback to the trainee through audio and visual cues, allowing the learner to appreciate tissue handling, as well as moments of increased patient discomfort or use of pressure at risk of causing perforation. They are significantly more expensive compared to the low-fidelity models.

Nippita and colleagues sought to understand the value of high- and low-fidelity models in the context of simulation education for clinical trainees inexperienced in IUD placement [12]. They recruited and enrolled senior nurse practitioner students as well as junior resident physicians in ob-gyn and family medicine, randomizing each trainee to standardized simulation training on either a high-fidelity virtual reality simulator or low-fidelity uterine disk model. They found that both groups improved in IUD placement skills following the training; however, improvement was similar between groups. They also found increases in self-perceived comfort and competence with various types of IUD placement, again similar between groups. Post-simulation knowledge assessment scores were also similar for both groups, both immediately post-simulation and at three months after simulation. Overall, the authors found that the benefits of simulation training for this group of novice trainees were similar, regardless of whether the trainee used a high- or low-fidelity simulator.

High-fidelity virtual reality IUD training systems have been found to be of higher educational value for more experienced clinicians. Dodge and colleagues surveyed 237 clinicians in a network of ambulatory reproductive health centers who used a high-fidelity virtual reality simulator in an IUD training [13]. These clinicians included mostly nurse practitioners (71%), physician assistants (12%), certified nurse midwives (10%) and physicians (4%). Most were relatively experienced with both levonorgestrel and copper IUD insertion. Despite high levels of perceived pre-training competency, the self-reported comfort level after training increased for all tasks. The participants rated video play-back, photos of the insertion path, varying axis of the uterus and IUD insertion activities as the most valuable components of the virtual reality simulator. These findings suggest that there is likely to be greater value added with more nuanced learning available through the high-fidelity trainers for more experienced clinicians compared to novice learners.

The insertion of an IUD into the uterus immediately postpartum or post-abortion is another skill that can be easily simulated and taught. Unlike the standard insertion of an IUD into a small nongravid uterus, there are multiple ways to place an IUD postpartum or post-abortion, including using the clinicians' hand, a forceps or an IUD insertion device. Each of these techniques can be simulated on a model. A commonly used simulator for postpartum IUD training is the Simulaids Obstetrical Manikin (Simulaids, Inc., Saugerties, NY) fitted with a simulated postpartum uterus, such as a fleece-lined stuff sac within a neoprene wine tote. The Mama-U Postpartum Uterus Trainer (Laerdal Global Health, Stavanger, Norway) is another low-fidelity model that was specifically designed to train on postpartum IUD insertion. The Mama-U has a transparent window into the uterus so that the learner can see the IUD location, while the use of an obstetric mannequin is somewhat higher fidelity, but less portable and more costly. Goldthwaite and colleagues developed and evaluated a postpartum IUD training curriculum, including a simulation component, which is available online [11,14]. A total of eighty-four physicians and certified nurse midwives participated in the training, and were evaluated pre-training, immediately post-training and at six months after training. The participants demonstrated sustained improvement in knowledge and comfort with insertion skills immediately and at six months after training.

22.2.3.2 Contraceptive Implant

Contraceptive implants are placed subdermally in the arm, and insertion and removal are simple procedures that can be taught via simulation. The only commercially available contraceptive implant in the USA is the Nexplanon, a 68 mg etonogestrel implant (Merck & Co., Inc., Kenilworth, NJ). Clinicians are required to sit for a manufacturer-sponsored clinical training program prior to provision of any clinical services. The standard Nexplanon training includes a simulation component, with a model arm that includes layers simulating the skin, subcutaneous tissue and muscle. Additional single- and multi-rod subdermal contraceptive implant systems are available internationally, and their insertion and removal procedures can be taught via similar simulation trainings.

Occasionally, a contraceptive implant may be deep or non-palpable at the time of removal. Both a dry model and an animal model have been described as simulation-training opportunities for these more complex contraceptive implant removal procedures, and both are available online [11]. The dry model makes use of the Merck Nexplanon training arm but adjusts the model to insert the contraceptive implant deep into the muscle. The animal model is a higher-fidelity model making use of a turkey leg and ultrasound.

22.2.3.3 Sterilization

Laparoscopy is an essential surgical skill for gynecologists, and many surgeries are now performed via minimally invasive techniques. Most gynecologic surgical training programs in the USA and in many other countries have incorporated laparoscopic simulation into their educational curriculums. Many laparoscopic trainers exist, from low-fidelity box trainer to high-fidelity virtual reality simulators. Bilateral tubal ligation and salpingectomy are simple, common procedures and are generally performed laparoscopically. Training for these procedures can be easily incorporated into standard laparoscopic training programs. Integrating sterilization and family planning discussions into general laparoscopic training programs provides an effective means of integrating family planning skills and considerations into routine gynecology, reinforcing family planning as a component of comprehensive women's health care.

Bilateral tubal ligation is often one of the first laparoscopic procedures performed by gynecologic trainees, making it an excellent candidate surgery for evaluating the role of surgical simulation in operative performance. Banks and colleagues enrolled twenty first-year resident physicians into a study, randomizing them to either routine apprenticeship surgical training in the operating room, or training including time in a surgical simulator laboratory [15]. They found that those trainees assigned to the surgical simulator laboratory performed significantly better than those with apprenticeship teaching alone on all assessment tools utilized (a checklist, a global score and a pass/fail analysis), and scored significantly better on a knowledge post-test, validating the use of simulators to improve resident physician knowledge and operative performance.

22.3 Communication and Counseling

Simulation can be a powerful tool for both teaching and evaluating communication and clinical counseling skills. A common tool in medical education today is the use of the objective structured clinical examination (OSCE) to evaluate a medical student's performance when confronted with a structured clinical scenario. The OSCE tool can be used to evaluate performance of scenarios related to reproductive health.

Presenting a patient with a positive pregnancy result can be a daunting task to those in medical training. Many students do not have the opportunity to observe pregnancy options counseling while in their pre-clinical years. Learning and practicing communication around pregnancy options counseling lend themselves well to the simulated patient encounter. Lupi and colleagues have developed an online instructional module as well as a validated standardized patient exercise that can be integrated into medical training for this purpose [16]. In the online module, students learn basic epidemiology related to unplanned pregnancy, have the opportunity to explore their own values related to pregnancy options and then learn a standard approach to non-directive pregnancy options counseling. Students can then put these principles into practice and be evaluated through a standardized patient simulation. In the validated OSCE scenario, the patient is a twenty-four-year-old woman presenting to urgent care with nausea, who receives the diagnosis of an unplanned pregnancy. Students are rated on many clinical and counseling points, including their delivery of positive pregnancy test results, their response to the patient's emotional silence when hearing the news, their presentation and counseling on pregnancy options (parenting, adoption, abortion) and screening for intimate partner violence and reproductive coercion. The online module and OSCE scenario have been evaluated as a blended learning module [17]. The authors found that all students agreed that the online module helped prepare them for the OSCE exercise. Students with prior clinical experiences related to options counseling outperformed those without clinical experience. This example simulation utilized for counseling opportunities can be easily implemented in all medical education settings, including low-resource settings.

22.4 Emergency Response

Multidisciplinary simulation training for obstetrical emergencies is a well-recognized tool, which has been shown to improve clinical outcomes [18]. In 2012, a joint publication by seven medical societies, including the American College of Obstetricians and Gynecologists, titled "Quality Patient Care in Labor and Delivery: A Call to Action" was released, in which simulation training was recommended as part of a comprehensive strategy to improve outcomes in obstetrics [19]. Those providing abortion care know that clinical emergencies occurring at the time of abortions are similar, if not identical, to those that occur on a labor and delivery unit. Incorporating D&E hemorrhage scenarios into existing obstetric simulation-training infrastructure can lead not only to improved outcomes for abortion care, but also to improved awareness of family planning services within the broader field of obstetrics and gynecology. An example simulation curriculum utilizing the NOELLE model (Gaumard Scientific, Miami, FL) is available online, following a classic obstetric hemorrhage simulation algorithm, but in the context of a D&E for an

eighteen weeks' gestation intrauterine fetal demise [11]. Not only does this simulation allow for taking a multidisciplinary team through an emergency scenario, but it also allows for conversations related to team member comfort and reactions to the provision of abortion services.

22.5 Promoting Interest in the Field of Sexual and Reproductive Health

Simulation training can be an engaging, inspiring, and fun experience for both trainees and trainers. While simulation training for more senior clinicians can help refine surgical techniques, training for the more junior learners, such as medical students, can have different impacts. For example, simulation-training workshops can create an environment where students can interact with clinicians and learn about career opportunities. Unlike didactic learning where an educator is lecturing to a crowd, simulation training allows the trainer and trainees to engage more dynamically together, and discussions can occur organically. Students not only have the opportunity to ask questions relevant to the simulation activity, but they often take the opportunity to learn more about sexual and reproductive health in general, or about careers in the field. In a study evaluating gynecologic simulation training among medical students, Nitschmann and colleagues found that not only did the students improve in clinical confidence with procedural skills, but they also reported an increased interest in pursuing a surgical field, and an increased interest in women's health following the training [20]. Simulation training in abortion and contraception can be used, therefore, not only as a clinical tool, but also as a tool for advocacy, exposure and recruitment into the field of sexual and reproductive health.

References

1. Reznick RK, MacRae H. Teaching surgical skills – changes in the wind. *N Engl J Med.* 2006; **355**(25):2664–2669.

2. Learning Pyramid. Bethel, ME: National Training Laboratories.

3. Papaya Workshop. http://papayaworkshop.org.

4. Steinauer J, Preskill F, Robertson P. Training medical students in intrauterine procedures using papayas. *Med Educ.* 2007;**41**(11):1099–1100.

5. Paul M, Nobel K. Papaya: a simulation model for training in uterine aspiration. *Fam Med.* 2005;**37**(4):242–244.

6. Training in Early Abortion for Comprehensive Healthcare. Workshops for you to use.

www.teachtraining.org/training-tools/simulation-workshops

7. Baldwin MK, Chor J, Chen BA, Edelman AB, Russo J. Comparison of 3 dilation and evacuation technical skills models. *J Grad Med Educ.* 2013;**5**(4):662–664.

8. York SL, Migas S, Haag J, et al. Creation and initial assessment of a second-trimester uterine

model. *Simul Healthc.* 2014; 9(3):199–202.

9. Low-tech D&E model. Online video clip. www.innovating-education.org/2016/03/low-tech-de-training-model-instructional-video

10. York SL, McGaghie WC, Kiley J, Hammond C. Implementation and evaluation of a dilation and evacuation simulation training curriculum. *Contraception.* 2016;93(6):545–550.

11. Innovating Education in Reproductive Health. Simulations. www.innovating-education.org/category/simulations

12. Nippita S, Haviland MJ, Voit SF, Perez-Peralta J, Hacker MR, Paul ME. Randomized trial of high- and low-fidelity simulation to teach intrauterine contraception placement. *Am J Obstet Gynecol.* 2018;218(2):258 e251–258 e211.

13. Dodge LE, Hacker MR, Averbach SH, Voit SF, Paul ME. Assessment of a high-fidelity mobile simulator for intrauterine contraception training in ambulatory reproductive health centres. *J Eur CME.* 2016; 5(1):30416.

14. Goldthwaite LM, Sheeder J, Teal SB, Tocce KM. Comfort with skills and knowledge after immediate postpartum intrauterine device training. *Obstet Gynecol.* 2016;128(Suppl 1):6S–11S.

15. Banks EH, Chudnoff S, Karmin I, Wang C, Pardanani S. Does a surgical simulator improve resident operative performance of laparoscopic tubal ligation? *Am J Obstet Gynecol.* 2007;197 (5):541 e541–545.

16. Lupi CS, Ward-Peterson M, Castro C. Non-directive pregnancy options counseling: online instructional module, objective structured clinical exam, and rater and standardized patient training materials. *MedEdPORTAL.* 2017;13:10566.

17. Lupi C, Ward-Peterson M, Chang W. Advancing non-directive pregnancy options counseling skills: a pilot study on the use of blended learning with an online module and simulation. *Contraception.* 2016;94(4):348–352.

18. Deering S, Rowland J. Obstetric emergency simulation. *Semin Perinatol.* 2013;37(3): 179–188.

19. Quality patient care in labor and delivery: a call to action. *JOGNN.* 2012;41:151–154. doi:10.1111/j.1552-6909.2011.01317.x

20. Nitschmann C, Bartz D, Johnson NR. Gynecologic simulation training increases medical student confidence and interest in women's health. *Teach Learn Med.* 2014; 26(2):160–163.

Chapter

23

The Benefits of and Strategies for Supporting Residents' Partial Participation in Abortion Training

Jody Steinauer and Jema Turk

23.1 Introduction

Since 1996, the governing body for graduate medical education in the USA, the Accreditation Council for Graduate Medical Education (ACGME), requires that obstetrics and gynecology (ob-gyn) residency programs provide access to abortion training [1]. The policy states, "Programs must provide training or access to training in the provision of abortions, and this must be part of the planned curriculum." It goes on to describe that "residents who have a religious or moral objection may opt out, and must not be required to participate in training in or performing induced abortions." Further, training programs are allowed to opt out due to religious or moral objections, but they must find a training opportunity for their residents at another institution. Since 1996, additional family planning requirements have been added to the core ACGME requirements to now explicitly include routine training in abortion care for any indication, the management of abortion complications and all methods of contraception (see Chapter 3) [2].

In its 2014 committee opinion on abortion training and education, the American College of Obstetricians and Gynecologists (ACOG) recommends all ob-gyn programs provide opt-out abortion training where "abortion is routinely integrated into medical education as a critical element of women's reproductive healthcare." ACOG states programs should continue efforts to destigmatize abortion and integrate abortion education into medical school curricula [3]. Additionally, ACOG has defined clear expectations for an individual ob-gyn to claim the right to conscientious refusal, outlined in their committee opinion, "The limits of conscientious refusal in reproductive medicine" [4]. They define conscientious refusal as a time when a "clinician feels that providing indicated, standard health care for a patient would present for them a conflict of conscience" and therefore declines to provide that care. They go on to define appropriate limits around conscientious refusal, state that these clinicians must provide accurate and unbiased information and prompt referral to care and direct that in an emergency they have an obligation to provide medically indicated and requested care.

Abortion training can be integrated into residency programs in a number of ways. It can be fully integrated, which means that it is routinely scheduled for learners; individual learners who do not want the training can completely or partially opt out. This has been termed "opt-out" training as in the ACOG committee opinion, and "routine" training. The Ryan Program requires "routine" training to qualify for support. The training can also be available to learners but "optional" or "opt in," meaning that it is not routinely scheduled and a learner has to ask to be scheduled or to "opt in" to participate. Finally, it can be simply not available in the training program, and a motivated individual would have to learn the skills outside of the program without formal support.

Ob-gyn residency programs have increasingly integrated abortion training since the ACGME policy went into effect in 1996, with only 5% of programs in 2014 reporting no training [5]. This increase in training in the USA was in large part supported by the Ryan Program, described more fully in Chapter 3. However, in that same 2014 study, among the programs with training, the levels of integration varied; in 64% the training was routinely included in residents' schedules and in 31% it was optional. Seven program directors (4%) reported having been cited by the Residency Review Committee (RRC) for not meeting the abortion training requirement (six programs with optional training and one with no training) [5]. Some of the programs applying for the Ryan Program support do so because they have been cited by the RRC for inadequate training.

For family medicine, the ACGME states that residents must have experience with gynecologic issues, including family planning, contraception and options counseling for unintended pregnancy. Published in 1998, the American Academy of Family Physicians' "Core Educational Guidelines for Maternity and Gynecologic Care" included abortions up to ten weeks' gestation as an advanced skill that should be available within training programs for interested residents [6]. The more recent guideline for women's health and gynecologic care also includes abortion training in its advanced skills, but expands the gestation to include surgical and medication abortion in the first trimester [7]. Additionally, this guideline lists "dilation and curettage" as an advanced skill, and the guideline on maternity and gynecologic care lists 'dilation and curettage' for incomplete abortion as a core skill, but specifies that it may be considered "advanced" at some programs [6]. As a result of a number of training initiatives for family medicine residents, abortion training has increased over the last twenty years. This increase is important, but notably occured at a much slower rate than in obstetrics and gynecology programs. (See Chapter 15.) Currently only 8% of family medicine programs offer integrated, opt-out training, compared to more than 60% of ob-gyn programs. (See Chapter 15.)

Studies in ob-gyn and family medicine have documented resident participation in training. In ob-gyn, among 2,876 residents in 93 programs with routine training between 1999 and 2019, 83% fully participated and 17% partially participated [9]. Full participation in family medicine programs with abortion training has increased from 55% in 1996 [10] to 79% in 2017 [11].

23.2 History of Opting Out/ Partial Participation

Before the passage of the ACGME mandate, training varied widely. The Ryan Program, in order to evaluate training approaches and outcomes, including clinical competence and the opt-out experience, launched a separate, ongoing evaluation effort under the leadership of Dr. Jody Steinauer, and published its findings.

Early in its history, the Ryan Program simply defined its expectation for routine training as opt out, not opt in. This approach acknowledged that residents had a choice prescribed by the ACGME. Initially, this choice was presented as an either-or choice. Residents who did participate were assigned to another rotation and did not have the opportunity to learn about the public health, clinical or emotional aspects of the abortion experience. By 2009, the Ryan Program in its application required that all residents should participate to their comfort level with a clear opt-out policy and learning expectations of opt-out residents.

By 2014, the Ryan Program was consistently using the term *partial participation* instead of *opt out*. This shift was informed by findings from studies about opt-out experiences and site-visit feedback. The concept of partial participation acknowledges that residents, regardless of their personal or religious perspective about abortion, should be given an opportunity to learn about a woman's abortion experience, ideally by accompanying her through the visit, from intake, counseling and the procedure to post-abortion recovery and contraception.

In the program's early evaluations of residents who chose to opt out, it became clear that participation, even if only by providing post-abortion contraception, could lead to significant insights about women's need to have an abortion, the motivation and professionalism of those who do them and reflections about future professional responsibilities regarding the provision of abortion and referral of patients [12,13]. The shift of attitude and expectation for future practice could be drastic, moving from a refusal to step into an abortion clinic to accepting women's need for terminating a pregnancy, as illustrated in the words of a Ryan Program resident in 2011:

[I am] comfortable with IUDs and other contraceptive procedures. ... I can hopefully prevent another abortion from being done. ... It did open my eyes to the fact that this is a very difficult situation that they're in ... it made me grateful for not ever having to be in that situation, as a man. ... What would I do in this scenario? It did make me

Table 23.1 Proportion of sixty-seven partially participating ob-gyn residents indicating positive effects on family planning skills

Skills	% Indicating positive impact
Counseling skills	
Contraceptive counselling	92%
Pregnancy options counseling	88%
Counseling about aspiration abortion	86%
Early pregnancy loss counseling	82%
Counseling about medication abortion	81%
Pre-operative skills	
Ultrasound for pregnancy dating	74%
Preoperative assessment	62%
Procedural skills	
Pain management for transcervical procedures	72%
IUD placement	68%
Cervical anesthesia	63%
First-trimester uterine aspiration	57%
Postoperative management of complications	64%

Source: Summary of data from Steinauer et al. [15].

think about that a lot more. (from a partially participating male resident in the West, interviewed in 2011)

In addition to learners' personal beliefs about abortion, the culture of the training program environment also affects the resident's decision to participate. Studies of ob-gyn training in the USA have demonstrated that levels of resident participation are correlated with the program's expectations for and availability of training. For example, in 1987, Darney et al. documented that more residents fully participated in training in programs with integrated, routine abortion training compared with residents in programs with optional training [14]. Likely, the decision to opt in or out may not simply be based on personal beliefs but may also be influenced by the departmental culture and faculty attitudes that define the expectations for resident participation.

23.3 Definition of Opting Out/ Partial Participation

While the majority of ob-gyn residents in programs with routine training fully participate, some do not feel comfortable with all aspects of abortion care, depending on personal beliefs,

religious perspective and family and social background. When given an option to partially participate, residents often take and appreciate the opportunity to go beyond simply observing counseling or providing post abortion contraception. Typically, they want to learn about other aspects of care such as ultrasound, cervical block and dilation, long-actiing reversible contraception (LARC) placement and sterilization [12].

Learners who do not fully participate and opt out of doing uterine evacuation procedures for abortion often choose to do them for other reasons, for example early pregnancy loss or pregnancy complications [15]. Their level of participation sometimes changes during residency and during the rotation itself.

23.4 Benefits of Partial Participation

Participation in training to a level of individual comfort, rather than opting out of all family planning training, is highly beneficial. A quantitative study of ob-gyn residents in 2013 found that 92% of residents who opted out of at least some portion of the family planning rotation reported a positive impact and highly valued the skills they acquired, including the skills listed above and management of analgesia and anesthesia during procedures and rare post-abortion complications (Table 23.1) [15]. These residents also gained skills in uterine aspiration; 84% performed at least one abortion, typically for a pregnancy complication [15]. Another study found that residents felt prepared to use the skills in uterine aspiration for early pregnancy loss, emergency care and possibly abortion care for patients with pregnancy complications [13].

Qualitative research has given additional insights into valued skills: interacting with patients facing unintended pregnancies, improving counseling skills and learning to prioritize the care that their patients need over their own views or beliefs [13]. In in-depth interviews, residents described greater acceptance of women seeking abortions, abortion providers and abortion in general and greater comfort counseling about and referring for abortion [13]. Even learners who began their family planning training intending not to fully participate felt the training better prepared them for future careers in women's health, especially the ability to manage abortion complications and care for women experiencing miscarriage [13].

Hearing the stories of women seeking abortion care challenged interviewees' assumptions about who gets abortions and for what reasons. While none planned to integrate abortion into their post-residency practice, respondents described more favorable attitudes toward all aspects of the abortion experience.

23.5 Overview of Best Practices for Supporting Partial Participation

In this section, we describe the approach we have suggested that Ryan Programs use to support partially participating residents, which can be used as a guideline for other programs. In order to identify learners who may not want to fully participate in abortion training, the residency program leadership may disseminate their programs' partial participation policy before training commences. They may then introduce training details and the process of partial participation during orientation. (See Figure 23.1 for an overview protocol of introducing and supporting decision making around participation.)

The process of deciding about participation can be challenging for learners. Learners who want to partially participate may have different levels of comfort with different aspects of family planning care. Therefore, faculty need to have systems in place to help the learner make participation decisions. A study of twenty-six ob-gyn residents explored how they navigated partial participation in abortion training, how they weighed

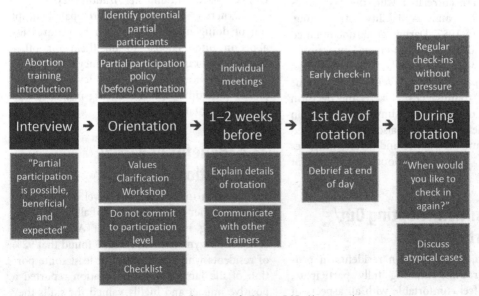

Figure 23.1 Partial participation overview for training facilitators D&E, dilation and evacuation

different factors and how they determined their limits [16]. Residents determined the extent of their participation at different times in training: some knew exactly what they would do (or not do) before residency began, others decided along the way. Those who determined the extent of their participation as training occurred were influenced by a variety of reasons. Some were affected by personal factors – perhaps their family wouldn't approve of them providing abortions – or by their sense of professional obligations – that is, they didn't want to burden their fellow residents or clinic staff if they opted out of providing care to certain patients. For others, their perception of support or pressure from fellow residents and or their supervisors had an impact on their decision making [16].

It is important for the residency leadership to be transparent about abortion training and the options for residents to partially participate. Faculty may find it difficult to find alternative learning experiences for partially participating residents. One study of family medicine residency programs found a variety of alternative curricula assigned to these residents [17]. For example, one program required residents to meet with faculty to review didactic curriculum, while other programs simply encouraged leaners to participate in non-abortion specific skills, such as options counseling, ultrasound and procedural skills, to the extent they were comfortable [17]. We recommend that faculty meet with the residents to review the learning objectives for the rotation and then work on a plan to meet the objectives and gain competence in skills while also respecting their personal limits.

As faculty work with residents to facilitate their decision making and learning on the rotation, they might be careful to clearly communicate and respect learners' boundaries. In one study, a small minority of partially participating ob-gyn residents felt disappointed in how expectations were communicated [16]. These residents wanted to opt out of all related training and care, but faculty expected them to participate in pre- and post-abortion care, such as counseling and ultrasound. While this is rare and the vast majority of partially participating residents participate in all aspects of care except doing the uterine aspiration, these finding show the importance of clear and early communication with residents,

and the tensions partial participation may provoke. Partial participation in family planning training is complex and "demands clear communication and acceptance between resident and attending as well as clinic staff" [13].

23.6 Protocols and Guidelines for Supporting Partial Participation

Tools are available for residency program leadership and faculty to help prepare learners for family planning training and to support their decision making about participation. A useful exercise to guide learners in decisions related to participation is a Values Clarification (VC) workshop focused on abortion. The workshop typically involves facilitated reflection and clarification of feelings about abortion. VC workshops range in length and content, but typically consist of small-group discussion, case studies, expressive activities and self-administered worksheets [18]. In VC workshops, facilitators work to create a safe environment in which participants are encouraged to engage in reflection. In an international study of more than 4,000 abortion providers in 12 countries between 2006 and 2011, values clarification workshops improved abortion knowledge, favorable attitudes and intentions to integrate abortion in care [19]. Freedman et al. [20] recommended that a values clarification curriculum should be an explicit component of abortion training, contending "such examination and awareness can improve professionalism in physician–patient interactions where unrecognized judgments might impact the provision of care." The Ryan Program recommends the use of VC exercises for residents, nurses and staff, and many programs incorporate these exercises into their resident orientation protocol.

As we have described, it is important to engage in discussions about participation early in resident training. In order to inform a practical guide for residency program leaders, the Ryan Program conducted interviews with family planning faculty at programs with abortion training about their experiences with residents who did not fully participate in training. In these interviews, the faculty members described their strategies regarding communication and flexibility in accommodating the resident. Their data reinforced findings from the 2014 qualitative study [16], which showed residents made decisions about their participation both before and during the family planning rotation, requiring faculty to be open minded and flexible. Regular, supportive communication led to a more positive experience.

We used these data to create a recommended protocol and guide to support partial participation. While this was generated by data within obstetrics and gynecology, we believe it could be modified for use in family medicine and other training programs. It includes suggestions for when to facilitate discussions, terminology to encourage transparency and clear expectations and suggested "check-in" questions during the training, with an overview shown in Figure 23.1.

Resources for facilitating Values Clarification workshops can be found on the website www.innovating-education.org and through organizations such as Catholics for Choice, the National Abortion Federation and IPAS.

The entire interactive guide and supporting resources for faculty to support partially participating learners can be accessed online at www.innovating-education.org/participation/.

This partial participation overview provides brief guidance for training leadership – residency program directors or other faculty who are responsible for family planning training – regarding specific points in residency. For example, introducing the rotation and expectations regarding abortion and family planning training is typically done during resident interviews, either by department chairs, residency program directors or Ryan Program directors. The specific mention of the availability of training reinforces not only the department's expectations, but also the acknowledgment of the departmental support of family planning and abortion. In turn, residents can use this information as they make their residency program decisions and have a clear understanding of whether their expectations match with the program.

With this overview (and full guide online) we make specific suggestions of when to introduce and discuss training and objectives. Many residents ask about the availability of family planning training and choose programs specifically because they are listed as Ryan Programs that have integrated family planning training. Transparency is essential – to the learners, faculty and clinic staff.

Some faculty find that it is helpful to understand residents' comfort levels before starting the rotation to support the learners and prepare the staff. For example, communicating with clinic staff that there will be a resident in the upcoming rotation who might be uncomfortable with some procedures would be helpful to planning appropriate resources and staffing. However, we recommend, as described below, that the faculty members be flexible and support the residents to change their participation levels throughout the rotation.

23.6.1 Interview for Residency

As early as the resident interview, the residency program director can introduce and describe the family planning rotation in the same way that other aspects of the training program are described. It is important to clarify that the training is routine, scheduled in their training and all individuals are expected to at least partially participate and learn the many skills taught on the rotation. It is important to normalize family planning and abortion training as an integral part of women's health care from the beginning of training – for example, by teaching about the public health aspects of abortion. A sample protocol for training and expectations is included (Figure 23.2) and additional templates can be found in the online guide.

One faculty member, in an interview study that informed this guide, described the experience in normalizing training:

> So we've tried to change the language, honestly, from "opt out" to "partial participation" . . . because I don't want any resident to ever think that they get to really opt out of women's health care in any kind of significant way.

23.6.2 Resident Orientation

We recommend messages about training be reiterated at orientation. It may be appropriate for program directors to schedule a values clarification during orientation, especially for programs during which first-year residents are scheduled to spend time in an abortion care setting. As previously mentioned, the Ryan Program considers a values clarification an important introduction to the rotation. Our interviews found that it is helpful to ask residents to look over the various skills

-PARTIAL PARTICIPATION PROTOCOL TEMPLATE-

PROCEDURE FOR OPTING OUT OF A PORTION OF RESIDENCY TRAINING

We have developed a mechanism for helping residents who are struggling with the dilemma of whether they hold a moral objection to a particular procedure, or whether they are just disturbed by or uncomfortable with the procedure itself.

It is the department's *expectation* that all residents will receive instruction in all aspects of residency training, including but not limited to:
- contraception including tubal ligation
- abortion counseling and techniques

It is not the department's policy that residents will be required to perform procedures that violate their beliefs.

1. The resident will meet with the key faculty member for the rotation and the program director. The purpose of this panel will be to be supportive and constructive and not directive and ooercive.

2. The resident will discuss their beliefs and concerns about this portion of their residency training.

3. The resident will delineate precisely what aspects of the rotation or training they do not want to participate in.

4. Faculty will help the resident identify key skills that are learned during this portion of their training, including career opportunities and limitations.

5. The resident will present alternative opportunities for obtaining these skills, if applicable.

6. Faculty will implement a process to ensure that the resident learns the critical skills via other opportunities.

7. A summary of the meeting with the faculty member and the program director will be signed by all three physicians and will be placed in the resident's file.

8. Permission to opt out of a portion of training will be approved by the program director after the above steps are taken.

Figure 23.2 Sample partial participation protocol. http://innovating-education.org/cms/assets/uploads/2016/03/1c3_PP_protocol_draft.doc

that can be learned in an abortion care setting and ask them to reflect on which aspects of care they would like to participate in and which they would not. It may be appropriate in some programs to provide learners a checklist of aspects of care and have a discussion about which are expected and explore the learners' plans for the others, either as early as residency orientation or later before the rotation starts. We recommend going through these details at a time closer to the rotation, although some programs prefer to review it well before the rotation begins. Figure 23.3 shows a sample checklist, and additional checklist templates can be found in the online guide.

If a program uses a checklist, it should be considered a dynamic document for residents and not a contract or final decision. This is also a convenient time to ask residents to review materials such as the ACOG Committee Opinion No. 385: "The Limits of Conscientious Refusal in Reproductive Medicine" [4] and the ACOG Committee Opinion No. 612: "Abortion Training and Education" [3], as well as their policy on training, and possibly to sign an acknowledgment that they understand the policy. This latter aspect of orientation is not required, but some programs use it to clarify their expectations, the professional obligations of the specialty and options for partial participation in training.

One faculty interviewee described the importance of discussing expectations at orientation as one way to help orient learners and prepare them more adequately for what is to come:

ABORTION AND FAMILY PLANNING ROTATION PARTICIPATION CHECKLIST

	Expected	Comments
Pre-operative care	X	
Pre-operative history and physical	X	
Ultrasound dating	X	
Pregnancy options counseling	X	
Abortion counseling / consent	X	
Contraceptive counseling	X	
1st-trimester ultrasound	X	
2nd-trimester ultrasound	X	
Cervical preparation		
Administration or misoprostol or mifepristone for cervical preparation		
Osmotic dilator placement		
Administration of medication abortion		
Intra-abortion care		
Analgesia management		
Local anesthetic block placement		
Mechanical dilation pre-procedure		
1st-trimester manual vacuum / uterine aspiration		
1st-trimester electric vacuum / uterine aspiration		
2nd-trimester dilation and evacuation		
Induction termination		
Specific circumstances		
1st-trimester uterine aspiration for medically complicated pregnancies		
D&E for medically complicated pregnancies		
Induction termination for medically complicated pregnancies		
1st-trimester uterine aspiration for pregnancy loss	X	
D&E for pregnancy loss	X	
Induction termination for pregnancy loss	X	
Post-abortion care / recovery	X	
Contraception		
IUD insertion	X	
Implant placement	X	
Sterilization	X	

Figure 23.3 Sample abortion rotation partial participation checklist. http://innovating-education.org/cms/assets/uploads/2016/03/2e1_PP_Recommended_Checklist_Template.pdf

I really feel, especially for the opt-out and partially participating, that residents feel overwhelmed and intimidated because they have these preconceived notions of themselves and their feelings and their ideas of how they want to participate and to what extent, and even engaging in conversation perhaps makes them feel that they should do more than what they're comfortable with, that they should stretch their limits. ... But I think that it would be perceived better if we're talking about this in the same way that we're talking about everything else, that we are doing this orientation because I just want to be clear beyond what's written in the syllabus about what the expectations are and this is how you can excel in this.

Similar recommendations from other faculty informed our recommendations to present the abortion training at orientation, to make the expectations clear and to inspire the residents to reflect on their participation early.

23.6.3 Before the Rotation

A short time before the rotation begins, the faculty member in charge of abortion training should reach out to residents again to reiterate training options and to clarify their intended level of participation, potentially review the checklist and review the expectations for the rotation. Again, this should not be considered a final decision, as many learners change their levels of participation during the rotation. However, if a resident is planning to opt out of some aspects of the training, it is important for the lead faculty member to inform other faculty and staff so they can prepare to support the learner and ensure adequate staff to provide care. One faculty interviewed described communicating with residents before training as a way to encourage self-reflection:

And the point of this is not an interrogation but it's to start to explore the resident's feelings about why they're thinking about not participating as much, trying to tease out what exactly it is that makes you uncomfortable and what you're having a problem with. The thing we're trying to avoid is "I'm just not comfortable." That's like that magic phrase of well there's a lot of things most of us aren't comfortable with. It doesn't mean we don't get to do it. And so we want the residents to have kind of embarked on some self-reflection about what this means and encourage them to do that.

This faculty member's and others' experiences informed our recommendations to make sure the resident understands the many skills they could learn on the rotation and to support the residents' reflection on their comfort with and intentions to participate in abortion care, so that the resident makes informed decisions to maximize the learning on the rotation.

23.6.4 During the Family Planning Rotation

On the first day of the rotation, the faculty member should orient the learner in the usual ways that learners are oriented to new training sites. This may include introduction to the clinical space and staff, review of the learning objectives on the rotation, following a patient through the abortion care experience, observation of counseling, and orientation to clinical practices such as ultrasound, preoperative assessment, consent and procedures. In addition, we recommend a debrief at the end of the first day to support reflection about their experience. We also recommend regular, similar check-ins during the rotation, not intended to pressure the residents to change their participation level, but to support their learning and growth. It is also the faculty member's responsibility to make sure the resident is meeting the learning objectives of the training and gaining the skills required to be competent in practice. This may require finding alternative ways to gain uterine aspiration skills, for example, by assigning the resident to a different unit to provide uterine aspiration care for patients experiencing pregnancy loss. Faculty also might assign topics for the residents to research and present as another avenue to support knowledge attainment in lieu of doing procedures.

Our interviews found that residents change their views and expectations over the course of residency. While it may be impractical considering the challenges of scheduling, insisting on early commitment does not allow residents to modify their participation as their comfort level and perspective change. One faculty member interviewed described how participation levels can change over the course of training:

[One] resident ... was incredibly anti-abortion when she started residency and looked with dread toward the reproductive health rotation. And so I met with her at the start – this was not a particularly touchy-feely resident ... I gave her my usual "spiel" and I said, "I'd like you to be there for a little while, as long as you're okay walking in the building, but we'll never push you." And by the end of her rotation not only was she in the room with me, handing me instruments, ... she was really assisting.

We heard about many similar experiences from other faculty members. These experiences are not uncommon and have helped inform our recommendation to communicate with residents throughout the rotation, to be flexible and try to accommodate changes in their participation plans and to help achieve maximal benefits, especially overall competence and attitude about the many aspects of abortion care during the family planning rotation.

23.7 Conclusion

Abortion training is a required component of US ob-gyn graduate medical education training and is recommended in family medicine training. While individual residents may choose to opt out of training, the Ryan Program's expectations and these recommendations emphasize the importance of facilitating the participation of residents to their comfort level to learn the many important and transferable skills for women's health-care providers.

Partially participating residents enjoy the rotation, appreciate the procedural skills they learn and their improved knowledge about all aspects of abortion and contraception, and feel more comfortable counseling and referring patients for care. Depending on which setting, institution and state, they will likely also have an understanding of the consequences of restrictions to care and the sometimes dire consequences of lack of access. After training, these learners will be better prepared to support the autonomy of and provide high-quality care for patients seeking abortion services, and they will acquire complementary skills for outpatient surgical procedures, routine and perhaps complex contraceptive care and pregnancy loss.

References

1. Accreditation Council for Graduate Medical Education. ACGME Program Requirements for Graduate Medical Education in Obstetrics and Gynecology; 2014.

2. ACGME Review Committee for Obstetrics and Gynecology. Clarification on Requirements Regarding Family Planning and Contraception; 2017.

3. ACOG Committee Opinion No. 612: abortion training and education. *Obstet Gynecol.* 2014;124(5):1055–1059.

4. ACOG Committee Opinion No. 385 November 2007: the limits of conscientious refusal in reproductive medicine. *Obstet Gynecol.* 2007;110 (5):1203–1208.

5. Steinauer JE, Turk JK, Pomerantz T, Simonson K, Learman LA, Landy U. Abortion training in US obstetrics and gynecology residency programs. *Am J Obstet Gynecol.* 2018; 219(1):86.e81–86.e86.

6. Maternity and gynecologic care. Recommended core educational guidelines for family practice residents. American Academy of Family Physicians. *Am Fam Physician.* 1998;58(1):275–277.

7. American Academy of Family Physicians. Women's health and gynecologic care. Recommended curriculum guidelines for family medicine residents. AAFP Rpt. No. 282; 2018.

8. Steinauer JE, Turk JK, Fulton MC, Simonson KH, Landy U. The benefits of family planning training: a 10-year review of the Ryan Residency Training Program. *Contraception.* 2013;88(2):275–280.

9. Landy U, Turk JK, Simonson K, Koenemann, Steinaurer J. Twenty years of the Ryan Residency Program in Abortion and Family Planning. *Contraception.* 2021;103(1) 305–309. doi:10.1016/j. contraception.2020.12.009.

10. Talley PP, Bergus GR. Abortion training in family practice residency programs. *Fam Med.* 1996;28(4):245–248.

11. Summit AK, Gold M. The effects of abortion training on family medicine residents' clinical experience. *Fam Med.* 2017;49(1):22–27.

12. Goodman S, Shih G, Hawkins M, et al. A long-term evaluation of a required reproductive health training rotation with opt-out provisions for family medicine residents. *Fam Med.* 2013; 45(3):180–186.

13. Steinauer JE, Turk JK, Preskill F, Devaskar S, Freedman L, Landy U. Impact of partial participation in integrated family planning training on medical knowledge, patient communication and professionalism. *Contraception.* 2014;89 (4):278–285.

14. Darney PD, Landy U, MacPherson S, Sweet RL. Abortion training in U.S. obstetrics and gynecology residency programs. *Fam Plann Perspect.* 1987; 19(4):158–162.

15. Steinauer JE, Hawkins M, Turk JK, Darney P, Preskill F, Landy U. Opting out of abortion training: benefits of partial participation in a dedicated family planning rotation for ob-gyn residents. *Contraception.* 2013;87 (1):88–92.

16. Turk JK, Preskill F, Fields A, Landy U, Steinauer JE. Exploring how residents who partially participate in family planning training determine their level of participation. *Womens Health Issues.* 2017;27(5):614–619.

17. Brahmi D, Dehlendorf C, Engel D, Grumbach K, Joffe C, Gold M. A descriptive analysis of abortion training in family medicine residency programs. *Fam Med.* 2007;39(6):399–403.

18. Turner KL, Page KC. *Abortion Attitude Transformation: A Values Clarification Toolkit for Global Audiences.* IPAS; 2014.

19. Turner KL, Pearson E, George A, Andersen KL. Values clarification workshops to improve abortion knowledge, attitudes and intentions: a pre-post assessment in 12 countries. *Reprod Health.* 2018;15(1):40.

20. Freedman L, Landy U, Steinauer J. Obstetrician-gynecologist experiences with abortion training: physician insights from a qualitative study. *Contraception.* 2010;81(6):525–530.

Chapter 2

Stigma and Abortion Care
Implications for Training

Meghan Seewald, Lisa A. Martin and Lisa H. Harris

24.1 Abortion Stigma: Conceptual Background

Stigma was first defined in 1963 by sociologist Erving Goffman as an attribute that is "deeply discrediting." Those stigmatized cease to be "whole and usual" people, becoming instead "tainted" and "discounted" [1]. Other sociologists later clarified that stigma is an interpersonal process, requiring both a stigmatizer and one stigmatized. It is a process of distinguishing and labeling difference, stereotyping and discrimination [2]. Stigma can result from one's work. Sociologist C. Everett Hughes named stigmatized work "dirty work" and the people who do it "dirty workers" [3]. Dirty workers perform work that is socially necessary, but is nevertheless physically disgusting, socially degrading and/or morally dubious [4]. Examples include gravediggers or garbage collectors. Stigma is a global phenomenon; however, local dynamics shape its manifestations.

While stigma is a decades-old sociological concept, attention to abortion stigma is more recent. Here, we provide a brief overview of the impact of abortion stigma on those who seek care, then focus on stigma and the abortion-providing workforce. While abortion care teams often include advanced-practice clinicians, nurses, counselors, medical and surgical assistants and administrators, our focus is the impact of abortion stigma on doctors and medical trainees specifically.

24.1.1 Stigma and Patients

In 2009, Kumar, Hessini and Mitchell defined abortion stigma as a "negative attribute ascribed to women who seek to terminate a pregnancy, that marks them, internally or externally, as inferior to the ideals of womanhood" [4]. There are many reasons why abortion is stigmatized, including that it is not universally legal and may carry a taint of being illegal, religious traditions that do not permit abortion, the belief among some that abortion is morally equivalent to killing a born person and that it allows women to deviate from traditional maternal, life-giving roles. Stigma both comes from and reinforces stereotypes of women who have abortions as selfish, promiscuous, irresponsible and in violation of gendered expectations of women and motherhood [5]. These negative stereotypes can be a source of loss of self-esteem and social isolation. They also generate reluctance to disclose abortion experiences to others, and since abortion is a "concealable" stigma, it can be hidden. Concealment of abortion offers some protection from social judgment and ostracism, discrimination, loss of status and/or exclusion from social groups and institutions [5].

Abortion stigma adversely impacts care logistics and paths. For example, if women do not wish to disclose their abortions to others, they may find it difficult to negotiate time off work, ask for help with childcare or obtain a referral from a primary care physician. In the face of these difficulties, some women may find it easier to conceal their pregnancy and desire to end it from those around them; others may choose to self-manage their abortion, or seek care outside of the formal medical sector [6]. While some people are able to self-manage abortion safely (in particular those with access to evidence-based medication regimens), others are not, and health consequences can be devastating [6]. Stigma also indirectly impacts women seeking abortion care by contributing to shortages in the physician workforce, and difficulty finding a nearby provider, discussed below.

24.1.2 Stigma and Caregivers

Stigma and negative stereotypes about abortion-providing physicians are ubiquitous, including that they are greedy, immoral, incompetent "butchers", or "hacks" [7]. Abortion work is a type of dirty work, involving physical taint (blood, fetal parts), social taint (close contact with women seeking abortion, who are themselves stigmatized), and moral taint (the belief, among some, that abortion is morally equivalent to murder or is life-ending) [3]. Abortion caregivers are socially needed, yet are looked down upon by many for doing their work.

24.1.3 Stigma Is Everywhere: The Socio-Ecological Model

Abortion caregivers experience stigma at all levels of a socio-ecological model, a theoretical framework for understanding the multiple social levels that generate experience. We consider abortion caregiver stigma at each of these levels in Table 24.1.

Individual-level abortion stigma includes experiences of internalized, perceived and enacted stigma – meaning the ways stigma affects one's self-perception, beliefs about the perceptions of others and actual experiences of discrimination or unfair treatment. For abortion caregivers, individual-level stigma commonly manifests in feeling "marked," or defined solely by their abortion work, overwhelming all other parts of their identity. Physicians also describe feeling judged, isolated and like "outsiders" within medicine.

At a community level, many caregivers experience judgment and disapproval from others: family members, friends, church or school acquaintances and even patients. As with people seeking abortion, this leads to constant disclosure negotiations; many choose not to disclose their abortion work to avoid difficult conversations or negative consequences, such as violence or harassment.

Institutional-level stigma includes the marginalization of abortion and abortion-providing physicians within medicine and medical

Table 24.1 Abortion stigma in a socio-ecological model

Quotations come from abortion caregivers who participated in Providers Share Workshop research around the world, discussed later in this chapter.

Level	Definition	Example
Individual	Experiences of stigma by individuals, including people who have abortions and their caregivers.	*"I feel very judged. . . . [Even] patients think we're bad people even though we're doing what they want us to do."*
Community	Social and cultural norms, attitudes and behaviors toward abortion (including women and providers) that exist in communities.	*"If something bad goes wrong here and everyone in the world knows I am an abortion doctor, will I still be able to go to church?"*
Institutional	How policies and practices within health-care institutions, professional societies and medical education can marginalize abortion within mainstream medicine.	*". . . the ER staff will invariably say some crap about 'the jokers over at the abortion clinic.' There is this implied stereotype that doctors [who] do abortions can't do any other part of medicine."*
Structural	How laws and policies introduce barriers to abortion and serve to discriminate against women and caregivers.	*". . . There are government representatives who are religious leaders. . . . And they've become the biggest obstacle in [defending] abortion rights. We've been plagued by archaic laws. [In some situations] the police come in all the way into the operating room."*
Public Discourse	How abortion, people who seek care and caregivers are portrayed in media and popular culture, and referred to in dominant discourse.	*"I could see this bumper sticker and it just said 'abortion' on the top. . . . I was dying to see what it said underneath. . . . What it said was, 'abortion: one dead, one wounded.' . . . That is so unfair. Why do I have to take this?"*

Source: Adapted from LeTourneau [11]; Harris et al. [7]; Kumar et al. [4].

education. Around the world, most abortions are performed in freestanding outpatient clinics [8], physically separating abortion from the rest of medical care and perpetuating the stereotype that abortion is not health care. Such physical separation can complicate the process of referring patients for care or follow-up treatment.

Structural-level abortion stigma permeates law and policy. Many countries have laws restricting abortion access, which often specifically target physicians. In some places, performing abortions carries criminal penalties; in others, physicians face burdensome regulatory standards such as requiring hospital admitting privileges at a nearby institution. These and other laws are often justified as necessary to protect women's health and safety, but often rely on stereotypes of abortion-providing physicians as unconcerned with patient safety and requiring additional oversight compared to other doctors [9].

Finally, public discourse is filled with stereotypes of physicians who provide abortion care as incompetent and dangerous. An analysis of abortion as portrayed on American television found that legal abortion providers were often depicted as providing unsafe care, perpetuating stereotypes of abortion as dangerous [10].

24.1.4 Consequences of Stigma: Important Conceptual Ideas

24.1.4.1 Stigma's Vicious Cycles

Stigma generates vicious cycles; that is, stigma results in an outcome, and that outcome generates further stigma, which then further reinforces the outcome. We describe several of these cycles below.

24.1.4.1.1 Stigma and Silence

As described earlier, silence around abortion experiences is a consequence of stigma for both physicians who provide abortion care and their patients. Silence feels like a more manageable, even desirable, choice for many, allowing experiences with abortion to remain invisible. However, when neither people who have abortions nor those working in abortion care talk about their experiences, abortion comes to seem unusual or deviant, reinforcing its stigmatized status.

Kumar, Hessini and Mitchell described a vicious cycle of stigma and silence for people who have abortions, called the "prevalence paradox" (Figure 24.1) [4]. As they describe it,

widespread stigma prevents people who have abortions from discussing their experiences or reporting them in health-care settings. As such, abortion is thought to be rare or unusual. A social norm is then created that abortion is deviant. As a result, people who have abortions face judgment and discrimination. Fearing these outcomes, individuals choose not to speak about their abortion experiences, perpetuating the cycle.

A similar cycle, the "legitimacy paradox," exists for physicians (Figure 24.2) [12]. Due to stigma, many doctors who provide abortion care do not routinely disclose their abortion work, including their motivations for doing their work. As a result, abortion work comes to be understood as unusual or an abnormal kind of care for physicians to provide, and that abortion-providing physicians are guided by moral deficiencies, rather than moral conviction. A social norm is then generated that abortion caregivers are not "regular doctors," or are illegitimate and substandard. This leads to judgment, harassment, discrimination and, sometimes, harassment and violence. Fearing this, physicians remain silent about their work and their motivations for doing it, further perpetuating the cycle. A paradox exists then, as many highly trained, skilled physicians provide abortion care, yet are often depicted in public discourse as deviant and illegitimate.

24.1.4.1.2 Stigma and Restrictive Law and Policy

Even in settings in which abortion is legal, abortion stigma may lead to abortion restrictions, and those restrictions may in turn reinforce stigma. In particular, stereotypes of abortion-providing physicians may be used to justify restrictive abortion laws and policy, and those restrictive laws perpetuate stigmatizing stereotypes of physicians. For example, a 2012 US bill in the state of Michigan (HB 5711) required that abortion-providing physicians purchase extremely high levels ($1 million) of malpractice insurance coverage, and that abortion-providing facilities be subject to unique licensing and state oversight, among a range of regulations to which other doctors were not subject [9,12]. Proponents of the bill deemed such requirements necessary to remedy, as they alleged, "decades of documented abuses at abortion clinics which demonstrate a pattern and practice of gross violations throughout the industry" [13]. Embedded in this law is the stereotype that abortion-providing physicians

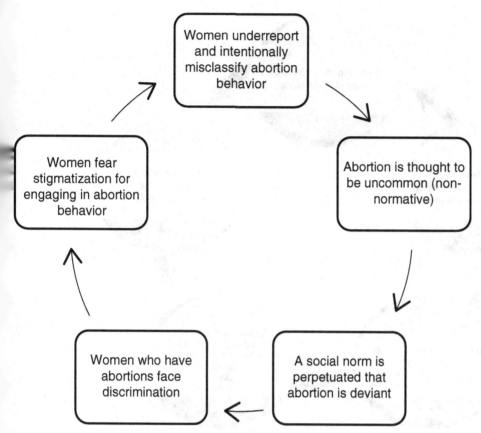

Figure 24.1 The prevalence paradox: the social construction of deviance despite the high incidence of abortion. Reprinted with permission from Taylor & Francis Publishing

are uniquely dangerous, likely to harm their patients, and in need of unique state oversight. This in turn generates further stigma, reinforcing ideas of abortion-providing physicians as technically deficient "butchers" [9,12]. In this particular case, physicians and advocates were never allowed to provide counterevidence to the legislature, thus leaving negative stereotypes unchallenged and permanently embedded in policy [12].

24.1.4.1.3 Stigma and Abortion Complications

Stigma and abortion complications also reinforce each other in another vicious cycle. Stigma can lead to abortion complications when, for example, a desire for privacy leads someone to seek care from an inadequately trained provider, choose an unsafe method of self-induction, or to delay seeking care for a complication. In addition, stigma can make complications more difficult to treat, for example if physicians are reluctant to transfer a patient to a hospital, fearing judgment or poor treatment of their patient, thus leading to care

delays. In turn, complications from abortion – rare as they are – contribute to the notion that abortion is unsafe, and that physicians who provide abortion care are poorly skilled, further generating stigma.

24.1.4.2 Dangertalk

In some cases, physicians' reluctance to disclose abortion work may stem not only from fear of judgment, harassment, violence or legal risks, but also from fear of harming pro-choice movements. Many providers describe a tension between pro-choice discourse and their lived experiences of their work. For example, pro-choice rhetoric does not typically recognize ways in which abortion raises questions about life and death, and can often devalues or does not acknowledge the fetus [14]. However, some abortion workers may feel that the fetus has moral significance, for patient and doctor alike, and that it is disingenuous to consider it like any other piece of "tissue." But when spoken aloud, especially publicly, these

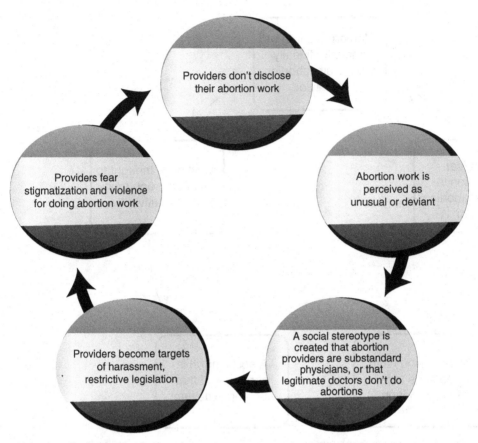

Figure 24.2 The legitimacy paradox cycle. Reprinted with permission from Elsevier Publishing

kinds of experiences seem threatening to pro-choice causes and risk contributing to stigma, and therefore constitute "dangertalk" [15]. Dangertalk, then, is speech that is true to one's lived experience, but that is potentially threatening to social movements that one cares about and considers themselves to be a part of.

24.1.4.3 Stigma as a Human Resource Issue

Stigma must also be understood as a human resource issue for the abortion care workforce. Stigma contributes to professional burnout and compassion fatigue: as experiences of stigma increase, feelings of work-related exhaustion (burnout) and indifference to the trauma of others (compassion fatigue) increase. Further, there is an inverse relationship between stigma and compassion satisfaction: as experiences of stigma increase, gratification from caregiving decreases [16]. Therefore, addressing and fostering resilience to stigma is an important component to sustaining a robust abortion-providing workforce.

24.2 Abortion Stigma: Issues for Training

Abortion stigma has important implications for clinical training – both for trainees (undergraduate medical students, residents and fellows) and those who train them. First, it can impact whether and how abortion is taught within preclinical or clinical curriculum. Second, it may impact trainees' decisions to participate in abortion training, even when opportunities are available. And finally, it affects trainee experiences once in clinical settings. Trainee needs for stigma education and management tools may vary dependent on their level of involvement in abortion care and regions where they work. For example, a Family Planning fellow who devotes two additional years to advanced training will have different needs than a medical student on a week-long rotation. Here, we outline shared needs across a range of training settings and learners.

24.2.1 Stigma and Medical Student Curriculum

Comprehensive undergraduate medical education on abortion is often limited. In a 2009 study, one third of medical schools surveyed in the USA and Canada reported no coverage of abortion-related topics [17]. Among those that did include abortion education, time dedicated to the topic varied widely, with one third of schools reporting less than thirty minutes spent [17]. In some settings, abortion is discussed exclusively as a moral and ethical issue, rather than a clinical one [17], which places abortion outside of the medical realm and centers it as a socially fraught, politicized issue instead of a clinical one. This impacts students' clinical knowledge and understanding of abortion, which other studies show is limited [18]. Stigma is likely a barrier to including abortion in medical education, as some institutions, faculty, administrators or other students may not want to be "marked" by involvement with abortion.

24.2.2 Stigma and Training Opportunities

Once someone is in residency, exposure to and training in abortion can be limited, despite studies showing that residents are interested in receiving such exposure [19]. In one US-based study, 64% of residency programs surveyed offered routine instruction in abortion (meaning hands-on training is standard, with the option to opt out). Such programs were likely to be in regions supportive of abortion [20]. Another 31% offered optional, opt-in training and 5% did not offer any training [20]. The study also identified sources of resistance to routine training, which included opposition among nurses, other physicians, hospital administration, community members and some medical residents [20]. The lack of uniform training is at odds with the fact that 97% of obstetrician-gynecologists will see women seeking abortion care [21], and thus may be ill equipped to help them.

24.2.3 Stigma and Training Decisions

Even when training opportunities are available, stigma can play a role in decisions to participate. Trainees may consider the impact of their participation on their relationships, professional status and aspirations, future practice opportunities, and whether they feel equipped to manage the various logistical and regulatory barriers that are involved in abortion practice [22]. These obstacles can be a larger deterrent to abortion provision than even fear of violence or harassment [22]. Much has been written about conscientious objection and abortion – a refusal to participate in abortion care on religious or moral grounds [23]. However, it is likely that stigma plays a role as well: that anticipation of judgment, status loss, social isolation or simply not wanting to carry a negative "mark" of abortion may be the underlying reason for declining participation, not conscience. However, to date there are no tools for helping trainees or their supervisors determine whether participation decisions are based in conscience, stigma, or a combination. Stigma also interferes with recognizing conscience as a motivation for abortion provision, as the idea of abortion care as a moral calling is in tension with centuries of depictions of abortion caregivers as morally deficient [23].

Once decisions to participate in training have been made, many trainees will begin to wrestle with issues of disclosing their abortion work to others. For some, telling others that they are training in women's health or reproductive health care, without naming abortion, may feel more manageable. Trainees may question whether to list abortion training on their curriculum vitae when pursuing job opportunities, or may be asked about potential abortion provision in an interview setting. Some institutions explicitly ban abortion provision as a condition of employment [22]. Trainees may struggle with obtaining additional, ongoing training in abortion, particularly if they work in hostile settings. Some may fear retaliation from their departmental administration and/or colleagues if their abortion work or desire to perform abortions becomes known. Instances of blacklisting and threats of revoking medical licenses or firing have been documented [23].

24.3 Stigma and Abortion in Practice

Clinical settings are where stigma most comes to life, and thus trainers and trainees need to be equipped to manage it.

24.3.1 Medical Marginalization and Clinical Care

As discussed, many abortion-providing physicians feel marginalized within broader health care, and feel judged by their colleagues who do not provide abortions. While research indicates that many physicians who do not provide abortions actually hold favorable views of their colleagues who do [24], even limited encounters with physicians who are judgmental or stigmatizing can leave lasting scars. For example, when abortion care providers need to transfer patients for follow-up or emergency treatment, some are met with resistance or flat-out rejection by hospital staff, who might refuse admission to their patients, admonish transferring doctors or patients or behave in ways that suggest patients transferred for abortion-related reasons are their last priority [25]. Stigmatizing attitudes about abortion among emergency department and inpatient hospital staff are likely influenced, among other reasons, by their disproportionate exposure to complications of abortion care. Although rare, serious abortion complications requiring hospital transfer and admission do occur [26]. Hospital staff never see the vast majority of patients, whose care proceeds uneventfully, giving them a markedly distorted view of abortion safety, and potentially a distorted view of the skill of abortion care providers. To the extent that trainees may be the first point of contact between abortion care facilities and hospital emergency departments, they may be significantly impacted by stigma when they attempt to facilitate transfers of care to hospital staff who are unwilling to help or who do so only begrudgingly, or uniquely vulnerable to developing erroneous stigmatizing stereotypes of abortion care providers or abortion itself when they are on the receiving end of transfers from abortion care centers.

24.3.2 Caregivers as Stigmatizers

While abortion caregivers experience stigma in a variety of settings, they are not immune from stigmatizing their patients. Many caregivers, after all, are socialized with the same kind of negative ideas about abortion and abortion providers as everyone else, including those stemming from religious teachings and upbringing. This may lead some caregivers, even those who identify as pro-choice, to feel frustration about or judge patients who have more than one abortion, who do not use contraception, who "waited too long" and seek abortion care in the second or third trimester, who have difficulty paying for their procedure or who have abortions for reasons that a caregiver feels is not "good enough." Some caregivers may judge for other physicians who provide abortion care later in pregnancy, beyond gestational ages they feel personally comfortable with. Trainees may bring these attitudes to their abortion learning experiences, or they may observe them in the people training them. Because negative attitudes likely impact patient care [27], trainees and those who instruct them must recognize these attitudes within themselves and in others.

24.3.3 Stigma and Trainers

Trainees and trainers may feel pressure to disrupt common stigmatizing depictions of abortion-providing physicians – that they are unskilled, and that abortion care centers are gloomy or dangerous places. They may feel pressure to be especially cheerful when interacting with other medical colleagues. They may feel as if there is no room for clinical complications or errors, as they are already widely depicted as technically deficient. Trainers may feel that it is important to demonstrate their clinical competence in other settings, like the operating room or on labor and delivery, in order to prove that they are indeed "regular doctors," or they may be self-conscious when learners observe them, feeling that they are under a moral or technical microscope. In other words, abortion caregivers may feel at every turn that they need to disprove negative stereotypes of "abortionists" that trainees might bring with them.

24.3.4 Stigma and Trainees: Psychosocial Impacts

Not uncommonly, trainees report difficult emotional reactions or experiencing complicated moral ambiguities when first observing an abortion procedure, especially those procedures later in pregnancy. Some report feeling nausea, faintness or weakness in their knees. Others may wonder about the questions about life and death abortion raises. Trainees may wonder if it is acceptable to talk about such complexities, given the already embattled and stigmatized state of abortion in many regions. Such speech would constitute "dangertalk," as described earlier.

Superimposed on these feelings and questions might be additional questions about what these reactions mean for a trainee's "pro-choiceness," and whether such reactions in themselves are stigmatizing. However, many trainees are able to hold these feelings and experiences and go on to provide care; they are able to "hold the tension of opposites," a psychological capacity to manage feelings and experiences that are true to one's lived experience, yet seem to be in conflict. [28]. Abortion may be experienced by trainees as life-ending, and also as vital for women's autonomy, and as such "life-beginning." An important part of teaching clinical abortion care is to also provide mechanisms for reflection about that care, including its complexities and ambiguities, and including reflection on learners' emotions and reactions. Teachers may wish to share times when they felt similar emotions or tensions, such as how they may have reconciled their abortion provision with their own religious beliefs. Acknowledging complexities or difficulties is not in and of itself stigmatizing, but rather recognizes that lived experience of abortion varies for caregivers, something that is also true for the patients. Stigma does its social work by reducing people to their one stigmatized attribute, rather than their full, robust lived self. Therefore, acknowledging varied lived experiences affirms the wholeness of a person, and as such may work to counter the reductive effects of stigma.

24.3.5 Stigma and Trainees: An Education in Structural Competence

While abortion stigma can be detrimental to training and care, there are ways in which it may also help trainees build an important skill: structural competence, or the ability to understand and manage the legal, social and economic structures and inequities that form the context for their patients' experiences and abortion practice, many of which stem from stigma [29]. For example, the stigma to which patients are subjected may create logistical or financial barriers to their care, as discussed above. Abortion caregivers become experts in helping their patients navigate such barriers – for example, identifying funding for procedure costs, securing transportation, travel

assistance or childcare support or facilitating referrals or additional medical care for patients with complex underlying illnesses. Training in abortion care, therefore, involves not only developing clinical skills but also developing the "extra-clinical language of structure" that defines structural competence [30].

24.4 Strategies for Managing Stigma

There are strategies for addressing and managing stigma. Because stigma breeds silence, self-censorship and potential social isolation, strategies for managing stigma are often rooted in reflection, connection and sharing. Here, we focus on four strategies for stigma management among abortion care providers and trainees: values clarification attitudes transformation), the Bissell Consultant Abortion Access Program, the Fellowship in Family Planning Psychosocial Workshop and the Providers Share Workshop.

24.4.1 Values Clarification Attitudes Transformation (VCAT)

A number of organizations have developed values clarification exercises that provide opportunities for individuals to reflect on their own values and beliefs around abortion, with the aim of encouraging more supportive attitudes [31]. Values clarification attitudes transformation (VCAT) focuses on attitudes and beliefs that caregivers hold about abortion and women who seek abortion, not on caregivers' personal experiences of stigma. VCAT can be implemented with many different populations, but is commonly used with clinicians beginning their work in abortion care.

There is a variety of different VCAT activities, and most involve discussion of hypothetical scenarios or reflection on personal experiences and views. The structure of the activities is variable. Some modules can be implemented as stand-alone activities; some organizations may choose to implement several activities over the course of a one- or two-day workshop.

Studies of VCAT have found that it can have a favorable impact on participants' knowledge of abortion and improve abortion attitudes, particularly for participants who begin the workshop with less favorable attitudes [32]. Many organizations find the exercises helpful to use during trainings of new staff, to clarify their own values and attitudes and to communicate organizational values around abortion. The long-term impacts of VCAT are unknown.

24.4.2 Bissell Consultant Abortion Access Program

The The Bissell Consultant Abortion Access Program (BCAAP) is a pilot demonstration project at the University of Michigan. BCAAP established a group of subspecialist consultants from various medical disciplines who are supportive of abortion care and whom family planning specialists can contact directly when they have questions about patients' medical eligibility for outpatient abortion care. It was established primarily for clinical access reasons – to reduce barriers to subspecialist expertise and facilitate efficient care. While it has done this effectively, it has also better integrated family planning specialists into the broader medical community in the area.

Early analysis of BCAAP's impact shows that one main consequence of the program is to reduce feelings of marginalization, isolation and stigma among family planning specialists. The impact has been particularly significant on trainees, as they are often the first point of contact with subspecialist consultants. BCAAP shows promise as a program that can be implemented in a range of settings, which could have important implications for trainees on both clinical patient-care and provider psychosocial levels.

24.4.3 Fellowship in Family Planning (FFP) Psychosocial Workshop

Since 2007, the US-based Fellowship in Family Planning (FFP) has offered a two-day Psychosocial Workshop for current Family Planning fellows, graduated fellows and Fellowship directors. The workshop offers a safe space for discussing and reflecting on experiences working in abortion care, including experiences with stigma. Previous topics have included abortion complications, managing challenging trainees or colleagues, abortion and religion, strategies for discussing the work with family members and combatting compassion fatigue. It is a sought-after FFP workshop, particularly by current fellows, and considered an important intervention for both educations about abortion stigma and managing its impacts.

24.4.4 Providers Share Workshop (PSW)

The Providers Share Workshop (PSW) is a facilitated group workshop and research initiative where abortion caregivers meet to discuss their work experiences, including abortion stigma [7,33]. The PSW was developed in 2007 and has since expanded across the USA, South America, Africa, southeast Asia and Europe. More than 1,500 abortion caregivers have participated.

Typically, participants meet for five sessions, each guided around a specific theme designed to address the unique rewards and burdens of doing abortion work. Workshops are led by trained facilitators and can be implemented over the course of a two-day retreat or spread out over several weeks. In order to encourage sharing of emotions and personal narratives, PSW employs symbolic and arts-based methods, such as photography and collage, which can facilitate communication around sensitive and difficult topics. Session themes have included "What Helping Women End Their Pregnancies Means to Me" and "Managing Stigma: The Decision to Disclose," among others (see Appendix 24.1).

PSW has been shown to reduce participants' experiences of stigma and professional burnout [16]. It has also been shown to reduce stigmatizing attitudes toward women seeking abortion [28].

While the PSW was initially designed for caregivers who have worked at their organizations for some time, it has been successfully adapted for trainees, which involves a didactic curriculum, case studies examining the impact of abortion stigma on disclosure of abortion work and on abortion complications and a one-day, interactive workshop focused on coping and resilience. It culminates in a full, two-day PSW. The goal is to foster resilience to stigma and help create a more robust and strengthened workforce. Readers interested in the PSW and/or related curriculum are encouraged to contact the corresponding author.

24.5 Conclusion: Why Addressing Stigma among Trainees Matters

While the phenomenon of stigma has received scholarly attention for several decades, abortion stigma and its impact on the abortion-providing workforce has only recently gained attention. Abortion stigma impacts virtually all areas of caregivers' lives and has a unique impact on clinical trainees. Stigma impacts trainees' exposure to abortion and their decisions to seek out or participate in training. Finally, it impacts clinical experiences once in practice.

Historically, the management of stigma has been left to individuals to navigate. As literature on abortion caregiver stigma has grown, tools to manage its impact have been developed, which may be particularly important for those in abortion training. Mitigating abortion stigma in public life, law and policy and within institutions is a long-term goal that requires significant cultural shifts in many settings. Until abortion is no longer a polarized, political issue, until abortion-providing physicians and their colleagues are understood as legitimate, respectable medical professionals and until abortion itself is understood as a standard part of health care, abortion stigma will persist. While reducing abortion stigma is a vital goal, caregivers, including trainees, need strategies to manage the experience of stigma. Making education and support mechanisms available to trainees is important in educating and supporting an abortion care workforce.

Appendix 24.1 Managing Stigma: The Decision to Disclose

The Providers Share Workshop

For most people, talking about their work hardly registers as a decision. For others who work in a stigmatized area, such as abortion providers, researchers and activists, doing so usually involves assessment of consequences for oneself (and family members). Negotiation of disclosure is not unique to abortion or abortion work; people with any stigmatized but invisible attribute engage in disclosure negotiations. Managing and negotiating disclosure takes energy, and can result in anxiety and fatigue and can impact relationships whether disclosure or non-disclosure is chosen.

Disclosure negotiations may include considerations of the following:

- *Degree* of disclosure – "Do I say I work in 'women's health care' or 'family planning' or that I work in abortion care?"
- *Persistence* of disclosure – "Do I continue to talk about my work after an initial disclosure, or do I let it recede into the background?"
- *Relative risks and benefits* of both disclosure and non-disclosure – "Will this disclosure cost me this friendship?" "If I don't disclose, will the relationship be less intimate, or will this person be hurt that I didn't trust them?"
- *Context* of disclosure – "Can I talk about my work at my partner's work party?" "Is it okay if the person sitting next to me on the airplane can see my slides on my laptop?" "Do I include abortion work/research on my résumé?"

- *Temporal* issues – "When is it appropriate to tell my kids what I do?" "Now that I know someone's politics, is it too late to tell them what I do?"

Goals of This Exercise

- Deepen awareness of ways disclosure is negotiated (or not negotiated) in your life.
- Evaluate the risks and benefits of the decision to disclose *and* the decision to not disclose.
- Provide increased awareness and control over disclosure decisions.

Exercise Instructions

1. In Part 1, select a relationship in which issues of disclosure arise and note important details about the relationship itself/its context.
2. In Part 2, explore the risks and benefits of both disclosure and non-disclosure (to you, the relationship, to others involved, to hopes for the relationship).

Part One: Relationship and Contextual Details

Part Two

Disclosure	Risks	Benefits
Non-disclosure		

References

1. Goffman E. *Stigma: Notes on the Management of Spoiled Identity*. New York: Simon & Schuster; 1963.

2. Link BG, Struening EL, Rahav M, Phelan JC, Nuttbrock L. On stigma and its consequences: evidence from a longitudinal study of men with dual diagnoses of mental illness and substance abuse. *J Health Soc Behav.* 1997 Jun;**38**(2):177–190.

3. Hughes CE. Good people and dirty work. *Soc Problems.* 1962;**10**(1).

4. Kumar A, Hessini L, Mitchell E. Conceptualising abortion stigma. *Cult Health Sex.* 2009;**11**(6):625–639.

5. Cockrill K, Nack A. "I'm not that type of person": managing the stigma of having an abortion. *Deviant Behav.* 2013;**34**:973–990.

6. Izugbara C, Egesa C, Okelo R. "High profile health facilities can add to your trouble": women, stigma and un/safe abortion in Kenya. *Soc Sci Med.* 2015;**141**:9–18.

7. Harris L, Martin L, Hassinger J, Debbink M. Dynamics of stigma in abortion work: findings from a pilot study of the Providers Share Workshop. *Soc Sci Med.* 2011; **73**(7):1062–1070.

8. Jones RK, Witmer E, Jerman J. *Abortion Incidence and Service Availability in the United States, 2017.* Washington, DC: Guttmacher Institute; 2019.

9. Harris LH, Martin LA, Youatt E, Bonnington A, Hassinger J, Debbink M. Michigan's HB5711: a case study of the role of abortion provider stigma in anti-abortion legislation. *Contraception.* 2013 Sep;**88**(3):443.

10. Sisson G, Kimport K. Doctors and witches, conscience and violence: abortion provision on American television. *Perspect Sex Reprod Health.* 2016;**48**(4):161–168.

11. LeTourneau, K. *Abortion Stigma around the World: A Synthesis of the Qualitative Literature. A Technical Report for Members of the International Network for the Reduction of Abortion Discrimination and Stigma (inroads).* Chapel Hill, NC: inroads.

12. Harris L, Martin L, Hassinger J, Debbink M. Physicians, abortion provision and the legitimacy paradox. *Contraception.* 2013;**87**:11–16.

13. Right to Life of Michigan. Abortion abuses and state regulatory agency failure. November 2011, revised March 2012. www.lifesitenews.com/ images/pdfs/MichiganRTL-03152012-Abortion_Clinic_ Abuses_March_2012.pdf

14. Kissing F. Is there life after Roe? How to think about the fetus. *Conscience.* 2004–2005;**25**(3):10–18.

15. Martin LA, Hassinger J, Debbink M, Harris LH. Dangertalk: Voices of abortion providers. *Soc Sci Med.* 2017 Jul;**184**:75–83.

16. Martin LA, Debbink M, Hassinger J, Youatt E, Harris LH. Abortion providers, stigma and professional quality of life. *Contraception.* 2014;**90**:581–587.

17. Steinauer J, LaRochelle F, Rowh M, Backus L, Sandahl Y, Foster A. First impressions: what are preclinical medical students in the US and Canada learning about sexual and reproductive health? *Contraception.* 2009;**80**(1): 74–80.

18. Cessford T, Norman W. Making a case for abortion curriculum reform: a knowledge-assessment survey of undergraduate medical students. *J Obstet Gynaecol Can.* 2011 Jan;**33**(1):38–45.

19. Shotorbami S, Zimmerman F, Bell J, Ward D, Assefi N. Attitudes and intentions of future health care providers toward abortion provision. *Perspect Sex Reprod Health.* 2004 Apr;**36**(2):58–63.

20. Steinauer J, Turk J, Pomerantz T, Simonson K, Learman L, Landy U. Abortion training in US obstetrics and gynecology residency programs. *Am J Obstet Gynecol.* 2018 Jul;**219**(1):86.e1–86.e6.

21. Stulberg D, Dude A, Dahlquist I, Curlin F. Abortion provision among practicing obstetrician-gynecologists. *Obstet Gynecol.* 2011 Sep;**118**(3):609–614.

22. Freedman L, Landy U, Darney P, Steinauer J. Obstacles to the integration of abortion into obstetrics and gynecology practice. *Perspect Sex Reprod Health.* 2010;**42**(3):146–151.

23. Harris L. Recognizing conscience in abortion provision. *N Engl J Med.* 2012 Sep 13;**367**:981–983.

24. Martin LA, Seewald M, Johnson TRB, Harris LH. Trusted colleagues or incompetent hacks? development of the attitudes about abortion providing physicians scale. *Womens Health Issues.* 2019; **30**(1):16–24.

25. Seewald M, Martin LA, Echeverri L, Njunguru J, Hassinger J, Harris LH. Stigma and abortion complications: stories from three continents. *Sex Reprod Health Matters.* 2019 Dec; **27**(3):1–11.

26. Upadhyay U, Desai S, Zlidar V, et al. Incidence of emergency department visits and complications after abortion. *Obstet Gynecol.* 2015 Jan;**125** (1):175–183.

27. Seewald M, Martin L, Hassinger J, Harris L. Abortion providers as stigmatized and stigmatizing: findings from East Africa. *Contraception.* 2016 Oct;**94**(4):388.

28. Woodman M. *Holding the Tension of the Opposites.* E-book. Sounds True, Incorporated; 1994.

29. Metzl J, Hansen H. Structural competency: theorizing a new medical engagement with stigma and inequality. *Soc Sci Med.* 2014 Feb 1;**103**:126–133.

30. Tervalon M, Murray-Garcia J. Cultural humility versus cultural competence: a critical distinction in defining physician training outcomes in

multicultural education. *J Health Care Poor Underserved*. 1998 May; 9(2):117–125.

31. Turner K, Chapman Page K. *Abortion Attitude Transformation: A Values Clarification Toolkit for Global Audiences*. IPAS; 2008. https://ipas.azureedge.net/files/

VALCLARE14-VCATAbortionAttitude Transformation.pdf

32. Turner KL, Pearson E, George A, Andersen K. Values clarification workshops to improve abortion knowledge, attitudes and intentions: a pre-post assessment in 12 countries.

Reprod Health. 2018; 15(40):1–11.

33. Debbink M, Hassinger J, Martin LA, Maniere E, Youatt E, Harris LH. Experiences with the Providers Share Workshop method: abortion worker support and research in tandem. *Qual Health Res*. 2016;26(13):1823–1827.

Chapter 25

Emotional Support

A Key Component of Training and Service Delivery in Sexual and Reproductive Health Care

Alissa C. Perrucci

25.1 Introduction

Teaching, learning and providing emotional support in the sexual and reproductive health-care setting is a key component of successful and sustainable abortion and family planning programs for both patients and providers: medical and nursing students, residents, counselors, nurses, clinicians and physicians. Teaching emotional support skills to both staff and learners brings great rewards to both the teacher and the learner. Emotional support skills help promote providers' career longevity, job satisfaction and ability to prevent and cope with burnout. Working in sexual and reproductive health care brings the possibility of exposures to secondary trauma – patients' experiences of sexual assault, intimate partner violence, substance use, homelessness and psychological disorders alongside race, class and gender oppression – which can be overwhelming and disorienting to providers with little training on or support in how to be present to patients with these experiences [1]. Self-awareness of one's own biases and preferences, comfort with others' expression of emotions and respect for the rights of others to make their own decisions strengthen providers' defenses against burnout and trauma exposure response.

Teaching emotional support skills in family planning and abortion care entails a recognition of the histories that patients bring from the communities in which they live. Prejudice, whether racial-, ethnic-, religious-, class- or gender-based, informs aspects of many patients' lives; their pregnancy and contraceptive decisions are interwoven with the lived experiences of these oppressions. Providers proficient in emotional support are aware of their own experience within racial, ethnic, religious, gender and class dimensions and how these experiences – both privileged and non-privileged – inform and influence their work [2].

Research on psychological response after abortion consistently demonstrates that there is no evidence of widespread negative psychological sequelae of abortion [3,4]. Post-abortion psychological response is augmented when the patient has a positive framing of the abortion decision, positive support and the ability to cope with stressful decisions. At the same time, some patients do report that the decision to terminate the pregnancy was difficult [5,6]. In these circumstances, emotional support and decision counseling skills are essential for patient-centered care.

25.2 Emotional Support within the Graduate Medical Education Framework

Medical education has tended to emphasize the teaching of specific medical knowledge and skills over developing the archetype of the healer within each physician [7]. However, more attention is being paid to beneficial outcomes – for both patients and providers – that are tied to the skillful provision of emotional support and patient-centered communication [8]. The Accreditation Council for Graduate Medical Education (ACGME) general competency domains, which form the framework for twenty-first-century medical education, contain several constituent components tied to abilities within emotional support: caring and respectful behavior; respect, compassion and integrity; sensitivity and responsiveness to a diverse patient population; and the ability to create and sustain a therapeutic, ethical relationship with patients [9]. These components are also tied to priorities for improvements in health-care quality by the National Academy of Medicine, most notably patient-centered care [10].

An important, routine activity conducted within the specialty of family planning and abortion care is the communication of pregnancy test results and subsequent pregnancy decision counseling. This is an educational objective in undergraduate medical education [11] and in obstetrics and gynecology and family medicine graduate medical education [12,13]. This activity engages competencies from the domains of patient care, interpersonal and communication skills and professionalism. It also lends itself to the framework of milestones, which are stages in the development of ACGME competencies, organized from less to more advanced, such as from novice learner through expert [14]. It can also be considered an Entrustable Professional Activity (EPA), defined as observable and measurable tasks that an individual can be trusted to perform [15]. EPAs are described as "measurable units of observable work" that, when the individual is trusted to do them, can be performed "safely and effectively without supervision" [16].

Pregnancy decision counseling is an activity that involves many opportunities for provision of emotional support. This activity contains not only important behaviors such as listening skills, verbal and nonverbal skills, and styles of questioning, but also attitudes and self-knowledge. Medical education has begun to acknowledge the historical emphasis on knowledge acquisition over attitudes and emotion skills, and what has been lost in terms of empathy and the value of the patient–provider relationship [9]. In this chapter, I use the activity of pregnancy decision counseling to illustrate self-knowledge, attitudes and skills in which emotional support is applied. I use the terms *teacher* and *learner* throughout, irrespective of credentials, education or profession.

25.3 Patient-Centered Communication

The fundamental principle that is the foundation for skillful emotional support in sexual and reproductive health care is the belief that "the patient has the answer" [17]. No matter the health-care decision or dilemma that a patient is facing, the provision of nonjudgmental guidance, without an agenda for the outcome, is key. In the context of pregnancy decisions, the proficient learner leads with firm resolution that each pregnancy alternative is equally moral – one is not a better person when one decides

to have an abortion versus make an adoption plan or parent. Furthermore, the proficient learner comes to recognize that people making pregnancy decisions ground their decision in their own moral values – care, compassion, mercy, justice, fairness and love. They also deserve to be respected for the individual, societal and historical context in which they are making a decision.

Practicing this fundamental principle as a proficient learner requires embracing these attitudes and beliefs:

- Letting go of an investment in the outcome of a patient's decision
- Creating a space for feelings; not interpreting a patient's expression of positive or negative feelings as a reflection on one's own success or failure
- Accepting that feelings or beliefs do not need to be fixed, that is, can be fluid and contradictory

These important attitudes and beliefs can be illustrated in a three-pronged approach to patient-centered communication: active listening, not assuming and self-reflecting. Each of these attitudes and beliefs can be translated into behaviors that can be observed in a teacher, practiced by a learner and evaluated through feedback.

25.3.1 Active Listening

A crucial aspect of emotional support in the family planning and abortion care setting is active listening. How is active listening demonstrated? Silence, curiosity and openness, and the use of open-ended questions are three attitudes and skills that we'll use to illustrate active listening across five milestones.

Let's use an example of a patient-learner interaction that happens in the clinic: a patient who begins to cry during an abortion visit. The timing could be any point in the clinic flow: registration, ultrasound, counseling, immediately pre-procedure or after the abortion in recovery. First, let's look at some examples of a learner's reaction to a patient who begins to cry that are illustrative of possessing *less* of an ability than required or *lacking* in the ability [18].

- Handing the patient a box of tissues and then leaving the room
- Commanding the patient: "Don't cry!"
- Demanding an explanation: "Why are you crying?"

These examples reveal a strong discomfort on the part of the learner with the expression of emotion. The consequence is the communication that the expression of feelings in the abortion care setting is unacceptable. Table 25.1 illustrates the progression of skills and attitudes for the emotion skill **active listening** across five milestones. To illustrate a learner who lacks basic competence, I created a level 0 milestone. Level 0 can be compared and contrasted with the subsequent milestones to more finely differentiate the behaviors involved in active listening.

A novice learner who is working at level 1 has good intentions such as providing comfort and reducing suffering, yet is still uncomfortable with the expression of emotion. Examples of level 1 behavior are handing the patient a box of tissues as soon as the patient starts crying or rushing to get the patient a drink of water. Instead, make it a habit to have tissues visible and accessible in the consulting room, within the patient's visual field, so that they may reach for them as needed.

When reaching level 2, the learner experiences growing comfort with bearing witness to emotions without the need to deny them. At level 3, the learner is introducing verbal techniques such as validating and normalizing, two key skills for creating a space for patients to express emotions by indicating that feelings are acceptable and manageable (Table 25.2). Validating statements communicate to the patient that you have seen and heard them.

They are affirming and supportive. Normalizing statements communicate that the patient is part of a human family, unique but not alone. These statements are a key part of the operationalization of the fundamental principle that the patient has the answer.

As the level 4 learner sits alongside the crying patient, a gentle validation can be offered: "It's okay to cry." After crying subsides, this learner shows an interest in hearing about the patient's personal experience by the use of an open-ended question. Open-ended questions allow the patient to express feelings and beliefs. In and of themselves, they can be normalizing and validating; they demonstrate the questioner's openness to the answer, no matter how controversial, inflammatory or provocative one may experience it. Some examples of open-ended questions include the following:

Table 25.2 Validating and normalizing statements

Validate	Normalize
It's okay to cry.	It's normal to be scared.
It's okay to not know the answer.	Lots of people have asked me that question.
I see your point; that makes sense.	This is a clinic where it's okay to talk about that.
That's a good question.	Other patients have expressed that, too.

Table 25.1 Milestones for skills and attitudes for active listening when a patient cries

Active listening	Milestone Level 0*	Milestone Level 1	Milestone Level 2	Milestone Level 3	Milestone Level 4
Skill	Demands an explanation: "Why are you crying?" Commands: "Don't cry!"	Quickly offers tissues or a glass of water.	Practices silence. Pauses before offering tissues.	Practices silence. Validates: "It's okay to cry."	Practices silence. Validates: "It's okay to cry." Asks open-ended questions: "What feelings are coming up for you?"
Attitude	Strong discomfort with the expression of emotion.	Desire to fix the problem and reduce exposure to emotions.	Turns the focus from personal experience onto the patient's experience.	Comfort and confidence with creating a space for emotions.	Open to learning more about the patient's experience.

*Milestone 0 represents a level at which the learner lacks basic competence.

- What feelings are coming up for you?
- What is that like for you?
- How so?
- (Can you) say more about that?

The proficient learner, through the use of silence, validation and one open-ended question, has achieved an essential milestone in creating an environment where patients feel supported. At level 5 (not pictured), the expert's countenance and body language communicate comfort and interest without being overbearing: arms uncrossed, slightly leaning in, with a facial expression that conveys attitudes such as thoughtfulness, equanimity, sincerity and respect.

25.3.2 Not Making Assumptions

The second component of our approach to patient-centered emotional support is not making assumptions. Making assumptions means taking shortcuts and jumping to conclusions, sometimes based on our explicit or implicit biases. How is not assuming operationalized?

Let's use the example of delivering positive pregnancy test results. This is a common activity in both the family planning and abortion care settings. It is accomplished through a urine pregnancy test, blood test, or even an ultrasound, especially in the emergency medicine setting. First, let's look at some examples of *initial* statements to patients after diagnosing pregnancy that are illustrative of a learner who lacks basic competence, a level 0 milestone:

- Congratulations!
- I'm sorry.
- Children are a blessing.

These statements reveal assumptions on the part of the learner and a disregard for the *patient's* appraisal of the pregnancy diagnosis. They may also reveal bias on the part of the learner, which presents an important opportunity for self-reflection: Do I find that I am more likely to say "congratulations" to patients who I think would make good parents and "I'm sorry" to patients who I think would not? Do my statements differ depending on my perceptions of the patient's age, gender, race, ethnicity or class? Do I react differently when the patient is homeless or abusing substances?

In the third example, the learner is labeling the pregnancy with the learner's own beliefs, which

may or may not be shared by the patient, but will certainly give the patient information about which topics of conversation, information or referrals are off limits with this learner. None of these examples presents the learner as a potential source of unbiased, non-judgmental information on pregnancy options.

Table 25.3 illustrates the progression of skills and attitudes for the emotion skill **not making assumptions** across five milestones. At level 1, the novice learner is more comfortable with talking than listening; has a basic understanding of abortion, adoption and parenting; and stays in that comfort zone, independent of the patient's preferences, which are not assessed. At level 2, the learner is growing more comfortable practicing silence and validating emotions. If a patient expressed a desire to pursue a particular pregnancy alternative, the level 2 learner would tailor information provision to fit the patient's stated intentions.

In the following dialogue, a level 3 learner defines the meaning of test results and asks an open-ended question to assess the patient's appraisal of the pregnancy diagnosis. The learner would then use the patient's responses to tailor the conversation about options, referrals or appointments:

LEARNER: I have the results of your pregnancy test. The result came back positive. That means you are pregnant.

PATIENT: [*Silence, thinking*]

LEARNER: [*Gently*] How are you doing with that information?

Assessing the patient's experience of being pregnant is a key question that can be used at any time, not just at the moment of pregnancy diagnosis. Proficient learners may employ this question even during a prenatal care visit in order to demonstrate openness to hearing about the patient's experience, determine the need for additional care or referrals or discover that the patient is considering abortion (Table 25.4).

After disclosure of a pregnancy diagnosis, patients may immediately express emotion, such as sadness, joy or anger. When that is the case, create space for those feelings. Practice silence, validate and ask open-ended questions. When a patient does express emotion, don't assume how they feel or what they plan to do. Sometimes, expression of emotion is coupled with certainty

Table 25.3 Milestones for skills and attitudes for not making assumptions after communicating a diagnosis of pregnancy

Not making assumptions	Milestone Level 0*	Milestone Level 1	Milestone Level 2	Milestone Level 3	Milestone Level 4
Skill	After imparting results, exclaims: "Congratulations!" Or: "I'm sorry."	Conducts basic conversations about pregnancy options.	Tailors information to the patient's stated pregnancy intentions.	Assesses patient's experience of learning about the pregnancy. Responds to patient's emotions.	Assesses patient's experience of learning about the pregnancy. Responds to patient's emotions. Asks a series of open-ended questions.
Attitude	Assumptions about the patient's appraisal of pregnancy.	Stays in comfort zone of imparting information.	Acknowledgment of patient's preferences.	Patient's feelings and beliefs about options are central. Growing comfort with emotions.	Open to learning more about the patient's experience. Comfort with emotions.

* Milestone 0 represents a level at which the learner lacks basic competence.

Table 25.4 Examples of how to assess the patient's experience of being pregnant at three different stages of pregnancy

Stage of pregnancy	Assessment question
After the disclosure of a pregnancy diagnosis	What is that like for you, finding out that you are pregnant?
During an options counseling visit	Take me back to the time when you first learned that you were pregnant. What did you think? How did you feel?
During a prenatal care visit	How have you been feeling about being pregnant?

about the pregnancy alternative that they will pursue. Other times it's not. When a patient is clear about the decisional path, ask how you can be of assistance by providing information on options, making referrals or scheduling appointments. But when a patient's appraisal of the pregnancy is not apparent, don't assume – ask: "What is that like for you, finding out that you're pregnant?" Follow the feelings that you see and hear. Then, ask how you can be of assistance.

At level 4, the proficient learner uses a series of open-ended questions to assist an uncertain patient to embark upon a decision-making path:

- What are your thoughts about what you might do?
- What have you heard about abortion/adoption/parenting?
- When you've thought about abortion/adoption/parenting before, what did you think?

The first question opens the conversation. The next two questions explore feelings and beliefs about abortion, adoption and parenting. Their intent is to promote reflection on what is getting in the way of certain options, what is facilitating others and what would be good or not good about each particular path.

25.3.3 Self-Reflecting

Self-reflecting is the third component of the approach to patient-centered care that provides the opportunity for self-regulated learning. This can be conducted on an on-going basis throughout one's career. Self-reflecting on one's values and beliefs, preferences, and judgments and biases toward others in the health-care setting is a first step in the quest to provide patient-centered care. We have expectations and preferences about our own behavior and the behavior of others. Our level of clarity around these expectations and preferences affects our comportment toward patients and our reactions to their decisions. We must also be aware of the role of implicit bias in our work and how it affects how we treat and counsel patients differently because of race, class, gender, ethnicity or religion [19].

Thinking about the specialty in which you work, answer the questions about patient decision making below. Write your responses down in a journal. Revisit your answers over the course of your career. How have they changed? Have you become more flexible or less flexible? What impact has this had on your satisfaction with your work?

- Which types of decisions do I prefer that patients make?
- Which patient decisions are hard for me?
- If I'm honest, which patient decisions do I find foolish?

It is also essential to reflect on the expectations that you have had for *yourself* concerning pregnancy, abortion, adoption and parenting. Did you make plans? What life circumstances facilitated or hindered achieving those plans? Were there things that you said you would never do? How has that worked out? It is important to be aware of how assumptions about the superiority of planning as well as its achievability and desirability fail to take into account the structural inequities that permeate many people's lives, which reduce the resonance of this concept [20].

25.4 The Overall Skill of Pregnancy Decision Counseling

The overall skill of decision counseling brings together the knowledges, attitudes and skills of emotional support. This could be considered an EPA that could be entrusted to the learner to do with little supervision and then, when ready, with no supervision or independently. I describe skills for relevant ACGME competencies by milestone level as an example of how one could assess the learner's growth before determining when they are competent (Table 25.5). In this table, I use

milestones level 1 to 5. It contains skills and attitudes that we have seen before in active listening and not assuming. It also highlights several key concepts that are essential for fulfilling our fundamental principle that the patient has the answer.

Pregnancy decision counseling often involves imparting knowledge about community organizations that provide additional practical and emotional support for pregnancy, abortion, adoption and parenting [21]. It is imperative to connect with your local abortion fund; abortion funds make access to abortion a reality by providing financial and logistical assistance [22]. Adoption organizations that you refer to should be patient centered and comfortable providing counseling for all options, including abortion. Parenting organizations should connect people with financial assistance and resources for parents. Knowledge of these organizations is critical for patients with fewer resources or patients who need additional decision counseling that your team may not be able to provide.

25.5 Teaching Emotional Support Skills

How do we teach and learn these new attitudes and skills? Much of the initial groundwork we can do on our own, through self-reflection exercises and readings [17]. Attending workshops, webinars and online learning modules provides a second source of knowledge and examples of skills that can be practiced [23]. The third path of learning is through deliberate practice [24]. Proficiency in the provision of emotional support involves observing others who have gained this expertise, being observed in turn by them and receiving and discussing feedback from their observations.

Cognitive apprenticeship is an instructional model for teaching and learning in the real-world setting of the medical environment [25]. Cognitive apprenticeship involves six teaching methods: modeling, articulating, coaching, self-reflection, scaffolding and explorating [26].

During **modeling**, learners are assigned to a teacher whom they can shadow throughout the workday; ideally this takes place with the same teacher for several days or weeks in a row. That way, the teacher becomes familiar with the learner's abilities, limitations and goals, and they

Table 25.5 Examples of milestones related to Pregnancy Decision Counseling and linked to ACGME Competencies

ACGME Competencies	Milestone Level 1	Milestone Level 2*	Milestone Level 3*	Milestone Level 4*	Milestone Level 5*
Patient care Communicates effectively; demonstrates caring and respectful behavior.	Defines medical terms for test results.	Always uses an interpreter in the patient's preferred language. Uses multiple modalities (verbal, visual and auditory) to make information accessible.	Acquires skillful ways of explaining procedures that are accessible, truthful, comforting and empowering.	Demonstrates openness, flexibility and nonjudgment. Tailors approach to each patient based on the patient's unique needs and preferences.	Expert level of patient-centered communication, de-escalation, emotional support skills.
Patient care Provides patient counseling and education.	Conducts basic conversations about pregnancy options.	Growing competence in counseling for all pregnancy options. Responds to and respects patient preferences.	Competent in counseling for all pregnancy options. Knows state-specific laws and restrictions.	Proficient in counseling for all pregnancy options and state-specific laws. Connects patients to organizations that provide support for all options.	Teaches others about counseling for all pregnancy options and how to identify patient-centered and reproductive justice-aligned organizations.
Interpersonal and communication skills Communicates effectively using listening, verbal, nonverbal, questioning, explanatory and writing skills.	Strives to reduce patient suffering.	Practices silence when the patient is expressing emotions.	Practices silence. Validates and/or normalizes.	Practices silence. Validates and/or normalizes. Uses open-ended questions to learn about the patient's experience.	Incorporates body language and countenance to convey sincerity, equanimity, respect.
Professionalism Demonstrates sensitivity and responsiveness to diverse patient population.	Begins to examine personal preferences around pregnancy decisions.	Engages in self-reflection exercises to identify preferences and biases around pregnancy decisions.	Identifies own biases and preferences, impact of own privilege and authority when applicable, on interactions with patients.	Knowledge of how racism and oppression within different communities inform one's approach to patient–provider communication in family planning and abortion.	Is a leader in teaching about racism and oppression, reproductive justice, or is an expert ally teaching about privilege and the impact of racial bias on patient–provider communication.

* Each milestone level builds on the one below.

can track progress together. Modeling emotional support requires that the learner remain silent and simply observe the teacher during patient–provider interactions. The learner should write notes immediately after the interaction is over.

Before embarking on an observation of a patient–provider interaction, the teacher can prompt the learner to pay attention to specific components of the interaction and to look out for specific emotional support and communication skills that the teacher will use. This helps give structure to what the learner is observing so that they are better able to follow the conversation. As they progress in training, the teacher asks the learner to **articulate** the specific skills that they observed, what they liked or didn't like and their perceptions about the patient's responses.

Coaching is the phase of cognitive apprenticeship when the roles are reversed: the teacher observes while the learner puts a skill into practice. After an observation, the teacher and learner meet. The teacher provides written and verbal feedback. The teacher may propose different ways of phrasing questions or statements or have suggestions for improvements on word choice, tone and timing. As they progress in training, the teacher asks the learner to **self-reflect** on and evaluate performance during specific moments in the conversation.

In **scaffolding**, the learner takes on simpler tasks first. Communicating aftercare instructions is a great place to start because the learner is simply reading from a patient handout. Describing the visit, including describing the nature of the abortion procedure, is another task for novice learners because it also involves imparting information to the patient. Preparation for this task can be achieved by studying written scripts.

All learners, no matter their level of competence, can identify areas in which they wish to improve or **explore**. Even after proficiency is obtained, a teacher should continue to observe learners regularly. After implementing a change in practice, the teacher and learner return to modeling and coaching until learners are comfortable and confident with their new skills.

25.6 Conclusion

There is a movement within medical education to transform our attitude toward being in the role of the learner and to continuously strive to improve one's practice [27]. Medical educators are encouraging physicians to reconceive learning as taking place throughout the career trajectory, not just in medical school or residency. At the same time, with teaching, observation and feedback, novices can be entrusted to perform certain aspects of patient care early in their training. The goal is to normalize the state of being a learner at any stage in one's career, and that being an expert and being a novice can coexist within the same person. Emotional support lends itself to the cognitive apprenticeship model in the same way as other important, routine activities that are essential to providing high-quality, patient-centered care.

The provision of sexual and reproductive health care is one of the most rewarding contexts in which to provide service to others. Sexuality and reproductive health decisions and, as specifically discussed in this chapter, pregnancy decisions are a primary locus in which the individual's existential freedom is realized – these are central to each individual's humanity, personhood and subjectivity in the world. This is precisely why these types of decisions cannot be made by others for others. Pregnancy decision making is a context in which patients are contemplating their own moral values – care, compassion, mercy, justice, fairness – and taking the path that elevates the most good, given their life context. This path can bring out feelings – sadness, grief, guilt, regret, relief, tranquility, resolve and inspiration. All of these the learner must be ready to create space for, respond respectfully to and reflect upon.

References

1. van Dernoot Lipsky L. *Trauma Stewardship: An Everyday Guide to Caring for Self while Caring for Others*. Oakland, CA: Berrett-Koehler; 2009.

2. Gallardo ME (Ed.). *Developing Cultural Humility: Embracing Race, Privilege and Power*. Thousand Oaks, CA: Sage; 2014.

3. Major B, Appelbaum M, Beckman L, Dutton MA, Russo NF, West C. Abortion and mental health: evaluating the evidence. *Am Psychol*. 2009;**64**(9):863–890.

4. Biggs MA, Upadhyay UD, McCulloch CE, Foster DG. Women's mental health and

well-being 5 years after receiving or being denied an abortion: a prospective, longitudinal cohort study. *JAMA Psychiatry.* 2017;**74** (2):169–178.

5. Rocca CH, Kimport K, Gould H, Foster DG. Women's emotions one week after receiving or being denied an abortion in the United States. *Perspect Sex Reprod Health.* 2013 Sep;45(3):122–131.

6. Ralph LJ, Foster DG, Kimport K, Turok D, Roberts SCM. Measuring decisional certainty among women seeking abortion. *Contraception.* 2017;95(3):269–278.

7. Satterfield JM, Hughes E. Emotion skills training for medical students: a systematic review. *Med Educ.* 2007;41:935–941.

8. Levinson W, Lesser CS, Epstein RM. Developing physician communication skills for patient-centered care. *Health Aff.* 2010;29(7):1310–1318.

9. Swing S. The ACGME outcome project: retrospective and prospective. *Med Teach.* 2007;29(7):648–654.

10. Institute of Medicine. *Crossing the Quality Chasm: A New Health System for the 21st Century.* Washington, DC: National Academy Press; 2001.

11. Association of Professors of Gynecology and Obstetrics. *APGO Medical Student Educational Objectives,* 10th ed. Crofton, MD: APGO. www .apgo.org/students/apgo- medical-student-educational- objectives/. Accessed July 28, 2019.

12. American College of Obstetricians and Gynecologists. *CREOG Educational Objectives: Core Curriculum in Obstetrics and Gynecology,* 11th ed. Washington, DC: ACOG; n.d.

www.acog.org/education-and- events/creog/curriculum- resources/creog-educational- objectives

13. American Academy of Family Physicians. *Recommended Curriculum Guidelines for Family Medicine Residents. Women's Health and Gynecologic Care.* Reprint No. 282. Leawood, KS: American Academy of Family Physicians; n.d. www.aafp.org/ dam/AAFP/documents/ medical_education_residency/ program_directors/ Reprint282_Women.pdf

14. Accreditation Council for Graduate Medical Education, American Board of Obstetrics and Gynecology & American College of Obstetrics and Gynecology. *The Obstetrics and Gynecology Milestone Project: A Joint Initiative of ACGME, ABOG and ACOG.* 2015. www .acgme.org/Portals/0/PDFs/ Milestones/Obstetricsand GynecologyMilestones.pdf. Accessed December 17, 2019.

15. ten Cate O. Nuts and bolts of Entrustable Professional Activities. *J Grad Med Ed.* 2013;5(1):157–158.

16. Carraccio C, Englander R, Gilhooly J, et al. Building a framework of entrustable professional activities, supported by competencies and milestones, to bridge the educational continuum. *Acad Med.* 2017;92:324–330.

17. Perrucci AC. *Decision Assessment and Counseling in Abortion Care: Philosophy and Practice.* Lanham, MD: Rowman & Littlefield; 2012.

18. Frank JR, Snell LS, ten Cate O, et al. Competency-based medical education: theory to practice. *Med Teach.* 2010;32 (8):638–645.

19. Maina IW, Belton TD, Ginzberg S, Singh A, Johnson

TD. A decade of studying implicit racial/ethnic bias in healthcare providers using the implicit association test. *Soc Sci Med.* 2018;199:219–229.

20. Callegari LS, Aiken ARA, Dehlendorf C, Borrero S. Reproductive life planning and patient-centered care: can the inconsistencies be reconciled? *Matern Child Health J.* 2019;23:869.

21. All-Options: Pregnancy, Parenting, Abortion, Adoption. www.all-options.org/. Accessed June 30, 2019.

22. National Network of Abortion Funds. https://abortionfunds .org/. Accessed July 18, 2019.

23. Innovating Education in Reproductive Health. www .innovating-education.org/. Accessed July 28, 2019.

24. Ericsson KA. Deliberate practice and the acquisition and maintenance of expert performance in medicine and related domains. *Acad Med.* 2004;79(10 Suppl):S70–81.

25. Stalmeijer RE, Dolmans DHJM, Wolfhagen IHAP, Scherpbier AJJA. Cognitive apprenticeship in clinical practice: can it stimulate learning in the opinion of students? *Adv Health Sci Edu.* 2009;14:535–546.

26. Collins A, Brown JS, Newman SE. Cognitive apprenticeship: teaching the crafts of reading, writing, and mathematics. In LB Resnick (Ed.), *Knowing, Learning, and Instruction: Essays in Honor of Robert Glaser.* Hillsdale, NJ: Lawrence Erlbaum Associates; 1989:453–494.

27. ten Cate O, Carraccio C. Envisioning a true continuum of competency-based medical education, training, and practice. *Acad Med.* 2019;94 (9):1283–1288. doi:10.1097/ ACM.0000000000002687

Chapter

26

Sexual and Reproductive Health (SRH) Workforce
National and Global Advances for Availability, Accessibility and Quality

Diana Taylor

26.1 Global and US Health Workforce Overview

26.1.1 Health Workers and Their Importance (UN 2000; WHO 2006)

According to the World Health Organization (WHO), the definition of the health workforce includes "all people engaged in actions whose primary intent is to enhance health" and improve population health outcomes.[1] This includes not only physicians, nurses and midwives, but also laboratory technicians, public health professionals, community health workers, pharmacists and all other support workers whose main function relates to delivering preventive, promotive or curative health services.

National and global efforts to achieve the health targets set by the United Nations (UN) are thwarted in many countries by shortages of health staff, their often-inequitable distribution and gaps in their capacity and performance. The UN 2030 Agenda for Sustainable Development Goals (SDG) expands the Millennium Development Goals (2000–2015) relevant to health workforce and women's health: SDG 4 – Ensure inclusive and equitable quality education and promote lifelong learning opportunities for all; SDG 5 – Achieve gender equality and empower all women and girls. Although low- and middle-income countries face the most severe challenges in ensuring a sufficient, fit-for-purpose and fit-to-practice health workforce, countries at all levels of socioeconomic development face the challenge of how to sustain the human capital required to guarantee universal access and universal health coverage (including the elimination of preventable maternal and child deaths and unsafe abortion (see Chapter 2) [2].

26.1.2 Commonalities across Countries Related to Human Resources for Health (WHO 2013)

According to the WHO Global Health Workforce Alliance, a global deficit of more than 12 million skilled health professionals (midwives, nurses and physicians) is estimated by 2035 and implies the need to rethink the traditional models of education, deployment and remuneration of the health workforce, long-term system-building, comprehensive labor market engagement and essential data systems [3]. Since 1991, commissions have been established in the USA and globally to address health professional education (HPE) and to stimulate educational and regulatory reform. Commission reports (Table 26.1) influence national and global health workforce goals and strategies to focus on fostering a health workforce to address current and emerging needs that ensure competent, well-trained, diverse health-care providers to deliver and facilitate needed care. A 1998 report of the Pew Health Professions Commission recommends 21 competencies for all health professions for the twenty-first century, and in 2010, the Lancet Commission recommended strategic reforms and actions for transprofessional education to transcend professional silos through collaborative, non-hierarchical health-care teams that classifies health professionals by competencies adaptable to local contexts.

In 2013, the WHO recommended that health begins with health workers and their empowerment (voice, rights, responsibilities), which play a central

Table 26.1 US and global commissions on the health professions stimulate reform on education and regulation (1991–2019)

Health workforce reports	Sponsor (year)	Reference
Healthy America: Practitioners for 2005 (1991) *Twelve Critical Challenges: Revitalizing the Health Professions for the 21st Century* (1995)	Pew Health Professions Commission (1991, 1995)[1,2]	Proposed essential competencies and a new approach to health professionals' licensure, certification and regulations.
Recreating Health Professional Practice for a New Century (1998)	Pew Health Professions Commission Fourth Report (1998)[3]	Offers recommendations that affect the scope and training of all health professional groups along with 21 competencies for all health professionals for the twenty-first century.
From Education to Regulation: Dynamic Challenges for the Health Workforce (2008)	Association of Academic Health Centers (2008)[4]	The US workforce capacity can be improved by aligning health professional practice laws and regulations with competencies.
Health Professionals for a New Century: Transforming Education to Strengthen Health Systems in an Interdependent World (2010)	The Lancet Commission (2010)[5]	A global forum, sponsored by an independent interdisciplinary commission of the Gates Foundation, the Rockefeller Foundation and the China Medical Board, reports on a common strategy for postsecondary education in medicine, nursing and public health reaching beyond national borders and professional silos.
Envisioning the Future of Health Professional Education (2015, 2016, 2019)	Institute of Medicine (2015)[6] US Dept. HHS/HRSA (2016, 2019)[7]	Expands education and workforce learning recommendations from 2010 Lancet Commission report to include strengthening health systems through national and global health workforce goals and strategies that ensure underserved communities have competent, well-trained, diverse health-care providers.

[1] Shugars D, O'Neil E, Bader J. (1991). *Healthy America: Practitioners for 2005, an Agenda for Action for U.S. Health Professional Schools.* Durham, NC: Pew Health Professions Commission. Abstract available at www.eric.ed.gov/ERICWebPortal/search/detailmini.jsp?_nfpb=true&_&ERICExtSearch_SearchValue_0=ED347896&ERICExtSearch_SearchType_0=no&accno=ED347896

[2] Pew Health Professions Commission. (1995). *Twelve Critical Challenges: Revitalizing the Health Professions for the 21st Century (Third Report).* http://futurehealth.ucsf.edu/Content/29/1995-12_Critical_Challenges_Revitalizing_the_Health_Professions_for_the_Twenty-First_Century.pdf
Finocchio LJ, Dower CM, McMahon T, Gragnola CM, and the Taskforce on Health Care Workforce Regulation. *Reforming Health Care Workforce Regulation: Policy Considerations for the 21st Century.* San Francisco, CA: Pew Health Professions Commission, December 1995. www.futurehealth.ucsf.edu/Public/Publications-and-Resources/Content.aspx?topic=Reforming_Health_Care_Workforce_Regulation_Policy_Considerations_for_the_21st_Century

[3] O'Neil EH, and the Pew Health Professions Commission (1998). *Recreating Health Professional Practice for a New Century (Fourth Report).* San Francisco, CA: Pew Health Professions Commission. http://futurehealth.ucsf.edu/Content/29/1998-12_Recreating_Health_Professional_Practice_for_a_New_Century_The_Fourth_Report_of_the_Pew_Health_Professions_Commission.pdf

[4] Holmes D. (ed.). (2008). *From Education to Regulation: Dynamic Challenges for the Health Workforce.* Washington DC: Association of Academic Health Centers; chapter 1 (Collier) and chapter 3 (Dower). http://www.aahcdc.org/policy/reports/From_Education_to_Regulation.pdf

[5] Frenk J, Chen L, Bhutta ZA, et al. *Health Professionals for a New Century: Transforming Education to Strengthen Health Systems in an Interdependent World.* A report of a global independent commission, titled "Education of health professionals for the 21st century," was published online at www.thelancet.com (doi:10.1016/S0140-6736(10)61854-5) on Nov. 29, and in *The Lancet,* Dec. 4, 2010, vol 376; pp. 1923–1958). www.healthprofessionals21.org/images/healthprofnewcentreport.pdf www.healthprofessionals21.org/

[6] National Academies of Sciences, Engineering, and Medicine. 2015. *Envisioning the Future of Health Professional Education: Workshop Summary.* Washington, DC: The National Academies Press. www.nap.edu/catalog/21796/envisioning-the-future-of-health-professional-education-workshop-summary

[7] US Department of Health & Human Services (DHHS), Health Resources Services Administration (HRSA). (2019). 2019–2020 Strategic plan: Goal 2, Foster a healthcare workforce able to address current and emerging needs (p. 6). www.hrsa.gov/sites/default/files/hrsa/about/strategic-plan/HRSA-strategic-plan-2019-2022.pdf; 2016–19 HRSA Strategic Plan available at https://www.hrsa.gov/sites/default/files/hrsa/about/strategicplan/strategicplan.pdf. US Department of Health & Human Services (DHHS), Health Resources Services Administration (HRSA). Bureau of Health Workforce Fact Sheet (2019). www.hrsa.gov/sites/default/files/hrsa/about/organization/bureaus/bhw/bhw-fact-sheet.pdf

role in developing and implementing sustainable strategies toward universal health coverage and the improvement of health services and population health outcomes. Common challenges across all countries include the following:

- Current and future *shortages of some categories of health workers*
- Replacement of an *aging health workforce*
- Insufficient use of *advanced practitioners, midwives, nurses and auxiliaries* in many settings
- *Difficulty in attracting and retaining workers* and the variability of enabling environments
- Adapting education strategies and the *content of pre-service education*
- *Performance assessment and quality of care* are not prioritized
- Human resource *information data and systems* require strengthening and investment

26.1.3 A Model for Addressing Health Workforce Challenges (2014)

To overcome health workforce challenges, the WHO applies a conceptual framework for considering the four critical dimensions of human resources for health – availability, accessibility, acceptability and quality – based on evidence from thirty-six low-, middle- and high-income countries [3].

- Availability – the sufficient supply, appropriate stock of health workers, with the relevant competencies and skill mix that corresponds to the health needs of the population;
- Accessibility – the equitable distribution of health workers in terms of travel time and transport (spatial), opening hours and corresponding workforce attendance (temporal), the infrastructure's attributes (physical – such as disabled-friendly buildings), referral mechanisms (organizational) and the direct and indirect cost of services, both formal and informal (financial);
- Acceptability – the characteristics and ability of the workforce to treat all people with dignity, create trust and enable or promote demand for services; this may take different forms such as a same-sex provider or a provider who understands and speaks one's

language and whose behavior is respectful according to age, religion, social and cultural values etc.; and
- Quality – the competencies, skills, knowledge and behavior of the health worker as assessed according to professional norms (or other guiding standards) and as perceived by users.

Even though all four dimensions are equally important, there is a logical sequence in addressing them. Without sufficient availability, accessibility to health workers cannot be guaranteed; and even if availability and accessibility are adequate, without acceptability, the population may not use health services; finally, when the quality of health workers is inadequate, the effects on services in terms of improving health outcomes will be suboptimal. The result of the causal chain means the reduction of people obtaining effective, high-quality care in relation to need.

26.2 SRH Workforce Development: Global and National Perspectives from the WHO, UK and the US SRH Workforce Summit

Since 2005, the WHO provides leadership for the delivery of essential sexual and reproductive health (SRH) care by competent health workers around the world. The WHO definition and conceptualization SRH care goes beyond maternal child health care to include the sexual and reproductive health of men and women throughout their life cycle, and adolescents of both sexes, and it is closely associated with sociocultural factors, gender roles and the respect and protection of human rights.

26.2.1 World Health Organization (WHO): Leading the Way for Delivery of Competent Sexual and Reproductive Health (SRH) Care around the World

At the 2005 World Summit, the UN adopted a resolution that all countries should strive to achieve universal access to reproductive health by 2015 calling on all national health care systems to increase their delivery of SRH services by a work force that has adequate knowledge, skill and appropriate attitudes to provide competent SRH care [4]. In 2009, the WHO also conducted an intercountry survey to identify SRH provision across *clinician type*, *setting* and *degree of SRH integration into primary health care*: antenatal, childbirth, newborn, family planning/infertility, abortion, sexually transmitted infections (STIs) and reproductive tract infections (RTIs), violence/cancer screening, and sexual health promotion/education. A summary of services by community health workers (CHWs), nurses, midwives, and doctors across six WHO regions and across seven areas of service provision is published in the WHO's *The Role of Primary Health-Care Providers in Sexual and Reproductive Health* [5] followed by a set of core SRH competencies for interprofessional primary health-care providers with the intent that these would be further adapted by individual countries to fit their unique national contexts [6].

According to the WHO, an expanded definition and conceptualization of SRH is central to the specification of SRH standards and competencies for health workforce capacity building. SRH extends before and beyond the years of reproduction, and it is closely associated with sociocultural factors, gender roles and the respect and protection of human rights. SRH services should be delivered as a collection of integrated services that address the full range of SRH needs. SRH must be part of the existing health-care system so that it is coordinated with public health and primary health care, and reflects human rights. The WHO SRH concept consists of six components: (1) improving antenatal, perinatal, postpartum and neonatal care; (2) providing high-quality services for family planning, including infertility services; (3) eliminating unsafe abortion; (4) combatting sexually transmitted infection (STI), including HIV, reproductive tract infections (RTIs), cervical cancer and other morbidities; (5) promoting sexual health; and (6) increasing workforce capacity and program development. The WHO thirteen core competencies "reflect the attitudes, tasks, knowledge and skills that health personnel in primary health care need to protect, promote and provide SRH in the community" [5, p1]. SRH competencies are grouped into four domains that encompass (1) essential behaviors and attitudes, (2) leadership and management competencies, (3) general competencies and (4) specific clinical competencies for frontline health-care providers, including nurses, midwives, nurse practitioners, physician assistants, physicians and community health workers (CHWs) [5,6].

26.2.2 SRH Workforce Capacity Building in the United Kingdom: Builds on the WHO Frameworks and Competency-based Education

In the United Kingdom (UK) (see Chapter 34), SRH care is provided to men, women and adolescents within a coordinated system of primary care and public health services. SRH service provision focuses on three areas: (1) the patient experience – ensuring that patients have access to a full choice of contraceptive methods and can see a competent health-care professional to discuss the full range of unintended pregnancy prevention options available to them without fear of harassment or stigma; (2) a well-trained workforce – assuring an optimal provider skill mix to cater to a wide population demand; and (3) the importance of integration – establishing clear referral pathways between services so that care can be integrated around the needs of the individual, not institutional or professional silos. SRH care applies across all health sectors where SRH is an element. Primary care and public health practitioners in particular are acknowledged to have a pivotal role to play in promoting high-quality SRH [7].

In addition, SRH education, training and certification have been established for RNs, advanced-practice nurses, midwives and nonspecialist physicians working in the National Health Service and builds on general prevention, public health and primary care competencies. As part of an effort to build health workforce capacity in SRH care across all settings, the Royal College of Obstetricians and Gynaecologists (RCOG) and the Royal College of Nursing (RCN) were tasked to develop standards and training guidelines for health providers including competency-based education in SRH.

The RCN independently developed SRH competencies specifically for nurses in primary, secondary, and community care settings.[8] Following this effort, the RCOG in conjunction with the Faculty of Sexual and Reproductive Healthcare (FSRH) established generalist and specialty training programs for physicians that were later expanded to include nurses and midwives [9]. Currently, FSRH offers several competency-based training pathways for a variety of clinicians. Competency-based education, training and certification in the specialty of SRH includes competencies in ten areas: (1) basic SRH services/skills; (2) contraception; (3) unplanned pregnancy care; (4) women's health/common gynecology; (5) assessment of specialty gynecology problems; (6) pregnancy care; (7) genitourinary conditions of men; (8) sexual health promotion; (9) public health, ethical, legal competencies; (10) leadership, management, technology, audit competencies. In this rational system, curriculum and training processes are coordinated across these ten components using a combination of teaching-learning and evaluation modalities for all categories of front-line health-care providers in the UK national health system [10].

26.3 SRH Workforce in the USA

Most people receiving SRH services in the USA are cared for by teams of providers that include administrative and clinical support staff as well as licensed health professionals and community-based health workers and educators (see Chapters 3, 5 and 9) [11]. With likely shortages of primary care physicians including obstetrician-gynecologists (ob-gyns), a shrinking proportion of nurse practitioners (NPs) prepared to provide women's health, and even fewer health professionals providing services in public health, community clinics and family planning, there is a need to consider the overall SRH workforce estimations and policy options.

Current trends in supply and demand for SRH services, particularly for low-income individuals, suggest a growing gap in the next decades, with demand outstripping supply of competent health professionals. The reasons for this gap are tied less to the production of clinicians overall and more to a reduced production of health professionals trained to deliver SRH care. The supply may be more than adequate to meet growing demands for SRH services if primary care clinicians (including nurses and pharmacists) were competent in SRH care and if there were incentives to choose this area of practice. Nurses, physician assistants (PAs), pharmacists and advanced-practice registered nurses (APRNs) which includes nurse-midwives and NPs, are all poised to increase their contribution to the promotion of SRH care, including abortion care. Nurses and APRNs have long-established reputations in women's health care, but pharmacists and PAs have been under-utilized to date in SRH services.

26.3.1 Challenges to SRH Workforce Capacity Development

Increasing the capacity of US clinicians to provide high-quality SRH care for all Americans has been declared an urgent public health priority. Implementation of the Affordable Care Act (ACA) in 2014 has added millions of individuals to the health-care system, stressing already limited resources to meet the SRH needs of these additional patients. The ACA's focus on primary care and prevention, which is defined by the US National Academy of Medicine as including family planning services, creates an obvious framework for building capacity.

There are multiple challenges preventing integration of SRH information into health professions education. Some of the limitations to engaging the entire health-care team in SRH care lie with inadequate preparation at the prelicensure level, the lack of graduate and post-graduate clinical training opportunities, a failure to recognize the potential distinctive contributions of all health-care professionals, including physicians, as well as political interference with the provision of SRH. The majority of providers worldwide of SRH clinical care are not physicians; they are nurses, nurse practitioners, nurse-midwives, PAs, pharmacists as well as unlicensed health workers, yet there are barriers to universal access to all of these providers that further limits efforts to reduce unintended pregnancies, births and sexually transmitted infections and improve SRH promotion. These challenges have been further complicated by political challenges to government involvement in the delivery of SRH care, especially the lack of adequate federal funding for unintended pregnancy prevention as well as state restrictions on abortion services (see Chapter 4). Regardless of the ultimate outcome of this political interference, preparation of and support for providers in all settings to deliver high-quality SRH care remain important.

26.3.2 Improving SRH Workforce Availability, Accessibility and Quality: Policy Options

The areas for immediate action require development and implementation of new ways to prepare future clinicians and front-line health workers, the further development of the existing primary care workforce, the incorporation of SRH into new models of health-care delivery and reimbursement and the leveraging of existing professional expertise to improve SRH care delivery [12]. A 2012 study by the RAND Corporation is the first US report focusing on the SRH workforce with analysis of supply and utilization combined with proposals for policy intervention [13]. The impact of the evolving health-care delivery system and expanding health insurance coverage is analyzed, which offers an opportunity to integrate the currently "siloed" system and bring it closer to the comprehensive system of SRH services across public health and primary care that the WHO recommends.

The findings and recommendations are relevant to all providers of SRH services including registered nurses, nurse practitioners, physician assistants, nurse-midwives, clinical pharmacists, primary care physicians (see Chapter 15) and ob-gyns. Short- and intermediate-term policy options and interventions spanning education, federal/state policy and emerging models of care delivery have the potential not only to close expected supply–demand gaps in the SRH workforce but also to improve the quality and efficiency of SRH service delivery, expand the provider base delivering SRH services and better integrate these services with other parts of the health-care system. Four major recommendations included the following:

- Apply a unifying definition of SRH as used by the WHO and implemented in a number of national health systems that includes a minimum package of SRH care accessible to all.
- Adopt a standardized, interprofessional curriculum for teaching core competencies in SRH that aligns competency-based SRH education, practice and credentialing standards within a coordinated system of primary care and public health.
- Integrate SRH education, clinical training, accreditation and credentialing across professions to better integrate SRH and primary care and health professions training and replace restrictive pathways to certification that currently impose barriers to obtain certification in SRH care.

- Respond to emerging models of care delivery, expand innovative models and create new policy options for increasing primary care clinician engagement in SRH service delivery. Several enabling actions could promote greater integration of SRH care into these models.

26.4 Advances/Progress in Availability, Accessibility and Quality of the SRH Workforce: Global and National Exemplars

Current and future shortages of skilled health professionals are especially critical in regions of the world that also have a high burden of unsafe abortion and related sexual and reproductive morbidity and mortality. Additionally, most countries, including many high-income ones, have subnational disparities in the availability of a skilled health workforce, with shortages being particularly high in rural areas or within the public sector. The 2013 WHO report on the global health workforce highlights the fact that advanced practitioners (eg, pharmacists, NPs, PAs), midwives, nurses and allied health workers are still insufficiently used in many settings. Involving such health workers makes it more likely that SRH services will be available to people when they need them.

In response to SRH workforce challenges and increased demand for SRH services in the USA, an interprofessional group of SRH experts from a wide range of educational, clinical and policy backgrounds came together to develop a shared agenda to address SRH workforce issues [12]. At the outset, the participants agreed on fundamental tenets of SRH care: comprehensive SRH that includes care of women and men throughout the life cycle with emphasis on adolescents and health equity; evidence-based prevention and management of unintended pregnancy, including abortion care; public health prevention models to address health disparities; and team-based, interprofessional models of care. Vulnerable populations have historically had limited access to SRH; therefore, strategies to improve access to care for all underlie all recommendations [14].

26.4.1 Advancing Workforce Quality: SRH Core Competencies for Primary Care Providers

As the US health system pivots to focus on primary care and prevention, the need for competencies and pathways to ensure that primary care providers are able to provide quality SRH care has emerged [15]. Building on efforts spearheaded by the SRH Workforce Initiative and the WHO SRH workforce competencies, studies were conducted to identify and refine core competencies in SRH for primary care providers in the USA [16]. The twenty-six core competencies encompass professional ethics and reproductive justice, collaboration, SRH services and conditions affecting SRH to inform education and training across professions, as well as to fill the gap between an established standard of care necessary to meet patient needs and the outcomes of that care. Of note, in contrast to the WHO and FSRH competencies, reproductive justice is referenced in this USA-focused set.

In addition, competency-based educational modules have been developed for health professional students to improve their understanding, clarify their values and learn of ways to integrate best practices for unintended pregnancy prevention and care into clinic settings [17]. Each module is based on essential unintended pregnancy prevention and care competencies to help students improve competency and hone their skills in defined areas – professional ethics, pregnancy options counseling, postpartum/post-abortion contraception, public health, quality and safety and global health. (See Chapter 19.)

26.4.2 Filling the SRH Workforce Gaps: Expanding Capacity and Accessibility of Abortion Care

In the USA, NPs, midwives and PAs have long played a vital role in providing SRH care, particularly in clinics and other settings that serve low-income patients. A 2004 study found that NPs, PAs and CNMs saw six times as many patients as did physicians for publicly funded family planning services; another found that "nurse clinicians" and PAs performed 73% of initial contraceptive exams in publicly funded clinics. In 2015, NPs, CNMs and PAs accounted for 63% of all clinical service providers delivering family planning services in Title X–funded care [18]. NPs, midwives and PAs are prepared in a wide range of procedures and skills that require a broad knowledge base and the development of specialized skills. Examples of such skills abound in specialty care (eg, cardiovascular procedures such as central venous catheter insertion), but clinicians who focus on SRH and/or primary care have also acquired numerous "advanced skills" that are now considered common practice: administering local anesthesia (including paracervical), inserting intrauterine devices, uterine aspiration for diagnosis or abortion, colposcopies and biopsies, performing and interpreting ultrasound exams, conducting intrauterine inseminations, performing and repairing episiotomies, suturing lacerations – the list goes on. They also prescribe a wide variety of medications, including hormonal contraception and, in many states, controlled substances. For many years, NPs, midwives and PAs providing SRH care have provided assessment and appropriate referrals as well as follow-up care for patients seeking pregnancy termination. Providing early abortion care is a natural extension of this practice. In fact, clinicians other than physicians have been providing safe abortion care to patients since 1973, the same year that *Roe* v. *Wade* made abortion legal throughout the USA [19].

26.4.3 Global Evidence for Safety and Quality of Abortion Provision

To ensure that women living in developing countries can readily access safe pregnancy termination procedures, WHO recommends that abortion can be provided at the lowest level of the health-care system. However, in many developing countries, even in settings where abortion is legal, access to abortion remains limited due to a shortage of trained physicians. A study by the Cochrane Collaborative concludes that most deaths and disabilities could be prevented through the provision of safe and legal induced abortion by qualified providers (nurses, nurse practitioners, ayurvedic practitioners, physician assistants, midwives, auxiliary nurse midwives and certified nurse midwives) in seven countries (Bangladesh, India, Nepal, South Africa, Sweden, the USA, Vietnam) [20]. (See Chapters 16, 29, 27 and 33.)

While two WHO reports highlighted that most SRH services including abortion care can be safely provided by properly trained health-care providers, they did not provide specific recommendations with respect to different types of health workers or the tasks for which task sharing are appropriate [21,22]. A 2015 WHO guideline fills this gap with evidence-based recommendations on the safety, effectiveness, feasibility and acceptability of involving a range of health workers in the delivery of recommended and effective interventions for providing safe abortion and post-abortion care, including post-abortion contraception [23]. The emergence of medication abortion (ie, non-surgical abortion using medications) as a safe and effective option has resulted in the further simplification of the appropriate standards and health worker skills and competencies required for safe abortion provision, making it possible to consider expanding the roles of a much wider range of health workers in the provision of safe abortion.

26.4.4 US Evidence for Safety and Quality of Primary Care Providers in Abortion Care

Between 2007 and 2013, the California Health Workforce Pilot Project (California HWPP-171) – a California-based, multi-site, six-year study of midwives, NPs, PAs and physicians as providers of early aspiration abortion care in community-based clinics – collected data from almost 20,000 patients and trained nearly 50 CNMs, NPs and PAs to competency in aspiration abortion care, resulting in conclusive evidence that abortion is very safe, whether it is provided by a nurse practitioner (NP), a certified nurse midwife (CNM), a physician assistant (PA) or a physician. Additionally, more than 2,500 patients surveyed at 25 separate facilities across the state of California rated the abortion care they received in this study as being extremely positive (9.4/10), regardless of whether the care had been provided by a NP, CNM, PA or MD/DO [24]. These conclusive results have been used to change anachronistic "physician-only" state laws which do not acknowledge the roles and experience of licensed NPs, CNMs and PAs, whose scope of primary and specialty practice includes management of conditions and procedures significantly more complex than medication or aspiration abortion [25].

26.4.5 Standardizing Competency-Based Abortion Training for Primary Care Providers

Although most women's health-care providers will interact with patients navigating issues of unintended pregnancy and abortion, abortion training is not universally available to primary care physicians or advanced-practice clinicians (NPs, CNMs, PAs) who intend to provide SRH services. While competency-based SRH training programs are available for nurses, midwives and physicians in countries with national health services (eg, UK FSRH – see Chapter34), evidence suggests that few US health professional education programs incorporate abortion training in didactic curriculum, and only a small percentage of residencies, regardless of type or specialty, with the exception of ob-gyn, offer integrated abortion training [26].

As part of the California Health Workforce Pilot Project Study, a standardized, competency-based curriculum and training guidelines were evaluated in the education and training of primary care clinicians in early abortion care [27]. Essential components of an evidence-based training program include education and training guidelines and textbook in early abortion for primary care providers and core competencies for entry-level primary care clinicians providing early abortion care, regardless of setting. In addition, a model for regulatory compliance of abortion provision for California clinicians is included.

26.5 Conclusion

Increasing the availability, accessibility and capacity of the national and global health workforce to provide high-quality SRH care has been declared an urgent public health priority and plays a central role in the improvement of population health outcomes. Despite challenges, there is significant progress to prepare future clinicians and front-line health workers, to develop the existing primary care workforce in SRH, to incorporate SRH into new models of health-care delivery and reimbursement and to leverage the existing global and national expertise to improve SRH care delivery. In this chapter, global and national examples describe the progress to align SRH practice, education and credentialing for improving SRH workforce capacity.

References

1. World Health Organization. *WHO Global Health 2030. World Health Report, Global Health Workforce Alliance.* Geneva: World Health Organization; 2006. www.who.int/workforcealliance/knowledge/resources/strategy_brochure9-20-14.pdf and www.who.int/workforcealliance/about/en/

2. United Nations. Transforming Our World: The 2010 Agenda for Sustainable Development; 2016. https://sustainabledevelopment.un.org/sdgs and https://sustainabledevelopment.un.org/post2015/transformingourworld

3. World Health Organization. *Global Health Workforce Alliance Report: A Universal Truth: No Health without a Workforce.* Geneva: World Health Organization; 2014. www.who.int/workforcealliance/knowledge/resources/GHWA-a_universal_truth_report.pdf

4. World Health Organization, Department of Reproductive Health and Research. Progress Report – Reproductive health strategy (2010–2015): To accelerate progress towards the attainment of international development goals and targets 2010;RHR 10.14. www.who.int/reproductivehealth/publications/general/rhr_10_14/en/

5. World Health Organization. *The Role of Primary Health-Care Providers in Sexual and Reproductive Health: Results from an Intercountry Survey* (Supplement 1). Geneva: World Health Organization; 2011. www.who.int/reproductivehealth/publications/health_systems/PHC_Supplement1.pdf

6. World Health Organization. *Sexual and Reproductive Health Core Competencies in Primary Care: Attitudes, Knowledge, Ethics, Human Rights, Leadership, Management, Teamwork, Community Work, Education, Counselling, Clinical Settings, Service, Provision.* Geneva: World Health Organization; 2011. http://whqlibdoc.who.int/publications/2011/9789241501002_eng.pdf

7. Faculty of Sexual and Reproductive Healthcare. SRH vision in the United Kingdom; 2015. www.fsrh.org/about-us/our-vision/

8. Royal College of Nursing. Sexual health competencies: an integrated career and competence framework for sexual and reproductive health nursing across the UK; 2009. www.nhsgrampian.org/files/sexual_health_competencies%20RCN.pdf

9. Wilkinson C, Halfnight D. (2013). The Faculty of Sexual & Reproductive Healthcare: 20th anniversary. *J Fam Plann Reprod Health Care.* 2013;39:78–79. http://dx.doi.org/10.1136/jfprhc-2013-100606

10. Faculty of Sexual and Reproductive Healthcare. Community sexual and reproductive health curriculum; 2012. www.gmc-uk.org/CSRH_Curriculum_27_November_2012_FINAL.pdf_51473364.pdf

11. Levi A, Burdette L, Hill-Besinque, K, Murphy PA (2013). The interprofessional sexual and reproductive health care team. *Contraception.* 2013;88:213–14. http://dx.doi.org/10.1016/j.contraception.2013.05.011

12. Nothnagle M, Cappiello J, Taylor D. Sexual and reproductive health workforce project: overview and recommendations from the SRH Workforce Summit, January 2013. *Contraception.* 2013;88(33):204–209. http://dx.doi.org/10.1016/j.contraception.2013.05.006

13. Auerbach DI., Pearson ML, Taylor D, et al. *Nurse Practitioners and Sexual and Reproductive Health Services: An Analysis of Supply and Demand.* Santa Monica, CA: RAND Corporation, 2012. www.rand.org/pubs/technical_reports/TR1224 (full report); www.rand.org/pubs/technical_reports/TR1224.html#recommendations (recommendations).

14. Cappiello J, Nothnagle M. SRH Workforce Summit: now is the time to bring sexual and reproductive health to primary care. *Contraception.* 2013;88:210–212. http://dxdoi.org/10.1016/j.contraception.2013.06.001

15. Simmonds K, Hewitt CM, Aztlan EA, Skinner E. Pathways to competence in sexual and reproductive health care for advanced practice nurses. *J Obstet Gynecol Neonatal Nurs.* 2017;46(5):e168–e179. https://doi.org/10.1016/j.jogn.2017.02.007

16. Cappiello J, Levi A, Nothnagle M. Core competencies in sexual and reproductive health for the interprofessional primary care health team. *Contraception.* 2016;93(5):438–445. http://dx.doi.org/10.1016/j.contraception.2015.12.013

17. Hewitt C, Cappiello J. Essential competencies in nursing education for prevention and care related to unintended pregnancy. *J Obstet Gynecol Neonatal Nurs.* 2015;44:69–76. www.jognn.org/article/S0884-2175(15)31762-7/fulltext (full text); https://rhnursing.org/resource/uppc-nursing-education-modules/ (education modules)

18. Taylor D, Safriet B, Dempsey G, Kruse B, Summers L. *Abortion Provider Toolkit*, 2nd

ed. San Francisco: University of California, San Francisco; 2018. www.aptoolkit.org

19. Taylor D, Maldonado L, Weitz TA. Policy Statement No. 20112: nurse practitioners, nurse midwives & physician assistants as abortion providers; 2011. www.apha .org/policies-and-advocacy/ public-health-policy-statements/policy-database/ 2014/07/28/16/00/provision-of-abortion-care-by-advanced-practice-nurses-and-physician-assistants

20. Barnard S, Kim C, Park MH, Ngo TD. Doctors or mid-level providers for abortion. *Cochrane Database Syst Rev.* 2015;(7)CD011242. www .cochranelibrary.com/cdsr/doi/ 10.1002/14651858.CD011242 .pub2/full

21. World Health Organization, Department of Reproductive Health and Research. *Optimize MNH: Optimizing Health Worker Roles to Improve Access to Key Maternal and Newborn Health Interventions through Task Shifting.* Geneva: WHO;

2012. http://www.optimizemnh .org/.

22. World Health Organization, Department of Reproductive Health and Research. *Safe Abortion: Technical and Policy Guidance for Health Systems,* 2nd ed. Geneva: WHO; 2012. www.who.int/ reproductivehealth/ publications/unsafe_abortion/ 9789241548434/en/

23. World Health Organization, Department of Reproductive Health and Research. *Health Worker Roles in Providing Safe Abortion Care and Post-Abortion Contraception.* Geneva: WHO; 2015. www .who.int/publications-detail/ health-worker-roles-in-providing-safe-abortion-care-and-post-abortion-contraception

24. Taylor D, Battistelli M, Anderson P. *California Health Workforce Pilot Project #171 Fact Sheet: Study Findings & Methods.* Advancing New Standards in Reproductive Health: UCSF; 2017. https:// rhnursing.org/wp-content/

uploads/2017/07/Fact2_ HWPP-Study-Findings-and-Methods.pdf; https://www .ansirh.org/research/hwpp-AB154

25. Barry D, Rugg J. *Improving Abortion Access by Expanding Those Who Provide Care.* Washington, DC: Center for American Progress; 2015. www .americanprogress.org/issues/ women/report/2015/03/26/ 109745/ improving-abortion-access-by-expanding-those-who-provide-care.

26. National Academies of Sciences, Engineering, and Medicine. *The Safety and Quality of Abortion Care in the United States.* Washington, DC: The National Academies Press; 2018. https://doi.org/10 .17226/24950

27. Taylor D, Battistelli M, Anderson P. Early abortion education and training guidelines for primary care providers. ANSIRH:UCSF; 2016. www.ansirh.org/ resources/training/early-abortion-education-training-guidelines

Chapter

27

Medical Education for Safe Abortion Services in Nepal

Swaraj Rajbhandari, Rajshree Jha Kumar and Sirjana Khanal

Ganga, 57-year-old mother, and Savitri, 23-year-old daughter, were serving life sentences in prison in Janana Jail, Kathmandu. We met them during one of our health camps for women prisoners. Savitri was already a mother to four children, and she did not want another child. Her youngest child was just 11 months old and Savitri could not handle another pregnancy. Her husband was working in India and would only come home once a year during the rainy season. She had to take care of the farm, house, cattle and her four children. Poor, never went to a school, unaware of any family planning options, she knew one thing: she could not have this baby. Out of desperation she reached out to her only hope: her mother, Ganga.

Ganga, herself a mother of seven children, did not want her daughter Savitri to suffer and agreed to help her. She prepared some homemade remedies and directed her daughter to apply them. After 3 days, Savitri aborted her baby, which survived for a few hours but then died; while making preparations to bury the baby, neighbors came to know about the abortion and seized this opportunity to call in the police. Both mother and daughter were arrested and later sentenced to life in prison for aborting a 7 months' gestation fetus (maximum punishment after the age of viability). Savitri was crying when she told us, "I did it for my family and now I cannot be with them [her youngest was with her in prison]. Don't I have the right to decide whether I want a baby or not?"

Janana Jail, Kathmandu, 1996

Janana Jail is the only female prison in Kathmandu. Prior to the legalization of abortion in Nepal in 2002, the majority of women there were jailed for abortion-related crimes: the more advanced the pregnancy, the longer the imprisonment. The old abortion law did not clearly distinguish abortion and infanticide, murder or homicide [1]. As a result poor, illiterate women would end up in prison for a long time. Prior to 2002, Nepali civil code (MulukiAin) did not allow abortion under any circumstances, even if the pregnancy threatened the life of the women [2,3,4]. Like other countries around the world where abortions were banned, women had no other option but to seek desperate measures. Sometimes it would be a family member, traditional birth attendants and, rarely, physicians who provided abortions. Since the law would punish both the person having the abortion and the service providers, incidence could not be measured. Those who had severe complications associated with abortion would either die at home or sometimes present to the hospital with sepsis, uterine perforation and shock. Accurate estimates of these events could not be made, as the majority died before reaching a hospital.

The World Health Organization (WHO) estimates that 25 million unsafe abortions occur worldwide each year. The majority of unsafe abortions, or 97%, occur in developing countries such as Africa, Asia and Latin America, accounting for almost 13% of the maternal deaths worldwide, and in some countries up to 60% [5,6]. (See Figures 27.1 and 27.2.)

Nepal is a landlocked country, and its diverse terrain creates geographic barriers that make the equitable distribution of health services difficult. In addition, a decade-long conflict in the country and an unstable political situation posed challenges in providing health care to its population of about 28 million. Nepal reported one of the highest maternal mortality ratios (MMR) in the world, with a high proportion of maternal deaths and injuries attributable to unsafe abortion [7]. In 1998, abortion and abortion-related complications contributed approximately 15% of maternal mortality in Nepal. Provision of safer abortion is associated with a reduction in MMR from 539 in

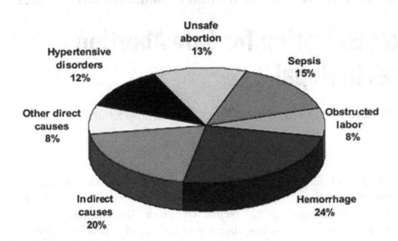

Figure 27.1 Global causes of maternal death: a WHO systematic analysis

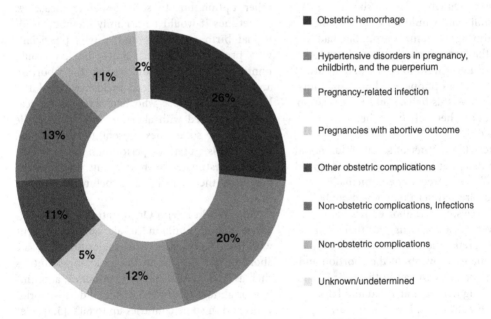

- Obstetric hemorrhage
- Hypertensive disorders in pregnancy, childbirth, and the puerperium
- Pregnancy-related infection
- Pregnancies with abortive outcome
- Other obstetric complications
- Non-obstetric complications, Infections
- Non-obstetric complications
- Unknown/undetermined

Figure 27.2 WHO Maternal and Perinatal Death Surveillance 2015, 2016, 2017, 2018

1996 to 259 by 2016. However, unsafe abortion still occurs and remains a significant cause of maternal morbidity and mortality despite legalization of abortion and improved access to care [8].

27.1 History of Abortion in Nepal

The Family Planning Association of Nepal (FPAN), an affiliate of the International Planned Parenthood Federation (IPPF), the largest nongovernmental organization in Nepal's health sector, laid the foundation in the 1970s to liberalize the abortion law. They brought key stakeholders together with the aim to discuss the relevance of and rationale for legalizing abortion: the laws were restrictive and, to make an impact on improvement of women's health, legalizing abortion was essential. The National Planning Commission on Population later recommended to the government that abortion should be made legal for pregnancies resulting from contraceptive failures. Other initiatives were taken by Nepal's Institute of Law to reform existing abortion law [4,9,10,11]. The Nepal Women's Organization, the only officially recognized women's organization prior to 1990, brought together representatives of the judiciary, public administration and social workers to develop a broader consensus for abortion legalization under certain conditions: if the pregnancy resulted as a result of rape or incest or if a pregnancy threatened a women's life [12]. Unfortunately, none of these issues was seriously considered by the national legislature.

There were several factors that made initial efforts unsuccessful: abortion was at that time too sensitive a political issue, and Nepal then received its major grants for family planning and health through the US Agency for International Development (USAID), which excluded (and still does) abortion services even if unsafe abortion was a major cause of maternal mortality: the 1980s saw the implementation of the Mexico City Policy (the first US "Global Gag Rule") [13]. By 1987, the Global Safe Motherhood Initiative had begun, and Nepal was committed to improving women's health. The Nepal Ministry of Health's Family Health Division (MOH/FHD) drafted its Safe Motherhood Policy in 1993 [14, 15]. Women's reproductive rights again became the focus after the International Conference on Population and Development (ICPD) and the Beijing Conference on Women.

It took almost three decades of reform before a law permitting abortion was passed. That would not have been possible if the law had been regarded as a fertility control measure. Instead, abortion was defined as a women's sexual reproductive health rights and empowerment issue. The 2002 reform permitted abortion as well as conferring on women other rights to self-determination in, for example, divorce and inheritance.

The new law allowed abortion on request up to twelve weeks of pregnancy; up to eighteen weeks of pregnancy as a result of rape or incest; anytime during pregnancy if the life, physical or mental health of the women is at risk or if the fetus is deformed. Abortion remained punishable only under two conditions: sex selective abortion and abortion without the consent of a pregnant woman. The law empowered women to choose to have an abortion without the consent of spouse or partner and without regard to present or past

marital status. It also ensured that adult women are not forced or deceived into having an abortion against their will or choice. In case of minors (less than sixteen years of age) or mental incompetence, a legal guardian must give consent. Privacy and confidentiality of the woman receiving abortion services are also guaranteed by the law.

In recognition of the importance of education and training, the law allowed only certified doctors or health workers specifically trained in safe abortion to provide it and only at an approved health facility. Only institutions and individuals certified by the government are eligible to provide abortion services under the Safe Abortion Service Procedure, which required the MOH/FHD to establish training programs and centers, first in teaching hospitals and urban clinics and later outside urban areas. The regulations governing the law specify that for pregnancy up to twelve weeks manual uterine aspiration (MUA) can be used, while beyond twelve weeks dilation and evacuation (D&E) can be used. Medical approaches are permitted at all gestations.

First-trimester surgical abortions were made available throughout the country in 2004. The services incorporated pregnancy testing, pre-counseling (for the woman's informed decision about the pregnancy termination and the method used, potential risks and consent), surgical abortion and post-abortion counseling (about follow-up care, signs of complications, prompt return of ovulation) and contraception of the woman's choice.

At the outset, the training program emphasized MUA as a safe and cost-effective approach in low-resource settings and encouraged public–private partnerships among academic institutions and nongovernmental organizations (NGOs) [16]. In a collaboration with Ipas and University of California, San Francisco, Kathmandu's Maternity Hospital had introduced MUA in 1995 for treating incomplete abortions so that some gynaecologists trained there had experience with it prior to legalization. After legalization, MUA training was offered to only twenty senior gynaecologists from central and regional hospitals and NGO and private clinics who had had previous training experience at an MOH/FHD "Training of Trainers" course in Kathmandu. Among these were four gynaecologists who the

US Packard Foundation sponsored to receive two months of abortion training at the University of California, San Francisco (two authors of this chapter – Drs. Jha Kumar and Rajbandari – Dr. Sabitri Kishore, who led the MOH/FHD abortion training program and Dr. Reeta Mandanhar who trained abortion providers at Tribuvan University Teaching Hospital). These gynaecologists began training additional physicians from both the public and private sectors. This "cascade" training initially included only MUA in order to foster rapid national scale-up of access to services. At the same time, Kathmandu's obstetrical teaching hospitals, CREHPA, and the Bixby Center at University of California, San Francisco, launched a ten-year evaluation of the effects of the new law on women's health [17] (Figure 27.3).

Despite rapid expansion of the services, many women in rural and remote areas remained out of reach. In 2006, a key strategy for improving access to safe abortion was developed to train staff nurses for MUA services. The Government of Nepal in 2008 further expanded services to include advanced-practice and midlevel providers. Staff nurses and auxiliary nurse midwives (ANM) certified as skilled birth attendants became eligible to perform MUA up to 8 weeks. Nepal now provides safe abortion service up to the community level through this "task-shifting" mechanism. As a result, there are currently MUA providers at nearly 1,600 sites in 75 districts across Nepal.

Overall, 5,600 women received abortion services from nurses at 42 facilities between June 2009 and April 2010. Complications were experienced by 68 surgical abortion clients (1.6%) and 12 medication abortion clients (1.2%), comparable to those of trained physicians; 67% of facility managers reported that clients preferred nurse providers over physicians or had no preference [18]. Basnett et al. observed that the trained nurses provided high-quality service delivery and recommended additional support of training, facility supervision and improvement in drugs and equipment supply (see Chapter 4).

27.2 Second-Trimester Abortion Care in Nepal

In 2006, a national facility-based survey found that 13% of women seeking abortion were turned away because they were more than twelve weeks

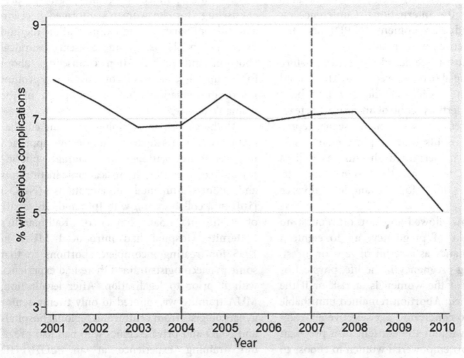

Figure 27.3 Trend in the percentage of abortion cases with serious complications presenting at four tertiary care hospitals in Nepal, 2001–2010, n = 23,493

pregnant [19]. The adverse effects of "turning away" are well documented [20]. With this evidence of the strong need for second-trimester care, advocates and policymakers developed in 2007 a "Strategic Plan for Second-Trimester Abortion" to offer medical abortion and D&E through tertiary care facilities. According to Nepal's "Second-Trimester Abortion Care Protocol," women can safely have abortions up to eighteen weeks of gestation in the case of rape or incest and at any gestational age for a life-threatening condition if the site providing second-trimester abortion care services meets the following criteria:

- Availability of comprehensive emergency obstetric care (24/7)
- Doctor/nurse willing to provide second-trimester procedures
- Support from hospital management
- Availability of first-rimester MUA 6 days/week
- Availability of ultrasound and blood products
- Adequate waste disposal system, for example, pit disposal

Training in D&E surgery was accomplished from 1993 to 2016 through NGOs, for example, IPAS, and US teaching hospital partnerships in which sixteen US Fellowship in Family Planning Fellowship–trained gynaecologists worked with Nepali colleagues to observe and demonstrate second-trimester abortion techniques under ultrasound guidance. They taught primarily in Kathmandu, but some also traveled to teaching hospitals and sites in outlying regions.

27.3 Medication Abortion Services

Medication abortion (MA) was added in 2009 on a pilot basis. In 2010, encouraged by that success, medication abortion services were expanded to 75 districts with the support of NGO and public–private partnerships and served more than 908,904 women. In 2016–17, 96,417 women received safe abortion services: 55.6% were medication, and 13.8% of safe abortion service users were adolescents (<20 years) [21]. Initially, MA services were provided by either physicians or staff nurses. Trainers were drawn from the pool of comprehensive abortion care providers who had received a Clinical Training Skills Certification from the National Health Training

Center (NHTC). Later, reflecting the government's emphasis on rapid decentralization, MA services up to 9 weeks of pregnancy were also provided by ANMs and allowed in all public and private hospitals and in some NGOs throughout Nepal's 75 districts, many of which are in remote, mountainous areas.

The credentials required for training are registration in the Nursing Council for nurses and ANMs who are already trained in intrauterine contraception and safe birthing and who work in a birthing center. The trainings are conducted for 5 days: 2 days theory and 3 days practical with real clients. The curriculum is endorsed by the MOH/FHD (now Family Welfare Division) and NHTC. Every year, a refresher workshop is offered to approximately 32 trainers to ensure skill standardization and knowledge update. By 2019, 1,582 ANM and 671 staff nurses were trained.

Medication abortion provision by ANMs has been demonstrated to be safe and effective at the primary health level in Nepal [22]. At the end of 2018, 1,582 ANMs and 825 sites were listed as providing MA services and, 1,656 doctors and 671 nurses were MVA service providers at 591 sites.

Beginning in 2013–14, the safe abortion program was amended to include the availability of modern contraceptive methods at all safe abortion sites. Samandari et al. concluded that advocacy, public–private and NGO partnerships, task shifting from gynaecologists to ANMs along with certification, availability of necessary equipment and drugs, inclusion of abortion in nursing, medical school, and residency education, and comprehensive planning and implementation efforts led to remarkable achievements in the availability and use of safe abortion in all 75 of Nepal's districts [23].

27.4 Medication Abortion Drugs

Mifepristone (200 mg) followed by misoprostol (800 mcg) for pregnancy terminations have been approved by the Department of Drug Administration (DDA) as MA drugs. At present, four companies' preparations are approved for MA, but pharmacy dispensing practices over the counter are a major challenge. Pharmacies are usually the first point of contact of clients in Nepal. Many midlevel health providers run their own pharmacies and offer medication abortion pills. Research compared two days' orientation on estimating pregnancy duration and dosing MA drugs for pharmacy workers in one district (Jhapa) with an untrained group in a second district (Morang). A pre-intervention baseline survey was carried out with 230 pharmacy shops in the intervention district and an equal number in the comparison district during June and July 2011. It showed that trained pharmacy workers were more knowledgeable and efficient about providing MA services than untrained ones. The MOH/FWD now makes MA training available to pharmacists using a curriculum adapted from this research [24].

27.5 Development of Policies, Strategies and Guidelines

After legalization, Nepal's MOH/FHD developed in 2003 a National Safe Abortion Policy and Procedure Order [25,26]. Similarly, a Medical Abortion Scale Up Strategy, National Safe Abortion Service Implementation Guidelines and MA Drug and Equipment Supply Guidelines were developed in 2008, 2011 and 2013, respectively [27]. In 2018, the national Safe Abortion Service Implementation Guidelines were revised to incorporate the free safe abortion policy.

27.6 Capacity Development of Service Providers

Under the leadership of the MOH/FWD, the NHTC developed systematic, comprehensive strategies for scaling up safe abortion services, including training in all recommended methods, supervision and monitoring. In technical assistance with its partner NGO (IPAS/Nepal), NHTC

developed safe abortion reference and training manuals and a curriculum. (See Tables 27.1 and 27.2.)

*Though 86 were trained, only 58 are providing services at present

Abortion service sites are selected based on the Criteria in Abortion Services Program Implementation Guideline, 2017 [28]. Evidence-based training of service providers in selected sites is by the Ministry of Health (MoH) in collaboration with development partners. The MoH also collaborates with partner organizations to arrange trainers' annual continuing education meetings.

Safe abortion services (MVA/MA) are included in the medical education curriculum for all obstetrics and gynaecology (ob-gyn) residents except at the Patan Academy of Medical Sciences. In 2006, safe abortion services were first offered in Nepal's first medical school, Tribhuvan University Teaching Hospital/Institute of Medicine (IOM). The curriculum has included training in safe abortion services for residents since 2010. Other ob-gyn residency programs are implementing abortion training rotations for their residents, which began in June 2019. Similarly, MOH/FWD, in coordination with NHTC, has integrated an abortion services curriculum in physician, midwifery and nursing education. The selection of service providers for clinical training requires that:

- Doctors should be registered in the Nepal Medical Council.
- Staff Nurse/Sr. ANM/ANM should be registered in the Nepal Nursing Council.
- For physicians who have completed an ob-gyn residency or hold a diploma in ob-gyn or general practice, abortion services training is

Table 27.1 Abortion method and trained services providers, Nepal, through 2018

Type of services	Trained providers		No of listed sites
	Type	No	
MVA	Doctors	1656	591
	Staff nurses	671	
MA	ANM	1582	825
Second-trimester services	Doctors only	58*	29

Source: Records; Ministry of Health/Family Welfare Division/IPAS, Nepal

Table 27.2 Milestones of Abortion Services in Nepal [29]

Year	Activities
2002	Legalization of abortion
2003	Developed National Safe Abortion Policy and procedural order
2004	Started the first legal abortion services in Kathmandu at Maternity Hospital
2004	First MVA training course for service providers
2006	Piloted and started comprehensive abortion services by staff nurses
2007	Second trimester safe abortion introduced
2008	Mifepristone and misoprostol registered by Department of Drug Administration
2008	Mid-level providers training started
2009	Scale up strategy approved. Piloted and started services by trained ANMs
2010	All 75 districts had at least one listed safe abortion site with at least one qualified provider
2011	Developed National Safe Abortion Service Implementation Guideline
2013	Developed MA Drugs and Equipment Supply Guidelines
2015	Developed National Safe Abortion Policy and procedural order
2016	Free abortion services guideline developed

provided in integrated form (both MVA/MA) in 3 days.

- Doctors at government facilities, private clinics or NGOs are provided training for 10 days.
- Staff nurses at government facilities, private clinics, or NGOs who are trained as Skilled Birth Attendants or trained for intrauterine device (IUD) insertion are provided training for 10 days.
- Senior ANM or ANM who are also trained as Skilled Birth Attendants and in IUD insertion from governmental facilities (Hospital/Primary Health Care Center/Health Post/Birthing Center) or from NGOs are trained for 5 days. They are allowed to provide MA services up to 63 days (9 weeks) only.

27.7 Selection for Training in Second-Trimester Abortion

Those eligible for the second-trimester abortion training are physicians who have been regularly performing first-trimester abortion at ten to twelve weeks and have been observed for second-trimester aptitude. They must then undergo training as follows:

- Physicians who have completed ob-gyn or general practice residencies and want second-trimester abortion training for D&E and medical induction require twelve days of training.
  - Physicians who want training for medical induction only require seven days.

At present, there are ten training sites in the government sector and some in nongovernment sites. From 2003 to 2018, around 3,900 different health-care providers were trained under NHTC.

27.8 Monitoring for Quality Assurance and Improvement

Monitoring tools were incorporated into existing health management information systems (HMIS) to measure the progress of abortion services and identify areas for improvement. All public-sector abortion care sites aggregate monthly data on the number of post-abortion care clients, induced abortion clients, clients accepting post-abortion contraceptives and clients with complications. Service statistics are reviewed monthly by site staff, quarterly at district review meetings with site facility managers and annually at both regional and national review workshops. The MOH/FWD also regularly reviews indicators on post-abortion complications and post-abortion contraceptive acceptance.

27.9 Free Safe Abortion Services

Nepal's government has promoted safe, legal and cheap (or free) abortion, but public health facilities did not uniformly offer abortion as a "choice" to all women. Even minimal "service charges" of Rs. 1000 (US$10) for MA and Rs. 850 (US$8.5) for MUA presented barriers for poor women. In 2015, the government declared that abortion services were free of charge at public health facilities. A "Free Safe Abortion Service

Guideline" (2013–2015) described the following conditions for free services:

- For all abortion <12 weeks or >12 weeks in all listed facilities
- For incomplete or continued pregnancy after abortion
- For other post–abortion complication management

During implementation of the free service, the government instituted payment to providers as follows:

- Rs. 800 ($8) per case for MA/MUA (<12 weeks)
- Rs. 2000 ($20) per case for (D&E/Medical Induction) (>12 weeks)

The incentives received by the institutions are distributed through the Health Facility Operation Management Committee for use as follows:

- 70% in managing combi pack, canulas and other supplies
- 20% incentive to service provider
- 10% for assistant of service provider

27.10 Post-Abortion Care Service

Complications arising from incomplete unsafe abortions, both spontaneous and induced, are a major cause of maternal mortality and morbidity. To improve maternal health, the MOH/FWD implemented prior to legalization of abortion a Post-Abortion Care (PAC) service. The first PAC service site at Kathmandu Maternity Hospital included as a priority post-abortion contraception. The National Safe Abortion Policy of 2003 also emphasized post-abortion contraception, but immediate provision at abortion sites remains low. The increase in first-trimester medication abortions poses special challenges for post-abortion contraceptive use in Nepal and worldwide because the abortion occurs in the absence of contraceptive providers.

Accordingly, in 2002–03, the -PAC On-the-Job-Training Program was introduced to provide quality PAC services for 24 hours a day, 7 days a week at sites with large numbers of service providers. This plan was considered a cost-effective way to train service providers in post-abortion contraception without disturbing daily routine work at the service site. PAC provision has played an important role in transition to universal safe abortion services in Nepal.

27.11 Abortion Awareness in the Community

Even though abortion is now legal in Nepal, women still suffer from serious health problems or even die due to lack of access to safe abortion. Legalization alone is not enough. Economic constraints, lack of awareness and stigma associated with abortion have been major factors hindering women from seeking abortion services. Abortion stigma plays a critical role, and it leads to negative health outcomes for women and girls of our communities. Clandestine abortion still causes complications, sometimes leading to long-term disability or death. The reasons why women choose to have a clandestine rather than safe abortion are often closely related to marital status, social stigma, age, family size and social, economic and health factors. Age-specific abortion rates are determined by at least three factors: when women are most likely to become pregnant, when pregnancies are most likely to be unintended and when women are most likely to resolve an unintended pregnancy by abortion rather than go on to have an unplanned birth. Because of restricted access to health facilities, poor awareness, costs and cultural prohibitions in many rural and remote areas, women still rely on untrained providers and use many types of traditional and nonmedical methods to end unintended pregnancies, ultimately leading to morbidity and mortality.

Knowledge of women on the availability of abortion in Nepal is still very poor. According to NDHS 2016, 59% of women of reproductive age do not know that abortion has been legalized, and 52% do not know about a place where safe abortion service is available to them. Female Community Health Workers (FCHVs), the grass roots health informants, can disseminate key messages of maternal, newborn and child health, and family planning including abortion. They share health information with adolescent, newly married and other women in their mothers' group meetings. "Community Dialogue Meetings" raise awareness of safe abortion and reduce its stigma. Women learn that everyone, including poor rural women, has the right to safe, accessible, acceptable, affordable and equitable abortion services.

References

1. Center for Reproductive Law and Policy and Forum for Women, Law and Development. *Abortion in Nepal: Women Imprisoned.* New York: CRLP; 2002.

2. Ministry of Law and Justice. *Muluki Ain, 2020 (Legal Code, 1963).* Kathmandu: Ministry of Law and Justice; 1963.

3. Shrestha GB. *Yek Tippani (Muluki Ain: A Commentary),* 7th ed. Kathmandu: Pairavi Prakashan; 2002.

4. Thapa S. Abortion law in Nepal: the road to reform. *Reprod Health Matters.* 2004; (24 Suppl):85–94.

5. Ganatra B, Gerdts C, Rossier C, et al. Global, regional, and subregional classification of abortions by safety, 2010–14: estimates from a Bayesian hierarchical model. *Lancet.* 2017;390(10110):2372–2381.

6. WHO and Guttmacher Institute. Worldwide, an estimated 25 million unsafe abortions occur each year. Joint news release; 2017.

7. Ministry of Health. *Family Health Survey 2016.* Kathmandu: Ministry of Health, New Era, ICF; 2017.

8. Pathak LR, Malla DS, Pradhan A. *Maternal Mortality and Morbidity Study.* Kathmandu: Ministry of Health; 1998.

9. Center for Reproductive Law and Policy and Forum for Women, Law and Development. *Abortion in Nepal: Women Imprisoned.* New York: CRLP; 2002.

10. Nepal Law Commission. *Nepal Law Commission Report, 1973.* Kathmandu: Nepal Law Commission; 1973.

11. Institute of Law. *Report on Law and Population Growth in Nepal.* Kathmandu: Institute of Law; 1979.

12. Law Reform Commission. *Law Reform Commission Report, 1982.* Kathmandu: Law Reform Commission; 1982.

13. Population Action International. *What You Need to Know about the Global Gag Rule Restriction: An Unofficial Guide.* Washington DC: PAI, 2001.

14. Ministry of Health. *National Health Policy.* Kathmandu: Ministry of Health, 1991.

15. United Nations. *Report on the International Conference on Population and Development, Cairo, September 5–13, 1994.* New York: United Nations, Department of Economic and Social Affairs, Population Division; 1994.

16. United Nations. Beijing deceleration and platform of action. In *Fourth World Conference on Women,* Beijing, September 4–15, 1995.

17. Henderson JT, Puri M, Blum Met al. Effects of abortion legalization in Nepal, 2001–2010. *PLoS ONE.* 2013;8(5):e64775.

18. Tasnim N, Mahmud G, Fatima S, Sultana M. Manual vacuum aspiration: a safe and cost effective substitute of electric vacuum aspiration for the surgical management of early pregnancy loss. *J Pak Med Assoc.* 2011;61(2):149–153.

19. Basnett I, Shrestha M K, Pearson E, Thapa K, Anderson KL. Evaluation of nurse providers of comprehensive abortion care using MVA in Nepal. *J Nepal Health Res Counc.* 2012;10(1):5–9.

20. Foster DG, Biggs MA, Raifman S, Gipson J, Kimport K, Rocca CH. Comparison of health, development, maternal bonding, and poverty among children born after denial of abortion vs after pregnancies subsequent to an abortion. *JAMA Pediatrics.* 2018;172(11):1053–1060.

21. Government of Nepal, Ministry of Health and Population, Department of Health Services, Family Health Division. National Facility Based Abortion Study Kathmandu; 2006.

22. Basnett I, Sharma SK, Bhusal CL, Parajuli RR, Anderson KL. Increasing access to safe abortion services through auxillary nurse midwives trained as skilled birth attendants. *Kathmandu Univ Med J.* 2011;9(36):260–266.

23. Samandari G, Wolf M, Basnett I, Hyman A, Anderson K. Implementation of legal abortion in Nepal: a model for rapid scale up of high quality care. *Reprod Health.* 2012;9:7.

24. Tamang A, Puri M, Lama K, Shrestha P. Pharmacy workers in Nepal can provide the correct information about using mifepristone and misoprostol to women seeking medication to induce abortion. *Reprod Health Matters.* 2015;(Suppl 44):104–105

25. *National Safe Abortion Policy and Strategy.* Ministry of Health, Department of Health Services, Family Health Division; 2002.

26. *Safe Abortion Service Procedure.* Kathmandu: Ministry of Health, Department of Health Services, Family Health Division; 2003.

27. Abortion Task Force. *Workshop Report – National Implementation Plan for Abortion Services.* Kathmandu: Ministry of Health, Department of Health Services, Family Health Division; 18–19 November 2002.

28. *Safe Abortion Services Program Implementation Guidelines.* Kathmandu: Ministry of Health, Department of Health Services, Family Health Division; 2011.

29. Shrestha DR, Regmi SC, Dangal G. Abortion: still unfinished agenda in Nepal. *J Nepal Health Res Counc.* 2018;16(1):93–98.

Chapter

28

Abortion Training and Integration in Ghana

Emmanuel S. K. Morhe and Vanessa K. Dalton

28.1 Introduction

Contraception and safe abortion services are particularly important in low-resource settings where complications of unintended pregnancy and unsafe abortion are a leading cause of maternal mortality and morbidity. Although contraception prevalence rates (eg, the percentage of women using contraception) have generally improved over the past decade, contraception use rates remain unacceptably low [1]. This fact is especially true in African countries where the contraception prevalence rate is 23.9%, which is half the rate of other poor countries [1]. Furthermore, when unwanted pregnancies do occur, too many women are unable to access safe abortion services, even in countries where abortion is legal [2]. The poor accessibility of quality contraceptive and abortion services in sub-Saharan Africa is attributed in part to inadequate resources, including a shortage of health-care providers [3,4]. As a consequence, African women suffer from high rates of unintended pregnancy and its consequences, including death [5]. Worldwide, sub-Saharan Africa has the highest burden of these preventable sexual and reproductive health-related deaths [6].

This chapter presents an overview of the International Family Planning Fellowship Program (IFPFP) in Ghana – one approach to increase women's access to quality contraception and abortion services by integrating family planning and comprehensive abortion care training and building a dedicated workforce. The Ghanaian experience provides a platform for the development of similar programs in the developing world.

28.2 The Setting: Ghana

Ghana is a low-middle-income country located in West Africa on the Gulf of Guinea and has a population of about 28 million people, most of whom live in rural areas. Ghana's economy is largely driven by agriculture and the service sector, and is the second fastest growing economy in Africa [7,8] (Figure 28.1).

According to the 2017 Ghana Maternal Health Survey, the total fertility rate has steadily declined from 6.4 in 1988 to 3.9 in 2017 [9]. Fertility is higher among women in rural areas, as compared to urban areas (4.7 vs. 3.3 children per woman), and is highest in the Northern Region (5.8 children per woman). Knowledge of contraception is widespread, with virtually all reproductive-aged women able to identify at least one method of modern contraception. Still, the contraception prevalence rate among all sexually active women between 15 and 49 years of age is about 25%, with 20% using a modern method of contraception [9].

While an estimated 10% of all pregnancies in Ghana end in induced abortion, many women are still unaware that abortion is legal [9]. According to the most recent Maternal Health Survey, over one quarter of women who had an induced abortion reported using a non-medication method (unknown tablets, herbal enema, inserting substance into the vagina, etc.) and fewer than half sought care from a health-care facility. Although complications from induced abortion are a common cause of maternal death, the proportion of cases fell from 11% to 4% in the past 10 years. Based on current fertility and mortality rates, it is estimated that about 1% of women in Ghana will die from pregnancy-related causes [9].

28.2.1 Family Planning and Reproductive Health Care in Ghana

Following independence, the Ghanaian government embraced family planning as a key strategy to address alarming population growth rates. Family planning services were introduced in 1961 by the National Association of the Orthodox Protestant Churches and were

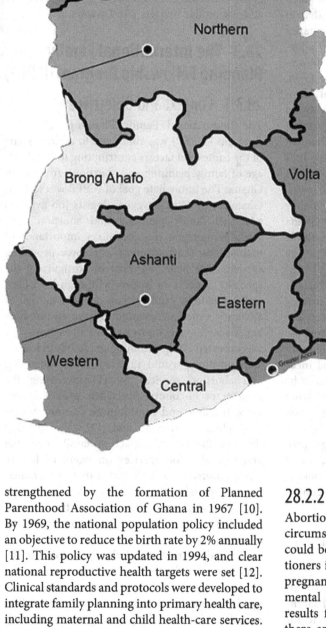

Figure 28.1 The regions of Ghana

strengthened by the formation of Planned Parenthood Association of Ghana in 1967 [10]. By 1969, the national population policy included an objective to reduce the birth rate by 2% annually [11]. This policy was updated in 1994, and clear national reproductive health targets were set [12]. Clinical standards and protocols were developed to integrate family planning into primary health care, including maternal and child health-care services. Provider training was mainly through in-service training workshops hosted by nongovernmental organizations (NGOs), such as the US Agency for International Development (USAID), and were heavily dependent on donor funding.

28.2.2 Abortion in Ghana

Abortion has been legal in Ghana under certain circumstances since 1985. Accordingly, abortions could be performed by registered medical practitioners in a registered health facility when (1) the pregnancy poses risk to the life or physical and mental health of the woman; (2) the pregnancy results from rape, defilement or incest; and (3) there are fetal malformations incompatible with life [2,12]. However, abortion was not formally introduced into Ghana's reproductive health policy until 2003, an event that paved the way for national comprehensive abortion care (CAC) standards and protocols development. Detailed national CAC standards and protocols were rolled out in 2006 by the Ghana Health Service (GHS) under monitoring and supervision of the Ministry of Health, when safe abortion was identified as one of the five components of the Ghana Health Service's objectives to reduce maternal morbidity and mortality [2,9,13]. Under this updated guidance, midwives were explicitly permitted to perform abortion services in order to enhance access to services. Midwives who provided abortion care were trained under task-sharing in-service training programs organized by the GHS. Skill training was carried out by national physician trainers. Training was sponsored by a number of NGOs including the American College of Nurse-Midwives (ACNM), Planned Parenthood Association of Ghana (PPAG), Ipas and Marie Stopes International, now MSI Reproductive Choices.

Even within a supportive legal and policy environment, rates of unsafe abortion in Ghana remain high, likely as a consequence of multiple factors. Women and providers are poorly informed about safe abortion services [9,14,15] and there is a lack of trained personnel, especially in rural areas of the country [16]. Cost, privacy concerns and limited access to existing services (which tend to be centralized) continue to pose serious barriers. As a result, many women still obtain abortion care outside of the formal medical system [9]. Finally, abortion continues to be stigmatized, which discourages women from seeking services within the medical system and deters health-care providers from providing services in many areas. As in other settings, providers that offer abortion services are often marginalized and professionally isolated, making it difficult to recruit other providers or clinical sites.

28.2.3 Human Resources and Abortion Care in Ghana

Attracting and retaining health-care personnel willing and able to provide abortion and family planning services are critical components to the availability of safe abortion. In Ghana, as in many other countries, abortion and family planning services are largely siloed and poorly integrated into primary care services, in part due to the stigma emanating from sociocultural norms and

years of restrictive abortion laws. This marginalization of services constitutes a formidable barrier to access to abortion care in the country [17] and is not a problem unique to Ghana. One idea was to create an academic track for physician family planning and abortion specialists, modeled after the successful Fellowship in Family Planning program introduced in the USA in the 1990s to address similar barriers (see Chapter 3).

28.3 The International Family Planning Fellowship Program (IFPFP)

28.3.1 Context and Objectives

The International Family Planning Fellowship Program (IFPFP) was conceived to address some of the contextual factors contributing to the shortage of family planning and abortion providers in Ghana. The immediate goal of IFPFP was to train Ghanaian obstetrician-gynecologists (ob-gyns) in advanced family planning and abortion care, while recognizing the enormous importance of maintaining the midwifery workforce providing services. The belief was that by formalizing the specialty, a cadre of leaders with high-level clinical, operational, and evaluation skills, as well as advocacy experience, would emerge and assume key leadership positions around the country. It was expected that positioning graduates in leadership positions would improve family planning and abortion services by (1) increasing the number of in-country specialists providing services, training, and consultation; (2) introducing new clinical services; and (3) disseminating data on the health impact of family planning and safe abortion services on women's health. Furthermore, it was anticipated that by formalizing the specialty, the specialty would be viewed as "legitimate," countering some of the isolation and stigma that deterred many from providing services.

To understand the underlying rationale for the approach taken by the Ghanaian institutions, the historical context of post-graduate training in ob-gyn in Ghana is important. Prior to 1989, medical school graduates seeking post-graduate training in obstetrics and gynecology had to leave the country to obtain training in the United Kingdom or Europe. Only about 10% returned to practice in Ghana, at a time that concerns about maternal mortality were at the forefront.

Ghanaian leaders, in partnership with the Royal College of Obstetricians and Gynaecologists, the American College of Obstetricians and Gynecologists and the Carnegie Corporation, introduced an in-country post-graduate training program in obstetrics and gynecology in 1989. Subsequent evaluations of this program have concluded that it successfully expanded the obstetrics and gynecology workforce in Ghana. As of 2010, eighty-five physicians were successfully certified in obstetrics and gynecology. Figure 28.2 shows the cumulative number of retained obstetrics and gynecology specialists in Ghana. Overall, retention of obstetrics and gynecology specialists has reached 98% [18].

A critical legacy of the Ghanaian post-graduate training program was the reinforcement of the long-standing partnership between the University of Michigan and the two largest Ghanaian universities. The University of Ghana and Kwame Nkrumah University of Science and Technology (KNUST) have collaborated with the University of Michigan for many years, spanning generations of physicians, students and specialties. These relationships were, and continue to be, characterized by a bilateral exchange of people, ideas and resources [19]. It was from within this context that the International Family Planning Fellowship program was conceived and developed.

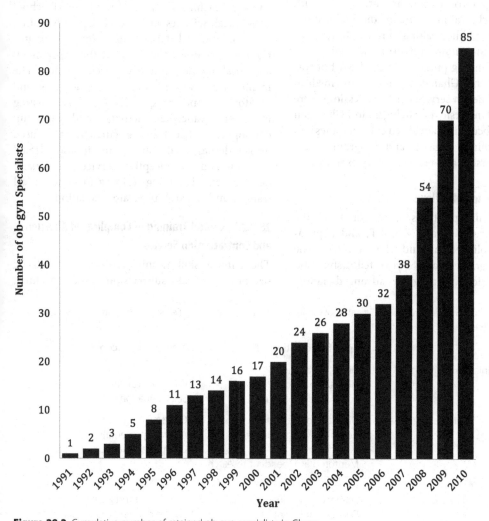

Figure 28.2 Cumulative number of retained ob-gyn specialists in Ghana

28.3.2 Training Program Content

28.3.2.1 Faculty Training

In preparation for the IFPFP, a three-week seminar was conducted at the University of Michigan in late 2007 to develop a training team, finalize the curriculum and develop a monitoring and evaluation plan. Seminar topics included complex contraception and abortion, competency-based educational approaches, clinical skills evaluation methods and program evaluation. Seminar participants consisted of an interdisciplinary group of faculty, including clinicians and academic faculty from Ghanaian medical and public health schools, and representatives from the Ghana Health Service and the Ghana College of Physicians and Surgeons.

The curriculum was developed with interdisciplinary input from seminar participants with expertise in clinical medicine, medical education, health policy, public health and research methodology. The curriculum drew from the Fellowship in Family Planning program in the USA but was adapted to the Ghanaian context of medical training and health service delivery. Sessions were led by both University of Michigan and Ghanaian faculty and focused on advanced clinical topics and clinical teaching, research and program evaluation, mentorship and team-building exercises.

28.3.2.2 Training of Fellows

The fellowship positions are posted at the University of Ghana and KNUST, and applications are solicited around the country. The training program is a two-year fellowship and includes clinical training in advanced family planning services, public health, evaluation and advocacy. Most fellows obtain a master's degree in public health at one of the two Ghanaian public health schools and complete a district placement. Table 28.1 summarizes the program's objectives, activities and evaluation approach. Upon completion, graduates of the program may apply for subspecialty certification in family planning and abortion from the Ghana College of Physicians and Surgeons, which requires the completion of a thesis and passing an oral examination. IFPFP was the first subspecialty certification program to be established in Ghana.

The first four fellows began the fellowship program in 2008; two were trained at Korle-Bu Teaching Hospital of the University of Ghana Medical School in Accra and two at Komfo Anokye Teaching Hospital of the KNUST School of Medical Sciences in Kumasi. Upon initiating the program, each fellow was assigned a mentor team that included the heads of the department, a clinical mentor and a research mentor. The mentor team was responsible for advising and mentoring, conducting evaluations and assisting in career advancement activities and leadership development. The training curriculum focused on key domains: clinical training in complicated abortion and contraceptive services, leadership development (including training to be a clinical trainer) and research/program evaluation.

28.3.2.3 Clinical Training in Complicated Abortion and Contraception Services

The clinical skill training consists of didactic sessions, clinical supervision and coaching,

Table 28.1 Objectives and measured outcomes of the International Family Planning Fellowship Program in abortion and family planning

Objective	Specific activities	Measured outcome
Improve clinical skills	Didactic training Simulation training Supervised procedures	Case logs Director evaluations Self-evaluations
Improve skills in clinical and health systems research	Didactic coursework Contribute to ongoing research project Mentored independent research project	Coursework grade Abstract presentations Completed manuscript
Improve leadership skills	Leadership seminars District placement Work with local nongovernmental organizations	Seminar attendance Log of nongovernmental or community-based work

documentation of case logs and competency assessment by the clinical mentors. The clinical training largely occurs at Korle-Bu and Komfo Anokye Teaching Hospitals.

28.3.2.4 Leadership Development

Leadership skill development training includes coursework, presentations at international family planning meetings and work with local agencies and NGOs engaged in family planning and reproductive health outreach. Fellows are encouraged to participate in existing leadership training programs offered at meetings or through their home institutions. The trainees are also expected to engage in volunteer services, including clinical care services, community outreach programs, public speaking engagements and post-graduate training events sponsored by various governmental and nongovernmental agencies.

28.3.2.5 Research and Evaluation

Fellows are required to obtain a master's degree in public health (MPH) during their fellowship. This degree program provides the framework for their research and evaluation skills training. Fellowship graduation requirements include a dissertation on a topic in family planning and reproductive health. Other research skill development activities include mentored and independent research projects. Abstract presentations at national and international meetings and manuscript publication in peer review journals are expected.

28.3.2.6 Certification Process

Final certification is awarded by the Ghana College of Physicians and Surgeons after submission of a dissertation and passage of an oral examination. Upon successful graduation, fellows are certified as specialists in Family Planning and Reproductive Health, the first subspecialty of obstetrics and gynecology recognized by the Ghana College of Physicians and Surgeons. The first cohort of fellows was certified in November 2011.

28.4 IFPFP Transition to Reproductive Health and Family Planning Fellowship Program (RHFPF)

The development and implementation of IFPFP was funded by a donor, but from conception, the goal was to transfer the program to the Ghanaian institutions as soon as feasible. After four years (two training cycles), program administration and leadership, as well as funding of the scholars, was transferred to the Ghana College of Physicians and Surgeons. With this transfer, some components of the fellowship were not maintained, including funding for fellows to obtain an MPH. Today, fellows often have to fund their degree program themselves. Fellow salaries are covered by the Ghana Health Service. Applications to the program continue to outnumber the available training spots.

28.5 Exchange with the US Fellowship in Family Planning Program

One of the goals of the IFPFP was to establish opportunities for Ghanaian specialists to engage with the global community of family planning providers and training programs to address the isolation and stigma experienced by many. These opportunities included participation in the US Fellowship in Family Planning meetings, where Ghanaian fellows presented their work, as well as attendance at other relevant meetings such as the annual meeting of the Society of Family Planning. During their visits to the USA, fellows also observed clinical services at high-volume abortion sites. In later years, graduated Ghanaian specialists hosted US fellows in Ghana for their international rotations and have served as consultants during the development of a similar training program in Ethiopia.

28.6 Fellowship Impact on Family Planning and Abortion in Ghana

Fellowship-trained specialists now work in a number of institutions and in positions around the country. They are engaged in pre-service training of medical students, midwives, physician assistants and residents in family planning and reproductive health. Specialists spend generally 30 to 50% of their time on activities related to capacity building, family planning and Comprehensive Abortion Care (CAC) service, research and advocacy. They play a critical role in increasing the availability of abortion services across Ghana by taking on significant leadership positions, establishing new clinical services and providing consultation and support for midwives who currently provide the majority of uncomplicated services around the country.

Pre-service clinical training of physicians and midwives in family planning and CAC is a critical role of specialists. Graduates and current fellows are assigned to reproductive health centers to provide clinical services and pre-service clinical training to a wide range of trainees. These include medical students, midwifery students, physician assistant students and residents. Prevention of unsafe abortion through use of contraception and provision of comprehensive abortion care has been included and continues to be revised in the curriculum for training of reproductive health-care professionals. The specialists organize and deliver the lecture series on abortion and family planning and provide training on long-acting reversible contraceptives (LARC) and sterilization procedures in simulation and real-time clinical settings. The specialists also serve as a resource for an array of post-graduate technical training programs in CAC, LARC and sterilization for ob-gyns and family medicine–trained providers.

Graduated fellows are taking on important leadership positions around the country. Several have taken positions in rural areas including in the Northern Region, which has the highest fertility rate in the country. A sample of positions is shown below:

- CEO, Tamale Teaching Hospital
- Inaugural Head of Department of Obstetrics and Gynecology, Ho Teaching Hospital
- Directors of Reproductive Health Units
- Head of Research and Development/Reproductive Health Center
- Faculty at University of Ghana
- Faculty at KNUST
- Faculty, University of Cape Coast

28.7 Discussion

It is widely recognized that access to safe abortion and contraception services is integral to efforts to decrease maternal mortality worldwide. Creating a formal professional pathway to specialize in family planning and abortion care is one approach to build and retain a skilled workforce. To date, Ghana's experience with IFPFP has achieved its immediate objective to train and place specialists in influential leadership positions, including in rural areas where the need is great. From these posts, they can not only influence the delivery of clinical services, but also can advocate for supportive policies and resources.

During the evolution of IFPFP (and subsequently RHFPF), several key lessons emerged:

- *The long-standing relationship between our institutions helped us successfully navigate challenges.* Inevitably, projects like IFPFP run into anticipated and unanticipated challenges. Navigating these issues can be especially difficult when partners come from high- and low-resource settings. This project certainly benefited from the fact that much time and reflection had already been invested in the relationship between the partners.
- *Identifying and engaging with other key stakeholders (hospital and medical school leadership, government agencies, NGOs) is important for sustainability and efficiency.* As in many settings, a range of organizations is heavily engaged in family planning and abortion advocacy, education and training. Engagement with this larger community helped the program identify gaps in service and training, and avoid inefficiencies or unnecessary duplication.
- *While the IFPFP was designed for subspecialty training in obstetrics and gynecology, we engaged with other health-care providers during program design and implementation to address gaps in training and service, including midwifery, medical and nursing students).* Non-physicians provide a large volume of family planning and abortion services in Ghana. Therefore, creating a specialty for physicians had the potential to threaten or exclude other providers or stakeholders. This engagement helped identify the critical roles fellowship-trained specialists play in supporting the entire workforce.

The Ghanaian experience demonstrates that in-country training of specialist physicians is feasible and can result in a high rate of retention. IFPFP, and now RHFPF, is contributing to the continued growth of a health-care workforce and educators with expertise in family planning and abortion.

References

1. Ahmed S, Choi Y, Rimon JG, et al. Trends in contraceptive prevalence rates in sub-Saharan Africa since the 2012 London Summit on Family Planning: results from repeated cross-sectional surveys. *Lancet Glob Health*. 2019;7:e904-e911.

2. Rominski SD, Lori JR. Abortion care in Ghana: a critical review of the literature. *Afr J Reprod Health*. 2014;18:17–35.

3. Creanga AA, Gillespie D, Karklins S, Tsui AO. Low use of contraception among poor women in Africa: an equity issue. *Bull World Health Organ*. 2011;89:258–266.

4. Stephenson R, Baschieri A, Clements S, Hennink M, Madise N. Contextual influences on modern contraceptive use in sub-Saharan Africa. *Am J Public Health*. 2007;97:1233–1240.

5. Lauro D. Abortion and contraceptive use in sub-Saharan Africa: how women plan their families. *Afr J Reprod Health*. 2011;15:13–23.

6. Ahman E, Shah IH. New estimates and trends regarding unsafe abortion mortality. *Int J Gynaecol Obstet*. 2011;115:121–126.

7. World Health Organization. WHO Country Cooperation Strategy, 2008–2011. Ghana; 2009. https://apps.who.int/iris/bitstream/handle/10665/136005/ccs_ghana.pdf;jsessionid=1AA40998E74F185484FAE1D73778C859?sequence=3.

8. The World Bank. The World Bank in Ghana; 2019 www.worldbank.org/en/country/ghana/overview.

9. Ghana Statistical Service. Ghana Maternal Health Survey; 2017. www.dhsprogram.com/pubs/pdf/FR340/FR340.pdf

10. Kwansa EV, Bentsi C, Anteson RK, Adofo CB. Integrated project plan for Ghana. *JOICFP Rev*. 1987;13:10–12.

11. Oliver R. Contraceptive use in Ghana: the role of service availability, quality, and price. Living Standards Measurement Study (LSMS) Working Paper no. LSM 111; 1995. http://documents.worldbank.org/curated/en/674821468771258900/Contraceptive-use-in-Ghana-the-role-of-service-availability-quality-and-price. Accessed July 29, 2019.

12. Government of Ghana National Population Council. *National Population Policy*, rev. ed; 1994. https://npc.gov.gh/wp-content/uploads/2019/01/National-Population-PolicyRevised-Edition-1994.pdf. Accessed July 29, 2019.

13. Ghana Health Service. Prevention & Management of Unsafe Abortion: Comprehensive Abortion Care Services Standards and Protocols; 2012. https://abortion-policies.srhr.org/documents/countries/02-Ghana-Comprehensive-Abortion-Care-Services-Standards-and-Protocols-Ghana-Health-Service-2012.pdf. Accessed July 29, 2019.

14. Morhe ES, Morhe RA, Danso KA. Attitudes of doctors toward establishing safe abortion units in Ghana. *Int J Gynaecol Obstet*. 2007;98:70–74.

15. Konney TO, Danso KA, Odoi AT, Opare-Addo HS, Morhe ES. Attitude of women with abortion-related complications toward provision of safe abortion services in Ghana. *J Womens Health (Larchmt)*. 2009;18:1863–1866.

16. Hill ZE, Tawiah-Agyemang C, Kirkwood B. The context of informal abortions in rural Ghana. *J Womens Health (Larchmt)*. 2009;18:2017–2022.

17. Lithur NO. Destigmatising abortion: expanding community awareness of abortion as a reproductive health issue in Ghana. *Afr J Reprod Health*. 2004;8:70–74.

18. Anderson FW, Obed SA, Boothman EL, Opare-Ado H. The public health impact of training physicians to become obstetricians and gynecologists in Ghana. *Am J Public Health*. 2014;104(Suppl 1):S159–165.

19. Anderson F, Donkor P, de Vries R, et al. Creating a charter of collaboration for international university partnerships: the Elmina Declaration for Human Resources for Health. *Acad Med*. 2014;89:1125–1132.

Chapter

29

Pre-service Integration of Abortion and Contraception Trainings in Ethiopia

Ferid A. Abubeker and Mengistu Hailemariam

29.1 Background

Since the International Conference on Population and Development (ICPD) Cairo conference in 1994, there has been increasing international commitment to sexual and reproductive health and rights, and there has been an expansion of sex education and reproductive health services globally. However, the efforts are far from sufficient to provide people with the means they need to make reproductive choices according to their wishes and their life situation [1,2].

The availability of modern contraception can reduce but never eliminate the need for safe abortion. Therefore, unintended and unwanted pregnancies remain a major challenge for girls and women worldwide [1,3]. Ending the silent pandemic of unsafe abortion is an urgent public health and human rights imperative. As with other more visible global health issues, this scourge threatens women throughout the developing world [4]. The estimated global abortion rate as of 2010–2014 was 35 per 1,000 for married women and 26 per 1,000 for unmarried women. According to recent estimates, at least 8% of maternal deaths worldwide are from unsafe abortion done by individuals without the requisite skills, or in environments below minimum medical standards, or both; at least 22,800 women die each year from complications of unsafe abortion. Almost all abortion-related deaths occur in developing countries, with the highest number occurring in those in Africa [5].

Access to safe, legal abortion is a fundamental right of women, irrespective of where they live. Ethiopia, in contrast to many other African countries, has a relatively liberal abortion law [6]. Prior to 2005, abortion was permitted in Ethiopia only to save the pregnant woman from "grave and permanent danger to life or health" with the approval of two physicians including at least one gynecologist. The revised law, enacted by Ethiopia's parliament in 2005, allows a woman to obtain a safe, legal abortion based on broad indications, including if she became pregnant through rape or incest, has physical or mental disabilities, if continuation of the pregnancy or the birth would endanger the health or life of the woman or fetus; if the fetus has an incurable disease or deformity; and if the woman is a minor who is physically or mentally unprepared for childbirth. The high maternal mortality rate due to complications of unsafe abortion framed the conversation for this legal reform [7].

Furthermore, the House of Representatives mandated the Ministry of Health to produce *Technical and Procedural Guidelines for Safe Abortion Services*, issued first in 2006 and later updated in 2013 [8]. These guidelines translate the law into actionable measures and aim to inform women, health professionals, law enforcement agencies and all sectors of society who care for the well-being of women and their families.

The guidelines, which are based on World Health Organization (WHO) standards, outline appropriate abortion methods at various stages of pregnancy. They also recommend the required trainings for different levels of health-care providers and set the standard regarding equipping health-care facilities vis-à-vis the task they are expected to perform, thus effectively implementing task sharing and shifting.

The Ministry of Health provided overall leadership and ownership of the program and sought technical guidance and support from other essential partners such as professional medical societies, nongovernmental organizations (NGOs) and relevant United Nations (UN) agencies. Professional medical societies and NGOs were important allies in formulating technical guidelines, training, and certification. In addition, international NGOs played a critical role in providing essential commodities and, at times, abortion services. The rigorously developed WHO guidelines for abortion services, as well as for task sharing, served as standards and provided legitimacy for advocacy groups. The Ministry of Health acted as a critical facilitator because of its authoritative and convening roles. Working within the one-system health framework, the commitment of the Ministry to the expansion of services was essential to increasing access, and this proved key to the successful establishment of the program.

Despite these reforms and the substantial progress made, clandestine abortions are still common, and unintended pregnancy is one of the main reasons for girls to drop out of school [9].

Access to abortion and contraception care requires consideration of a number of health system issues that include availability of clinical spaces with the necessary equipment and supplies, ensuring skills and performance of health-care providers, supportive and facilitative supervision and monitoring, evaluation and other quality-improvement processes. All levels of health-care professionals need specific training to guarantee a woman's right to privacy, to guarantee that they be sensitive to her needs and perspectives and to ensure that the services are rendered in a way that respects a woman's dignity.

Developing countries like Ethiopia with high burdens of maternal mortality, unsafe abortion and unmet need for contraception suffer from lack of trained health-care workers who can provide essential maternal health services including abortion and contraception care [10]. Despite expectations, most graduates of the health profession lack many of the competencies required to provide essential reproductive health services before they enter into practice. To fill this gap, the health sectors and development partners have relied on the traditional in-service trainings as the main practical solution [11]. Although this approach serves its function in terms of availing women of the service quickly (ie, promoting access), in-service trainings cannot be a substitute to address the graduates' lack of competencies for the future. Some of the disadvantages and challenges to the health system are training costs and service interruptions that occur when the health service providers must travel from their workplaces to training sites. We believe that our approach to educate and train students while they are still in school (in the pre-service period),

reinforcing the curriculum contents and making the training competency based will overcome these challenges.

Pre-service clinical health professional education programs should have consistent and progressive curricula that give adequate room for accommodating competency-based contraception and pregnancy termination training. It should be conducted in teaching facilities that promote evidence-based clinical medicine and that have committed and skillful faculties and sufficient client flow to provide all students with the requisite practice.

In this regard, with the generous funding from an anonymous donors and appropriate technical support from the University of Michigan, the Center for International Reproductive Health Training (CIRHT) has been implementing integration of contraception and pregnancy termination trainings in pre-service medical and midwifery education and obstetrics and gynecology (ob-gyn) residency programs in Ethiopia.

The following is a retrospective case study examining the CIRHT program designed for scaling pre-service trainings of comprehensive abortion and contraception care across ten Ethiopian schools of medicine and midwifery from July 2014–June 2019.

29.2 Integrating Comprehensive Abortion and Contraception Training into a Pre-service Education Setting

Encouraged by the successful implementation of a project she introduced and launched in 2011 to integrate contraception and abortion trainings into medical education at St Paul's Hospital Millennium Medical College in Ethiopia [12], Dr. Senait Fisseha, a University of Michigan professor of obstetrics and gynecology and medical director of Michigan's Center for Reproductive Medicine at the time, founded the Center for International Reproductive Health Training at the University of Michigan (CIRHT) in 2014. CIRHT envisions reducing maternal mortality and morbidity from unsafe abortion in developing countries by introducing a model that helps health professionals acquire knowledge and competencies needed for provision of abortion care and contraception before their entry into clinical practices.

On the basis of the lessons learned from St. Paul's Hospital Millennium Medical College, and inspired by the training models of the Ryan Residency Training and Fellowship in Family Planning in the USA, ten medical and eight midwifery schools in the following higher teaching institutions across the country have been targeted for the implementation of the CIRHT program: Addis Ababa, Gondar, Jimma, Hawassa, Mekelle, Haromaya, BahirDar and Debretabor universities, and Adama hospital medical college and St. Paul's hospital millennium medical college. The program included all levels of providers but focused initially on medical students, interns and ob-gyn residents and later included midwives. Therefore, the obstetrics and gynecology (ob-gyn) and midwifery departments were the primary targets for introducing the initiative.

29.2.1 General Description of the CIRHT Model

CIRHT designed an integration model that assures acquisition of knowledge and competencies for provision of contraception and abortion care in a pre-service education setting. It emphasized the premise that focusing on these components of reproductive health supports improvement of other aspects of women's health.

The CIRHT model strives to improve the capacity of partner universities to produce competent health-care providers who will deliver high-quality contraception and pregnancy termination services. Partner universities will achieve this by (1) ensuring that faculty members have the necessary clinical competencies as well as teaching and research skills; (2) delivering a curriculum that is comprehensive and competency-based for the students; and (3) creating adequate opportunity for simulation-based and hands-on clinical training.

The integration approach follows and is aligned with the three functions of academic institutions – education (training), clinical service and research. A framework (see Figure 29.1) has been designed to show the relation among CIRHT's strategic areas – namely, education, clinical service and research in producing a graduate to be sufficiently competent to give comprehensive abortion care (CAC) and contraception services.

29.2.1.1 Description of the Framework on Education

To reinforce learning of comprehensive abortion care and contraception services, CIRHT followed

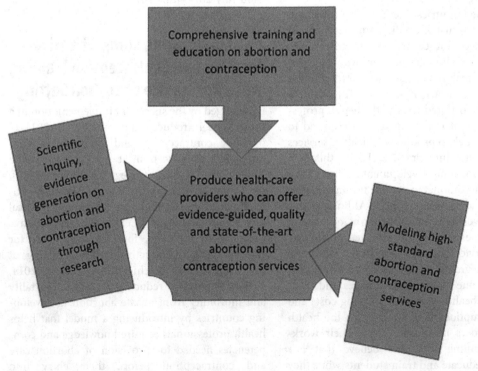

Figure 29.1 The relationship among CIRHT strategic areas

an approach that addresses the whole aspect of the curriculum, starting from reviewing the curriculum to monitoring and evaluation of its implementation. Reviewing the curriculum gave us the opportunity to make competency-based curricular changes.

Curriculum design: To assure acquisition of required skills on abortion and contraception, the competencies should clearly appear in the curriculum with a detailed course syllabus outlining the specific learning outcomes aligned with the appropriate teaching methods and assessments.

As part of the baseline study for the CIRHT's program implementation, the the learning and teaching activities of the implementing partner universities were assessed. Findings indicated that the undergraduate curricula of all medical and midwifery schools, as well as the ob-gyn residency training programs in these partner universities, did not have detailed syllabi that clearly outlined the learning outcomes or the teaching and assessment methods.

Through active engagement of the faculty, CIRHT supported the revision of curricula for trainings of undergraduate medical and midwifery students and ob-gyn residents to ensure the competencies required for provision of contraception and abortion care services are included.

Curriculum implementation: A well-written curriculum by itself would not guarantee its delivery as intended unless the necessary teaching resources are available and faculty are prepared to implement it. The faculty were oriented on the curriculum, and trained on how to use the teaching and assessment methods described in the curriculum.

Faculty then helped students acquire the skills in the safe environment of simulation before they were able to practice with live patients. Simulation enhanced their confidence, as they had multiple opportunities to make mistakes and learn from them as a means to ensure patient safety. To promote skills training, faculty skills teaching was not enough. Advocacy for the need for as well as setting up and equipping a skills lab with necessary mannequins were mandatory. For appropriate management of the clinical skills lab, individuals who oversee running the simulation lab were also trained on skills lab management.

Robust assessment methods are the best way to assure quality of education, as assessment drives learning. Faculty were trained on writing and applying context-dependent items that test students' abilities to apply concepts and principles rather than simply recall facts. They were also trained on how to develop and run an objective structured clinical exam (OSCE) to assess students' clinical decision making, communication and psychomotor skills. Partner schools were given exam blueprints and exam banks. To follow up on students' learning of skills at clinical sites, use of a log book was emphasized.

Curriculum implementation monitoring: In order to demonstrate results, training was followed up to measure impact. To accomplish that, a strong monitoring system was put in place using agreed-upon follow-up tools where data on curriculum implementation were monitored throughout the training process.

Leadership: Effective teaching and learning require positive educational leadership. Faculty at all levels of educational leadership were taught leadership skills along with continuous remote mentoring.

Partnership: Partnership with medical schools, Ministry of Health (MOH) and Ministry of Education (MOE) was key in implementing the curriculum and hands-on training. All three are in charge of establishing and implementing curricula and are responsible for administering the licensing exams. It was important to work with the National Board of Examination so that the competencies on contraception and abortion care services are included in the license examination (Figure 29.2).

Peer-assisted learning: Peer-assisted learning (PAL) is a form of academic support in which students mentor other students. The student mentors are trained in facilitation, coaching techniques and general mentoring principles, and meet regularly with mentees for study support sessions. The PAL scheme benefits students struggling with certain class content as well as mentors, reinforcing course material, developing learning and creative skills. Mentors are undergraduate volunteers who have strong academic records and good communication skills. CIRHT introduced PAL as a part of curriculum implementation, choosing to pilot the program at Addis Ababa University. Challenges experienced by the implementation team included recruiting and

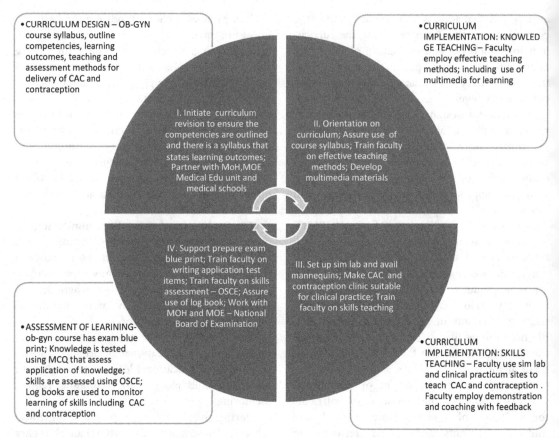

- CURRICULUM DESIGN – OB-GYN course syllabus, outline competencies, learning outcomes, teaching and assessment methods for delivery of CAC and contraception

- CURRICULUM IMPLEMENTATION: KNOWLEDGE TEACHING – Faculty employ effective teaching methods; including use of multimedia for learning

I. Initiate curriculum revision to ensure the competencies are outlined and there is a syllabus that states learning outcomes; Partner with MoH, MOE Medical Edu unit and medical schools

II. Orientation on curriculum; Assure use of course syllabus; Train faculty on effective teaching methods; Develop multimedia materials

IV. Support prepare exam blue print; Train faculty on writing application test items; Train faculty on skills assessment – OSCE; Assure use of log book; Work with MOH and MOE – National Board of Examination

III. Set up sim lab and avail mannequins; Make CAC and contraception clinic suitable for clinical practice; Train faculty on skills teaching

- ASSESSMENT OF LEARINING- ob-gyn course has exam blue print; Knowledge is tested using MCQ that assess application of knowledge; Skills are assessed using OSCE; Log books are used to monitor learning of skills including CAC and contraception

- CURRICULUM IMPLEMENTATION: SKILLS TEACHING – Faculty use sim lab and clinical practicum sites to teach CAC and contraception . Faculty employ demonstration and coaching with feedback

Figure 29.2 Model to assure competencies for CAC and contraception service delivery (the outcomes are listed in the rectangles and the activities are listed in the "pie" segments)

incentivizing mentors, as they are required to donate their free time to the program. One tactic used to recruit mentors was social media outreach, which was successful in spreading the word and raising interest. Both mentors and mentees reported positive experiences, strengthening knowledge on course subject matter and adjusting to university life.

Results: The first year of the program was spent on the preparation of the overall setup for the learning and teaching activities of the institutions using the reviewed curricula. As of the academic year of 2015/2016 (2008 Ethiopian academic year), all the partner medical schools that run undergraduate medical education and ob-gyn residency programs began implementing the new curricula, while that of the midwifery schools came to join a year later.

After the CIRHT intervention, ob-gyn and midwifery departments started using simulation to teach their students and assess skills learning through OSCE. Faculty not only have e-learning

resources they use for their flipped classroom but also developed the skills in producing e-learning materials.[1] They also recognized the need for locally produced videos for skills demonstration. CIRHT helped to develop seven audiovisual materials on CAC and contraception. An offline technology platform had been set up at all schools so that students could access e-learning materials on CAC and contraception, as well as other topics, without requiring internet connectivity. Approximately seventy student leaders were trained in PAL on how to coach their peers in taking responsibility for their learning.

---

[1] A flipped classroom is an instructional strategy and a type of blended learning where face-to-face interaction is mixed with independent study via technology. Students watch pre-recorded videos at home, then come to school to do the homework armed with questions and at least some background knowledge.

As an outcome of the program, all of the partner institutions have now technically equipped faculty and fully furnished and renovated skills labs. In addition, more than 4,500 medical and 1,480 midwifery students have managed to receive simulation-based and hands-on skill teachings. OSCE has become the primary method of skills assessment, and more than 2,100 medical and 500 midwifery students have been assessed using this standardized technique.

Although the CIRHT program targets competencies focused on abortion and contraception, the interventions had a broader positive effect and contributed to improving overall ob-gyn and midwifery teachings.

29.2.1.2 Description of the Framework on Clinical Services

Teaching hospitals in most developing and low-income countries are tertiary-level hospitals that are the only facilities able to manage complicated cases. They serve as referral centers where complex care is provided. Most of the time, such facilities have a shortage of rooms to care for the large number of routine cases, as they give priority to services that are not available in primary- or secondary-level health-care facilites. However, these facilities do not only provide patient services; they are also used as training centers for pre-service medical and other health science students. If a teaching hospital does not provide the services to be taught, faculties will not be kept abreast of the current evidence and students will lack adequate clinical exposure. As a result, students then graduate without the competencies they are expected to acquire.

This is especially true for family planning and abortion care services. As they are commonly provided at lower-level health-care facilities, even at the community level, teaching hospitals do not provide them, which in turn leads to lack of family planning and abortion competencies for graduating students.

In accordance with the findings of the CIRHT baseline assessment, hospitals designated for medical, midwifery and ob-gyn residency education in Ethiopia were not providing good-quality abortion and contraception services for a variety of reasons. Most faculty providers used to think that these services belong to lower-level facilities and not in tertiary care hospitals. As a result, the

teaching hospitals had given so little attention to the physical infrastructure needed for the two services that the CAC and contraception clinics, if at all available, were in shabby and hidden corners. Conversely, it was found that these hospitals had higher numbers of women presenting for deliveries. These women were also likely to seek postpartum contraception (PPC) care. However, because there were no active clinics in these hospitals to respond to the contraception demands, the women were referred elsewhere, leading to many missed opportunities for students and patients alike. Consequently, teaching about contraception remained largely theoretical and lacked hands-on practice in clinical settings. In addition, the students lacked exposure to those providers whom they could see as inspiring models of advocates and competent providers of abortion and contraception.

Considering all these prevailing facts, CIRHT introduced initiatives that improved the service quality and utilization of abortion and contraception services employing the interventions that follow.

Establishing a model reproductive health (RH) clinic: In order to improve the visibility and hence utilization of CAC and contraception services, teaching hospitals were supported to establish RH clinics that provide integrated services. Continuous dialogues with respective hospital administrations and MOH were conducted to find adequate spaces within the hospitals. New clinics were built or existing ones expanded and renovated to set up clinics conveniently named Michu clinics, which means "comfortable and friendly" in two of the commonly spoken languages. Faculty are assigned regularly in these clinics to provide the full range of abortion and contraception services, including dilation and evacuation (D&E) for second-trimester abortion and permanent methods of contraception. Medical interns and students, senior midwifery students and ob-gyn residents rotate working and learning in these clinics to boost the exposure of students to practical cases.

Quality improvement (QI) initiatives: Teaching hospitals were encouraged to introduce continuous RH QI initiatives. The initiatives are often implemented by a team led by the head of the ob-gyn departments and include at least two ob-gyn residents, nurses and midwives working in Michu clinics and labor wards. The team meets

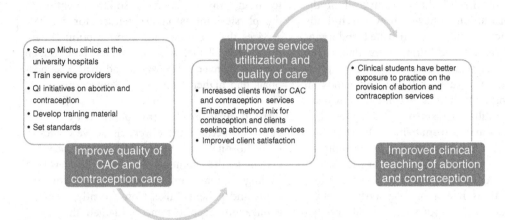

- Set up Michu clinics at the university hospitals
- Train service providers
- QI initiatives on abortion and contraception
- Develop training material
- Set standards

Improve quality of CAC and contraception care

Improve service utilitization and quality of care

- Increased clients flow for CAC and contraception services
- Enhanced method mix for contraception and clients seeking abortion care services
- Improved client satisfaction

- Clinical students have better exposure to practice on the provision of abortion and contraception services

Improved clinical teaching of abortion and contraception

Figure 29.3 Improving clinical services enhancing pre-service teaching of abortion and contraception

regularly, starting by assessing the quality of care at the respective institutions. Then members are supported in developing QI projects to improve the quality of services. This ensures collective work among faculty, residents, interns and midwives and helps them to get directly involved in improving the quality of RH services offered in Michu clinics. They work with other clinics in improvement collaborations, visit successful clinics for experience sharing, have ob-gyn residents present routine service data in their regular meetings and use data to monitor the progress of services (Figure 29.3). Faculty are often able bring about bold change ideas and thus become excellent role models to their students.

Results: Establishing Michu clinics in teaching hospitals after almost a year and six months since the launch of CIRHT in Ethiopia created a dramatic effect on the availability, uptake and quality of CAC and contraception services. CAC and contraception service utilization increased significantly, in most cases by 100%. The number of faculty supportive of CAC and contraception services increased dramatically due to CIRHT interventions. In the labor wards, PPC was provided across all partner schools. All sites had established QI teams, which guided QI projects to continuously improve CAC and contraception services. Several of these projects were connected to research and developed into reports or conference presentations.

As part of the service program, all new mothers were counseled on contraception options. Compared to the estimated national rates of PPC, the partner schools had a much higher rate of PPC. For all CAC and contraception services, it is important to note that none of the partner schools had quotas for uptake of specific services. Success was determined by access, availability and patient choice of CAC and contraception services by patients.

29.2.1.3 Description of the Framework on Research

Research support needs to start by exploring the status of research practice and its determinants. In order to design strategies to increase the practice of research, the faculty's lack of engagement in research needs to to be investigated as a part of the baseline assessment in order to improve CAC and contraception services and thus improve learning. The findings revealed that only a few clinicians in all partner institutions were ever engaged in research. Demands of clinical service, lack of research skills, poor inter- and intra-department collaboration, lack of funding and limited institutionalization of research were the common reasons cited for lack of research activities.

CIRHT created a research program aimed to strengthen and sustain a culture of research in reproductive health and build faculty research capacity in partner institutions by providing optimal research skills through a systematic and longitudinal approach. The overall approach was to focus on modeling a positive behavior, improving self-efficacy and social persuasion.

CIRHT created venues by inviting well-known clinicians who conducted research to share their experiences and challenge the prevailing belief that clinicians are too busy to do research.

A culture of developing research questions to generate evidence was initiated in the supported schools. Faculty were taught a systematic approach for conducting research by creating customized training schedules aimed to enable them to maneuver through the different stages of research.

The key principles that were followed include (Figure 29.4):

- Encourage on-site training: Because removing faculty and other health-care providers from their respective work stations creates service interruptions, all research-related trainings were done on site. The schedules were arranged with faculty convenience to minimize any service/teaching– learning disruptions.
- Team science: It was a requirement for a research team to have at least four members to be eligible for research support/grants by CIRHT. Meaningful engagement of investigators from different disciplines was actively encouraged to promote team-based research undertakings to overcome lack of collaboration.
- Convert all activities into learning opportunities: All the steps in research, including research topic selection, were converted into learning opportunities.
- Tapping into existing human resource: Faculty having research skills from the same institutions were made to engage.
- Mentoring: Content and method experts from the University of Michigan were assigned to mentor research teams.
- Tailor support: Customized supports to teams based on their needs and their pace were provided.
- Dissemination of research findings: Investigators who had their RH-related research papers accepted for oral and poster presentations were granted support to attend scientific forums.

Results: More than fifty proposals obtained from both ob-gyn and midwifery faculty that attempted to generate evidence to improve RH services were funded by CIRHT after rigorous review processes. While the ob-gyn research support has reached its goal, all of the midwifery research teams are at data analysis stage. Out of these supported research projects, many of them

were either presented in various international conferences or published in both local and international journals. CIRHT emphasized the need for keeping the momentum of inspired interests in research undertakings among faculty and worked hard from the outset to encourage and support institutions in having their own research and publications offices capable of competing and winning other grants.

29.2.1.4 Description of Monitoring and Evaluation of the Program

Having a simple and implementable monitoring and evaluation (M&E) strategy that adheres to site practicalities is crucial to continually improve program performance. For this reason, a comprehensive M&E strategy has been used during the course of the CIRHT program implementation. The CIRHT M&E strategy is designed to measure achievements systematically: to satisfy project information needs, to enable effective measurement of results, to prepare periodic reports and to allow analysis of why targets are or are not being achieved. This strategy details the various types and sources of data that will be collected and then used to evaluate measurable indicators. The M&E strategy elaborates a framework that comprises a range of indicators at various levels to measure, monitor and evaluate both implementation and outcomes of the CIRHT program in general. This framework is primarily based on the logical framework (LF) approach, with the idea that achieving specific results at different levels would lead to the desired impact.

Figure 29.5 depicts the logical sequence between inputs, outputs, outcomes and impact of CIRHT using LF, complemented by identification of data sources and interactive use of data through analysis and synthesis. This framework describes the components of CIRHT and the sequence of steps needed to achieve goals anticipated by CIRHT.

29.2.2 System-Strengthening Support

The CIRHT program in Ethiopia has not been operating in the conventional NGO fashion. It was specifically designed to work within the government system. It has been implemented under the aegis of the Ethiopian federal Ministry of Health through operational support of the St. Paul's Hospital Millennium Medical

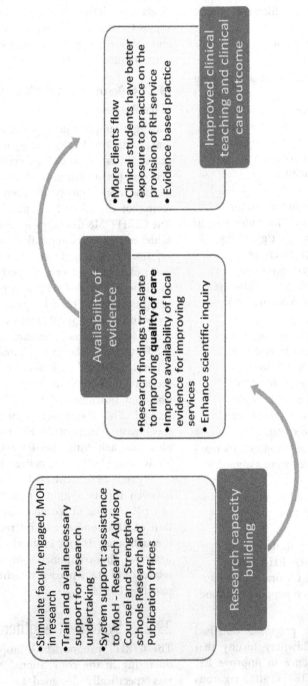

Figure 29.4 Improving faculty research undertaking, enhancing services and teachings of RH

- Stimulate faculty engaged, MOH in research
- Train and avail necessary support for research undertaking
- System support: asssistance to MoH – Research Advisory Counsel and Strengthen schools Research and Publication Offices

Research capacity building

Availability of evidence

- Research findings translate to improving **quality of care**
- Improve availability of local evidence for improving services
- Enhance scientific inquiry

- More clients flow
- Clinical students have better exposure to practice on the provision of RH service
- Evidence based practice

Improved clinical teaching and clinical care outcome

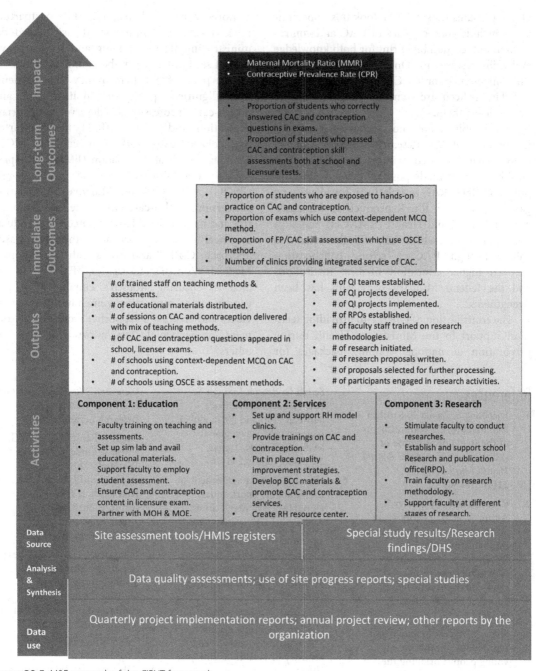

Figure 29.5 M&E approach of the CIRHT framework

College (SPHMMC). Furthermore, all planned activities were carried out onsite using the existing local operational structure and, in some instances, through a financial matching system. According to the results of the CIRHT program evaluation, this method and mechanism helped strengthen the existing government system in many ways and stimulate the institutions to

own all dimensions of the program in a sustainable manner.

CIRHT has provided continuous technical support to the Ministry of Health in the development of a licensure exam for medical graduates. It has supported the training of faculty representing most medical schools in writing context-dependent items, and developing and running

OSCE for skills tests. CIRHT took this opportunity to include competencies of CAC and contraception in the exam blueprint for both knowledge and skills assessment. Once students know that the competencies on CAC and contraception are tested in the licensure exam, they are likely motivated to learn them.

The establishment and continuous functioning of the National Research Advisory Council (RAC) that is based within the Ministry of Health has been made possible through the support of CIRHT. RAC is a platform for identifying gaps in evidence for Reproductive, Maternal, Neonatal and Child Health (RMNCH) and supporting research which help fill the identified gaps. Through RAC, a strong collaboration between higher education medical institutions and the federal Ministry of Health has been strengthened.

The contribution of CIRHT in providing technical support to the Ministry of Health during preparation of national training packages for comprehensive family planning (FP), postpartum FP and CAC was immense. It also helped the ministry initiate the training and service provision of second-trimester abortion using D&E.

As part of its firm policy that patients need dignified, quality and holistic care, and health-care professionals deserve appropriate protection and safety, CIRHT has supported the collaborative work between the MOH, Ethiopian Medical Association (EMA), Ethiopian Society of Obstetricians and Gynecologists (ESOG) and Ethiopian Midwives Association concerning health-care ethics, medical malpractice and medico-legal issues related to reproductive health services through the team-based approach. CIRHT also works with the Ethiopian Medical Women's Association (EMWA) in the area of ensuring women's empowerment and gender equity, supporting women health-care providers and creating a supportive working environment for women doctors, nurses, midwives and others.

References

1. Jejeebhoy S, Zavier F, Santhya KG. Meeting the commitments of the ICPD programme of action to young people. *Reprod Health Matters*. 2013; 21(41):18–30.

2. Chandra MV, Svanemyr J. Amim A, et al. Twenty years after International Conference on Polulation and Development: where are we with adolescent sexual and reproductive health rights? *J Adolesc Health*. 2015;56: S1–S6.

3. Shaw D. Access to sexual and reproductive health for young people: bridging the disconnect between rights and reality. *Int J Gynecol Obstet*. 2009;106: 132–136.

4. Grimes D, Benson J, Singh S, et al. Unsafe abortion: the preventable pandemic. *Lancet*. 2006;368:1908–1919.

5. Sedgh G, Bearak J, Singh S, et al., Abortion incidence between 1990 and 2014: global, regional, and sub-regional levels and trends. *Lancet*. 2016;388(10041):258–267.

6. Hilina B. Impact assessment of the Ethiopian abortion law. Unpublished master's thesis, Addis Ababa University; 2014.

7. *Technical and Procedural Guidelines for Safe Abortion Services*. Addis Ababa: Federal Ministry of Health of Ethiopia: 2006.

8. *Technical and Procedural Guidelines for Safe Abortion Services*. Addis Ababa: Federal Ministry of Health of Ethiopia; 2013.

9. Forum for African Women Educationalists. Female students in higher education institutions in Ethiopia: challenges and coping strategies. In *Strengthening Gender Research to Improve Girls' and Women's Education in Africa*. Nairobi: FAWE Research Series; 2010.

10. Singh S, Remez L, Sedgh G, Kwok L, Onda T. *Abortion Worldwide 2017: Uneven Progress and Unequal Access*. New York, NY: Guttmacher Institute; 2018. www .guttmacher.org/report/ abortion-worldwide-2017

11. Bongaarts J, Hardee K. The role of public-sector family planning programs in meeting the demand for contraception in sub-Saharan Africa. *Int Perspect Sex Reprod Health*. 2017;43(2): 41–50.

12. Gebremedhin LT, Nigatu B, Bekele D, Fisseha S. Gebremeskel BG. *Integrating Family Planning into Medical Education: A Case Study of St. Paul's Hospital Millennium Medical College (SPHMMC)*. Addis Ababa; 2016.

Chapter

30

Abortion Training and Integration into Clinical Practice in Colombia

Laura Gil, Oscar Marroquin and Maria Vivas

30.1 Global Perspectives of Legalization and Training

Chapter 30 outlines a case study of abortion training and integration into clinical practice in Colombia.

30.1.1 Historical Context of Abortion

In Colombia, abortion was completely banned until 2006, when the Constitutional Court partially legalized it [1]. This legalization was the result of forty years of work of several and diverse groups, feminist groups among them, who accomplished, through high-impact litigation, the decriminalization of abortion, enshrining it as a constitutional right, under the following circumstances: when the pregnancy poses a risk to a woman's health or life, is the product of sexual violence or there are fetal malformations incompatible with life.

Since then, Colombian policy has mandated the different actors in the health-care system to implement voluntary pregnancy termination (VPT) services throughout the country. Furthermore, the Constitutional Court has issued standards that require the different health institutions to offer services, and have available personnel resources. Such is the case of court sentence T-209/2008, in which it was determined that service provision institutions and the public network must guarantee an appropriate number of service providers [2]. Sentence T-388/2009 highlighted the importance of keeping patient confidentiality when providing voluntary termination of pregnancy services, and determined that women were entitled to ample and appropriate information in order to make the decision, and that all institutions must offer the service, even faith-based ones [3].

Regardless of the extensive legislation that aims to guarantee access to abortion services guaranteed by the state, only 11% of public and private institutions in the country have established abortion services or effective means to obtain an abortion [4]. Furthermore, the few services that are available are concentrated in the main cities, while the rest of the country faces geographic dispersion and low state supervision. In addition to this scenario, physicians, both general practitioners and specialists, who are the ones allowed to perform abortions by the regulation, are poorly prepared to face the complex aspects of delivering services. A study conducted by La Mesa por la Vida y la Salud de las Mujeres, demonstrated that several access barriers are imposed by the actual health-care system [5]. Specifically, health-care professionals including doctors, nurses and other support personnel, are unaware of the legal framework, such as the ruling that legalized abortion in Colombia, or later legislative developments. Professionals are not aware of the current regulations and impose unnecessary requirements on women, interpret legal exceptions in a restrictive fashion or obstruct services by claiming conscientious objection.

These circumstances are due, among other factors, to the lack of abortion training in medical schools. A review of the curricula of four medical schools in Bogotá, performed by the Andes University in conjunction with La Mesa por la Vida y la Salud de las Mujeres, found that education on abortion was not presented systematically. Only two of the reviewed schools gave students the opportunity to develop, albeit only partially and in a restrictive fashion, the necessary skills to perform a uterine evacuation to people who need a voluntary termination of pregnancy [6]. In two of the reviewed schools, students were found to have knowledge of sharp curettage, but not manual vacuum aspiration [6], which is the evidence-based method of choice for uterine evacuation. In Colombia, primary health care is provided by general practitioners who have complied with undergraduate training and a one-year internship program. Since abortion is partially decriminalized and included in the basic health plan covered by the social security system, abortion training should be part of medical programs. Nonetheless, universities are autonomous on whether or not include such content in their under- and post-graduate programs.

Thus, Colombian women, especially those particularly vulnerable as a result of poverty, illiteracy, ethnic minorities or residing in rural areas, still face multiple barriers and greater restrictions to safe services, some of those imposed by the health-care system. Furthermore, there is lack of acknowledgment of their rights, such as their rights to privacy, to dignity, to truthful, impartial and appropriate information for timely diagnosis and treatment, and to self-determination.

It is in this scenario of limited systems and human resources that Oriéntame, since its inception in 1977, has led the training, mainly of general practitioners on comprehensive management of unwanted pregnancy, which now also includes medical students. Originally, Oriéntame's own personnel, upon starting their employment, received training to develop specific skills related to the provision of abortion services. The uterine evacuation techniques used in the clinic when it first started were focused on the treatment of incomplete abortion and post-abortion care. After 2006, the clinic broadened its services to include voluntary terminations of pregnancy. Currently, the vast majority of abortions performed in Oriéntame happen because of the risk they pose to women's mental health due to an unwanted pregnancy. In order to ensure high-quality services, Oriéntame´s training prepares health-care professionals, including physicians, nurses and counsellors, to provide comprehensive abortion services in a setting that minimizes access barriers, in a low complexity primary care center.

Since the legalization of abortion, Oriéntame, in conjunction with the Ministry of Health (MOH), the office of the Government of Cundinamarca and the United Nations Population Fund (UNFPA), among others, has provided training services for health-care professionals in the public sector, which has contributed to the destigmatization of abortion services and a better understanding of the comprehensive management of unwanted pregnancy. However, the impact of this activity has been limited, since it is carried out within the scope of specifically funded projects, and thus limited by funding opportunities. Also, many of the trained providers are not in decision-making positions. When they return to their institutions, they are often unable to implement their abortion skills and knowledge.

To counteract the lack of education in medical schools, Oriéntame has been a practice facility for the Andes University School of Medicine since 2018. Students enrolled in the Public Health semester can opt for a six-week elective rotation, during which they are taught public health aspects of abortion and can observe counselling sessions and medical consultations.

These diverse training activities with diverse audiences has led Oriéntame to design a training model that adapts to Colombia's cultural context and its legal framework, increasing the odds that abortion services are actually provided and thus resulting in improved access to safe and legal abortion for Colombian women.

30.1.2 Initial Steps: Identifying Needs and Defining Content

Up to the time when abortion was partially decriminalized, all health-care professionals had been trained and had practiced under an absolute abortion ban; therefore, capacity building was pivotal to ensure the implementation of the new law. Three decades of work in the provision of high-quality sexual and reproductive health services within a comprehensive care model and a human rights framework ultimately led Oriéntame, at the time of the decriminalization, to play a key role for the implementation of legal abortion services in Colombia. Oriéntame's expertise was drawn from two perspectives: (1) as a service provider, Oriéntame normalized access to legal abortion by correctly interpreting the new law and ensuring services to women who are legally entitled to a lawful abortion under the health exception, specifically, by providing access to women with unwanted pregnancies who, by definition, face a risk to their health if they continue their pregnancies to term. And (2) as an academic authority, with the necessary experience to train health-care professionals in order to expand the provision of legal abortion beyond

Oriéntame and throughout the country, including the public health system.

30.1.2.1 The Oriéntame Approach to Training

Oriéntame's model of care was originally inspired by its founder, Dr. Jorge Villereal, who in turn was inspired by the outpatient service model of a group of abortion clinics in the USA after that country legalized abortion. To ensure the implementation of its model, Oriéntame has always trained its own team in intrauterine manual vacuum aspiration technique (MVA) – a method that practitioners are generally not familiar with, since sharp curettage is the most common practice despite its obsolescence, misoprostol prescription for medication abortion and its own counseling model. However, this training was always directed toward professionals willing to work at the clinic, and thus, sensitive to women's rights and abortion care.

In order to guarantee the implementation of services in a country with a strong Catholic base and high levels of stigma toward abortion, we needed to design a program that would provide the necessary technical knowledge, as well as address personal aspects that could interfere with the trainees' decision to provide, or refer women to, safe abortion services. Oriéntame's approach also sought to respond to the multiple access barriers that quickly arose in the early years after the partial legalization of abortion and to develop specific strategies on how to overcome them.

From very early on, Oriéntame has recognized the importance of having a multidisciplinary team. Both the team of trainers and the teams to be trained were composed of physicians, nurses and psychologists or social workers, so they would be prepared to reproduce this model of care at home with its multiple roles. The inclusion, since the decriminalization of abortion by the Constitutional Court, of general practitioners as main providers of abortion services was an important step to ensure access to services. The traditional view was that only the obstetrician-gynecologist (ob-gyn) specialists should be providers, a perception that would potentially limit access, especially in remote areas with few specialized professionals.

The second element of our training program was the conceptualization of abortion access from perspectives different from the traditionally moral or religious stands. Specifically, there was the need to raise awareness of the importance of access to safe abortion as a guarantee of basic human rights, as well as a medical act aligned with bioethical principles, and finally, abortion as a public health issue. These perspectives allowed and promoted personal reflection on the provision of services for reasons of conscience, as opposed to conscientious objection. Conscientious objection as a practice constitutes an access barrier when inappropriately exercised as a form of obstruction and the unjustified denial of services, causing dire consequences to women.

Personal reflection around these objective factors, however, is not always enough when trainees are faced with moral and religious principles and even cultural practices opposed to abortion. A third and crucial factor in our training program was to include a value-clarification process with standardized exercises, both individual and in groups, that allow the exploration of each trainee's feelings and ideas about abortion. These exercises allow individuals to express themselves in a nonjudgmental space, where all opinions are heard and valued, but also where the individual decision to have an abortion is acknowledged as worthy of respect and as the result of an exercise of conscience from each woman.

Finally, before proceeding to the clinical aspects, it was pivotal to provide trainees with arguments that allow them a liberal, legally correct interpretation of the exceptions for legal abortion. We use a comprehensive conceptualization of health and risk in accordance with the constitutional court ruling. This aspect of training prepares participants to apply the law in its full scope, allowing wide access to women in need of safe abortion and challenging the initial, restrictive interpretation that became one of the largest access barriers along with the misuse of conscientious objection.

Implementing this process of sensitization, together with the analysis of real and representative cases from the day-to-day operation of our clinic, and of cases that have set a legal precedent in our country, has been a successful strategy that allows trainees to reflect on the human and practical aspects of abortion, formerly eclipsed by prejudice and stereotypes. The time and effort invested in exploring each person's believes and points of view regarding abortion in a practical, experiential and interactive manner prior to the technical training have been shown to be of important value: this leads to openness of perspective and a much greater level of commitment compared to simply focusing on clinical and technical skills. The impact is evident in the change in attitudes and the diminishing levels of resistance that we observe among the groups throughout training each time we develop our program.

The technical content of the training follows a chronological sequence according to Oriéntame's model of care and comprises two main aspects of counseling and provision of the abortion itself.

The distinctive element of the counseling model developed by Oriéntame is its comprehensive focus. Far from being limited to simply providing information, but without becoming a therapeutic intervention, Oriéntame's woman-centered counseling model is a process of accompaniment based on communication and a structured reflection that involves the decision-making process, the concept of abortion as a right and the identification of special needs such as existing conflicts or possible emotional impacts that may require additional support or follow-up.

One of the main objectives of the training process in this regard is to deconstruct mistaken conceptions of abortion as a necessarily traumatic event, or about the need to question or argue against the decision. The training seeks to offer a simple and practical approach to support women through the process of abortion.

The training on the procedure to evacuate the uterus is based on the MVA technique, as well as the use of misoprostol and mifepristone. The need to employ models to teach MVA led us to look for practical and economic alternatives, realistic enough to show the trainees its ease of use and develop a certain level of confidence and skill in preparation for the actual procedure. In this search, we changed from the traditional pelvic model to fruit models. We found a particularly useful fruit, *pitayas*, also known as dragon fruit. This fruit is similar in size, consistency and shape to a first-trimester gravid uterus and allows simulating cervical fixation with a tenaculum, paracervical block, cervical dilation and aspiration of the cavity's content, reproducing the typical sensation of a complete evacuation. The training program in completed with post-abortion contraceptive counseling, and biosecurity, including appropriate sterilization of surgical instruments and infection prevention (Figure 30.1).

This content has been developed with an overall emphasis on the need to implement all of its components at the primary care level, challenging the mistaken and generalized conception that care must be centralized in highly specialized hospitals. Such views provide a false sense of security but in practice can become another access barrier.

In summary, the initial design of our training program for health-care professionals other than those working at Oriéntame was aimed at addressing and overcoming the most common access barriers. Those barriers were not simply limited to lack of technical skills, but encompassed social and personal aspects, such as the misuse of conscientious objection, stigmatization, discriminatory practices based on gender and even harmful medical practices rooted in years of witnessing the consequences of unsafe abortion, which resulted in the hyper-medicalization and treatment of abortion as a complex condition requiring care at tertiary hospitals and ob-gyn specialists.

In this sense, the objective was to create scenarios of sensitization and to provide training on basic theoretical and practical aspects. These first training experiences for health-care professional were carried out through programs organized by the MOH. Their aim was to bring together medical, nursing and psychology professionals from different areas of the country to the main cities to create teams that would implement an effective abortion service in the public institutions where they worked. However, even though important changes in perspective and attitudes about abortion took place, when these professionals returned home, they found resistance, stigmatization and accusations that prevented them from starting to work and develop effective care.

30.1.3 Lessons Learned along the Way: Evolving in Order to Achieve a True Impact

It is important to emphasize that regardless of the challenges faced, the first efforts bore fruit in that a critical mass of professionals became sensitized and motivated to provide abortion services. These efforts probably impacted the beginning of service provision, especially in larger cities, but they also demonstrated the need to develop a strategy that would incorporate operative, management and logistical elements to ensure the consistent

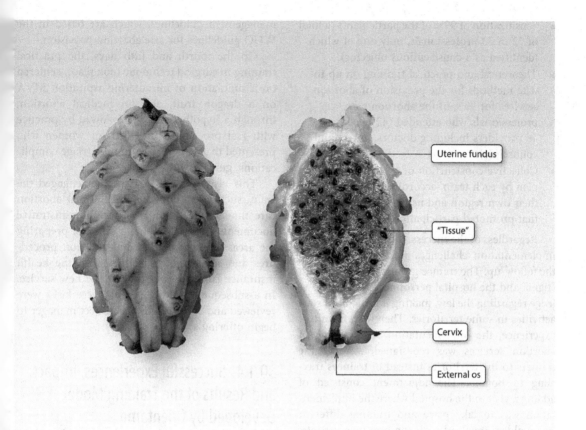

Figure 30.1 Biological model for MVA training with pitaya fruit

implementation of services and their growth in more remote regions.

The agreements between the Oriéntame Foundation, the MOH, and UNFPA, as well as with other nongovernmental organizations (NGOs), have played a fundamental role in supporting the implementation of abortion services in public institutions throughout the country.

In 2016, the Oriéntame Foundation, the MOH and UNFPA celebrated an agreement entitled "Incorporation and Operative Experiences of Practical Training Processes for the Implementation of Safe and Low Complexity VTP-Abortion Services (*Experiencias de incorporación y operatividad de procesos de entrenamiento práctico, para la implementación de servicios de IVE-aborto seguro en la baja complejidad*)." This project aimed at strengthening the technical institutional capacity for planning, managing, operating, and providing abortion services in fifteen low-complexity hospitals in the most vulnerable regions of the country. A total

of seventy-three professionals were summoned to Bogotá and organized into regional teams of five or six clinical and administrative workers to receive theoretical training on the legal, legislative, technical and ethical aspects of abortion in Colombia. They received practical training on evidence-based abortion techniques and service provision in accordance with the WHO Safe Abortion guideline [7] and the MOH guideline "Comprehensive Voluntary Termination of Pregnancy Care in Low Complexity Level Health Facilities" [8], developed in collaboration with Oriéntame.

As an innovative factor in comparison with past training initiatives, this agreement included an in situ follow-up component that would let us measure the progress of service implementation. Results showed that between 50 and 70% of the tasks to establish an abortion service were carried out in four hospitals, and over 70% in six of the fifteen facilities observed. The three most important achievements were the following:

- Sensitization of 99% of the participants (a total of 72 of 73 professionals, only one of which identified as a conscientious objector).
- Theoretical and practical training on up-to-date methods for the provision of abortion services for 93% of the abortion care professionals who attended (42 of 46 providers including doctors, nurses and counselors).
- Collective construction of an implementation plan by each team, according to the needs of their own region and using a methodology that promoted participation.

Regardless of the success, some difficulties and implementation challenges were evident during the follow-up. The trainee groups were faced with stigma and the hospital personnel's lack of knowledge regarding the law, making it difficult to start activities in some territories. Therefore, from this experience, the implementation and training of abortion services was redesigned, sending the trainers to the territories instead of trainees traveling to Bogotá. The adjustment consisted of adding a visit to the hospital where the implementation was to take place and training different stakeholders involved with the health-care route. In this manner, the aim was to have the training of multidisciplinary teams result in provision of services and not just the health personnel becoming familiarized with the issues surrounding unwanted pregnancy.

30.1.3.1 New Model of Training Executed in Four Phases

On the first day of training, all of the workers from clinical and administrative areas were included, regardless of whether they were in agreement or were going to be involved with providing abortion services. This initial activity was very important: it communicated to the staff the institution's commitment to abide by the law by opening a sexual and reproductive health service for women. Topics discussed included the Constitutional Court ruling and the regulation on abortion, statistics of unsafe abortion both globally and locally, conscientious objection and a special emphasis on the legal exceptions for health and life.

On the second and third days, the future institutional team that was to be part of the abortion services received theoretical training on the MOH management guidelines, which are based in the WHO guidelines for safe abortion provision.

On the fourth and fifth days, the practical training in surgical technique took place, centered on a simulation of intrauterine aspiration MVA on a dragon fruit, and on medical abortion, through a hypothetical case, followed by practice with real procedures provided for women who presented that same day with miscarriage complications, guided by the trainer.

This visit resulted in tasks that engaged the team, such as building an institutional abortion care model, generating necessary administrative documents to start providing services, preparing the areas for consultation and abortion procedures and/or planning meetings with the health insurance companies to present the new service. In a subsequent follow-up visit, these tasks were reviewed and approved by the project manager to begin offering services.

30.1.4 Successful Experiences, Impact and Results of the Training Model Developed by Oriéntame

In 2017 the Oriéntame Foundation made an agreement with the Latin American Consortium against Unsafe Abortion (CLACAI) called "Actions for the Improvement of Access to Voluntary Termination of Pregnancy (VTP) Services with an Emphasis on the Public Offer (*Acciones de mejora en el acceso a los servicios de Interrupción Voluntaria del Embarazo (IVE) con énfasis en la oferta pública*)." Following the new methodology and thanks to the exercise that had been carried out in 2016, two health-care centers of first level of complexity, the Hospital of Villavicencio and the Maternity of Soledad in the Caribbean region, were proposed as beneficiaries, given their low implementation level of services and the potential for advancing in the provision of abortion services.

Through this new initiative, a total of seventy-seven workers from both institutions were trained together with twenty professionals from clinical and administrative areas, including doctors, nurses and psychosocial support personnel. Teams of ten people each were grouped in each hospital to provide services. Thanks to the new methodology, service plan implementation increased from 50% in 2016 to 80% in 2017.

Currently, both public institutions provide medical abortion up to ten weeks, certify the health risks to women according to the legal exceptions and no longer pose access barriers, referring patients to comprehensive care, validating women's sexual and reproductive rights and recognizing them as human rights.

Thanks to the success of this agreement, two equally ambitious projects were undertaken in 2018. The first agreement was carried out in partnership with CLACAI, titled "Local Development and Implementation of Actions to Increase Access to Safe Abortion Services through the Legal Exceptions (*Desarrollo e implementación local de acciones para incrementar el acceso al aborto seguro a través de las causales de aborto legal).*" Its main goals were to increase sexual and reproductive health and rights (SRHR) knowledge at the local Hospital of Puerto Asís, Putumayo, and to strengthen the team of professionals caring for women who requested legal abortion services. For this new plan, the innovative strategy Information-Education-Communication (IEC)[1] was introduced to inform people in rural areas about the service, mainly indigenous and afrodescendant populations. A total of ninety-eight employees of the institution were trained along with fourteen service professionals, including health-care promoters who provided service information to the population, using promotional pieces financed by the project. As with the previous project, follow-up activities were carried out, verifying the successful implementation of the abortion service with remarkable institutional support, and promoting the service among the different health insurance companies covering the area. The project successfully started an integrated abortion service up to the fifteenth week of gestation in the municipality of Puerto Asís.

The second agreement was planned in conjunction with UNFPA to fulfill the need of strengthening and adjusting the abortion service in the Erasmo Meoz Teaching Hospital in Cúcuta, near the border with Venezuela. This specific city required an appropriately implemented service to respond to the humanitarian crisis, particularly the migration of the Venezuelan population into the country, and the high numbers of women with unwanted pregnancies who requested an abortion.

Although a previous training program had taken place, there were shortcomings subsequent to the training that prevented the full implementation of services. For example, some physicians wrongfully exercised conscientious objection in specific cases, only willing to perform procedures in cases of fetal malformation, which is in opposition to the constitutional mandate. In addition, we found a poor support network for patients in economic hardship as well as dehumanizing treatment, myths surrounding abortion and poor service promotion among stakeholders.

Oriéntame's training program was developed in three phases: first, assessment of the current level of participation of abortion services in the hospital; second, technical assistance to define and structure service delivery procedures; and third, monitoring and adjustment of service implementation.

We informed and sensitized forty-two clinical and administrative professionals, and trained eighteen professionals, including gynecologists, general practitioners, registered nurses and scrub nurses in modern abortion techniques (medication and surgical management), and supervised the provision of five MVA procedures. The existing route of care was modified, thus eliminating access barriers. Oriéntame demonstrated the importance of broadly interpreting the law to certify the risk to a woman's health, as well as the requirement of including it in the clinical records. Finally, the hospital's official document establishing the abortion service program was drafted, and the objecting and non-objecting professionals were identified.

Oriétame's training and follow-up experiences have been successfully translated to several countries in Latin America through its international program. Its aims are to meet the need for engaged and committed health-care providers, educating them about interpreting the law to its fullest extent, normalizing legal abortion and providing the best possible access to safe and legal abortion and post-abortion services among their communities.

---

[1] The IEC strategy's goal is to strengthen health promotion actions. The program generates a permanent information, education and communication campaign and at the same time formulates training strategies for health service professionals so they can refer and provide services to the population.

30.2 Conclusions

In many cases, after the liberalization of abortion, the health-care sector, far from guaranteeing women's rights to safe abortion, imposes access barriers to abortion services for a variety of reasons, which include not only lack of technical skills or knowledge, but also incomplete or misinformation about current laws, and the stigmatization of women seeking abortion. Recognizing these barriers over the years, Oriéntame has developed and updated its training model, initially meant for Oriéntame's personnel for the comprehensive management of unwanted pregnancy and incomplete abortion. Since 2006, when the partial legalization took place, the training model has been adapted to include voluntary termination of pregnancy services, expanding trainees beyond those who work at our clinics and including the personnel involved in service provision, even if not directly.

Our experience has shown that for the training of health-care professionals to translate into service provision, it is necessary to include a multidisciplinary team, perform values clarification, transmit a broad understanding of the legal exceptions and include logistical and administrative aspects of service provision, all within a human rights framework. It is in this context that technical skills and knowledge have meaning. Oriéntame's experience has demonstrated the need to adjust its training program to fit local health-care systems as well as to include all personnel involved. Monitoring and follow-up visits are also fundamental to measure and ensure implementation progress – all within the need of providing low-complexity services at the primary level of care.

Through collaborations with other institutions with the political commitment to ensure access to abortion care, Oriéntame has transformed the simple transmission of knowledge through training into a strategy for the normalization of abortion, the implementation of service provision and collaboration among health-care institutions.

References

1. Colombia Corte Constitucional, Sentencia C355–2006. Corte Consitucional Colombiana; 2006.

2. Colombia Corte Constitucional, *Sentencia T209–2008.* Corte Consitucional Colombiana; 2008.

3. Colombia Corte Constitucional, *Sentencia T388–2009.* Corte Consitucional Colombiana; 2009.

4. Prada E, Singh S, Remez L, Villarreal C. *Embarazo no deseado y aborto inducido en Colombia: causas y consecuencias.* New York: Guttmacher Institute. 2008. www.orientame.org.co/wp-content/files_mf/1418177246embarazon odeseadocolombia_2011.pdf

5. La Mesa por la Vida y la Salud de las Mujeres. *Barreras de acceso a la interrupción voluntaria del embarazo en Colombia;* 2017.

6. Hernández Flórez LJ, et al. *Revisión del plan curricular, los micro currículos, estrategias pedagógicas, y desarrollo de competencias en interrupción voluntaria del embarazo (IVE) de algunas facultades de medicina;* 2017.

7. WHO. *Aborto sin riesgo: guía técnica y de políticas para sistemas de salud.* 2nd ed. Geneva: WHO; 2012.

8. Ministerio de Salud y Protección Social and Fondo de Población de las Naciones Unidas. *Atención Integral a la Interrupción Voluntaria del Embarazo (IVE) en el primer nivel de complejidad: Documento técnico para prestadores de servicios de salud;* 2014.

Chapter

31

Medical Education in Sexual and Reproductive Health in Uruguay

Verónica Fiol, Maria Nozar and Leonel Briozzo

31.1 Establishing Integrated Training to Comply with the Law and Professional Mandates and to Ensure High-Quality, Evidence-Based Care

We begin this chapter with an overview of the elements needed to establish integrated training in abortion care in Uruguay. Uruguay has a unique abortion history because safe abortion care was initiated by asserting physicians' –specifically obstetrician-gynecologists' (ob-gyns') – professional obligations for mitigating risks to their patients. We will first describe the evolution of the legal framework on sexual and reproductive health, the history of training and how abortion care is provided in Uruguay. We then describe the role of community partners in establishing training, specifically the role of nongovernmental organizational (NGO) health intiatives. We close this section by describing the basic structures of training to care for women with unwanted pregnancy.

31.1.1 Legal Status of aBortion in Uruguay: Evolution of the Legal Framework on Sexual and Reproductive Health

Abortion has been legal in Uruguay since November 2012, during the first twelve weeks of pregnancy if that is the woman's wish [1] and during the first fourteen weeks if the pregnancy is the outcome of an officially reported rape. There are also exceptions to the law: situations of serious danger to the woman's life or health, and in case of fetal malformations incompatible with extrauterine life, with no gestational limit.

This legal change of 2012 was preceded by the development and implementation in the country of a risk reduction model on unsafe abortion. In

2001, a new NGO, Iniciativas Sanitarias (IS, Health Initiatives), designed an intervention program to decrease the incidence of unsafe abortion, and thus maternal morbidity and mortality from unsafe abortion [2,3]. The model was based on the conviction that even when health professionals are legally restricted from performing abortion, they have a duty to provide women who want to terminate a pregnancy with appropriate counseling and care both before and after a clandestine abortion.

To analyze the evolution of the legal framework and public policies in sexual reproductive health (SRH) in our country, we have defined three separate historical periods [4]: 1990–2001, 2001–2012 and 2012–2019.

31.1.1.1 1990–2001

During this period, abortion was illegal. The relevant legislation in force at that time was law 9763 dating back to 1938, which cites three grounds for exemption, none of which physicians complied with [5]. The unethical behavior of denouncing women seeking help for an incomplete abortion was common and prevented such women from seeking help. During that time, contraceptive methods were not universally available. In addition, medical education policies did not systematically include subjects related to SRH and women's rights. During those years, most maternal deaths in Uruguay resulted from unsafe, clandestine abortions [6].

31.1.1.2 2001–2012

This period is marked by the development and progressive implementation of the model for reducing the risk and harm of unsafe abortions called "Health Initiatives against Unsafe Abortion" [2,7]. The model was successfully put into practice with the support of the International Federation of Gynecology and Obstetrics (FIGO) as well as other national and international partners [8]. The program was based on the ethical responsibilities of medical professionalism [9], the basis and foundation of the Conscientious Commitment to Women's Health [10] that later led to implementation of the law decriminalizing abortion in 2012. During this period, in 2008, law 18.426 [11] on the Defense of Sexual and Reproductive Health was passed. This law constitutes an important milestone in SRH legislation, as it determines that the benefits of SRH are available to all, for example, contraception and approval of the risk and harm reduction model due to unsafe abortion in situations of unwanted pregnancy.

31.1.1.3 2012–2019

This period is characterized by the implementation of the law decriminalizing abortion established in November 2012. This extremely complex legislation was the result of intense political negotiation at the parliamentary level. Its principal characteristics are as follows:

- Voluntary termination of pregnancy (VTP) is no longer against the law under the following conditions: if the woman is a Uruguayan citizen and gestational age is no more than twelve full weeks or fourteen full weeks in cases of rape.
- The institutions belonging to the Uruguayan National Integrated Health System are responsible for implementing VTP services. Private, for-profit practice is not permitted in cases of VTP.
- A multidisciplinary consultancy team (composed of three members: a gynecologist, a professional in the area of mental health and another in social work) was mandatorily established by law to examine the medical and social aspects and advise women, with no decision power over women.
- An obligatory reflection time of five days was established between consultation with the health-care team and the pregnancy termination.
- Medical abortion (mifepristone and misoprostol) is established by the Ministry of Health as the procedure of choice for performing VTP within the framework of the law [12,13].
- The law recognizes the right to conscientious objection – although the concept is unclear – for both individual clinicians and for institutions linked to the Roman Catholic Church and other religions.

31.1.2 The History of Abortion Training in Uruguay

Uruguay's School of Medicine had long been a barrier to the development of a new sexual and reproductive rights agenda for residents and medical students. Our team, involved in the Medical School of the University of the Republic since the 1990s, needed to develop partnerships to promote a training curriculum in SRH. This was the only Public School of Medicine in Uruguay, until the creation in 2006 of the CLAEH University School of Medicine. This private university has a Doctor of Medicine degree but no post-graduate gynecology degree. As a result, a new integrated NGO for health professionals, Iniciativas Sanitarias (IS, Health Initiatives), was established in 2001, in conjunction with the association of midwives and other health professionals that began to bring together professionals committed to sexual and reproductive rights.

The Faculty of Medicine, the Gynecological Society and the NGO IS created a proposal for the implementation of the risk reduction model, which included an awareness and training curriculum for members of the health team. The first curriculum of professionalism committed to sexual and reproductive rights was developed. The first institution to support the implementation was the United Nations Population Fund in 2005. In 2006. funding was obtained from FIGO's initiative "Save Mothers and Newborns" to disseminate this model throughout the country.

By 2010, with the change in the directorate and head professor of the Gynecological Clinic A, the formal development of a university curriculum in SRH began.

31.1.3 Clinical Services and Training in the Teaching Hospital

The university training in SRH, both for medical students and post-graduate students in ob-gyn, covers three gynecological clinics (the equivalent of departments in other countries) of the School of Medicine of the University of the Republic (Clinics A, B and C). Our team is part of the

Gynecological Clinic A (GCA), located at the Pereira Rossell Hospital, which is responsible for training medical students and their dependent ob-gyn residents in SRH, contraception and abortion.

Post-graduate training in ob-gyn is carried out under the Medical Residencies regime. The Residency in Gynecology and Obstetrics is supervised by the Technical Commission of Hospital Medical Residencies, composed of two medical representatives of the Ministry of Health and three medical representatives of the University of the Republic, and is within the Faculty of Medicine. The Graduate School of the Faculty of Medicine is responsible for setting academic standards for training.

The Residency in Gynecology and Obstetrics is for a period of three years. To obtain the title of Specialist in Gynecology and Obstetrics, these three years must be satisfactorily completed and other academic requirements must be met (the completion of three scientific papers and passing a final test).

Residents can carry out their care practice in one of two hospitals where the clinics are located (Clinics Hospital and Pereira Rossell Hospital) or in the Associated Teaching Centers, public or private health centers, of Montevideo and the interior of the country. These centers must have previously completed the accreditation process at the Graduate School and must be associated with one of the Clinics.

31.1.4 Collaborations with Community Partners and Academic Community: Role of the NGO Health Initiatives

In the period 2001–2012, prior to the implementation of the VTP law, IS became one of the pillars in the dissemination and training in the model of reduction of harm caused by unsafe abortion. IS worked jointly with the Faculty of Medicine, the Gynecology Society of Uruguay and the Ministry of Health in the training of professionals and health teams.

To respond to changes in the legislation after the adoption of the VTP act, in 2012, IS designed a training plan for health professionals, which was presented to the Ministry of Health within the framework of a cooperation agreement to favor the implementation of the law.

The objectives of training included the following:

- Train the health teams and management teams of each health institution to act as a reference and develop an implementation plan for the VTP law.
- Train the SRH health teams around the country to proceed according to the guidelines in the technical guidance of the VTP law.
- Promote the participation of patients in the assessment of the quality of SRH services and adapt the characteristics of the services to their needs in real time through the dissemination of the VTP law.

Training includes the following: legal national framework; clinical care process; medical care; and institutional algorithms (critical path). This implies the recognition of the medical care steps in the VTP process, and the resources implemented by the health institutions to be able to comply with the clinical care process requirements: ministerial and institutional responsibilities; conscientious objection and ideology objection; methods for VTP; clinical implementation; medical records; confidentiality.

31.1.5 Training Methods

Training includes awareness workshops and clinical skills training courses. The workshops are aimed at all members of the Health Centers (medical professionals, non-medical professionals and service personnel) and aim to sensitize all workers of the Health Center regarding the reality of women with unwanted pregnancy. The courses are aimed at medical and non-medical health professionals who are directly involved in assisting women with an unwanted pregnancy: gynecologists, midwives, family doctors, psychologists, social workers and nurses.

Finally, there are also working days with patient organizations/user organizations: these are groups of patients/users of the health system that organize themselves to influence and improve the quality of care of the institutions.

In the period 2012–2018, a total of nineteen training courses were carried out by the Health Initiatives Training Center, both in Montevideo and in the interior of the country. A total of 1,260 professionals participated, including gynecologists, family doctors, midwives, psychologists and social workers.

These training activities are repeated regularly in Montevideo and the interior of the country based on the needs of the health teams and the Ministry of Health.

31.2 Designing and Implementing a Clinical Curriculum for Post-graduate Training Programs: Training Curriculum in Sexual and Reproductive Health

Training in sexual and reproductive health during the residency in ob-gyn depends on each of the three Gynecological Clinics (Departments). There is a training curriculum in gynecology common to the three Clinics, approved by the Graduate School of the Faculty of Medicine, but dates to 2003, and does not have specific training in SRH. The Gynecological Clinics have updated their training programs in recent years independently, having unevenly included different aspects of SRH.

In this section, we present the experience in training in SRH of Gynecological Clinic A (GCA), our gynecology department. Training in SRH is carried out as an integrated part of the Post-graduate Program on Obstetrics and Gynecology of the Gynecological Clinic A [14].

In this program, the profile of the gynecologist graduated from the GCA is outlined: "The gyne-cologist must be a competent specialist, capable of assuming the role of director in health care as well as consultant of the specialty with other specialties and professions. He is, conceptually, the woman's doctor at all stages of life."

31.2.1 Training Requirements for Obstetrician-Gynecologists

To be a specialist, the resident must demonstrate knowledge, skills and attitudes that enable him/her to adhere to the graduate profile of the GCA. Within these, we highlight some that are directly related to training in SRH:

- Ability to develop clinical skills to function independently in the emergency room setting and in the polyclinic, and with the ability to integrate health teams at all levels of care.

- Develop a vision of integrated bio-, psycho-, and social health, which addresses the main social determinants of health, with a gender perspective, in the defense and promotion of human rights and specifically of sexual and reproductive rights.

- Adhere to professional values, bioethics and confidentiality.

- Know and interpret health policies related to the specialty. Act competently in the health-care system, using resources responsibly and promoting health as a collective good.

The four training activities include the following:

1. Internship for SRH services. Residents are trained in the comprehensive consultation for unwanted pregnancy and VTP and experience with multidisciplinary teams. They become competent in the legal and technical aspects of VTP, incorporating the VTP consultation as another element of women's health.

2. Assistance to women seeking VTP during hospitalization. Residents must handle all technical aspects of VTP, medication abortion and electric vacuum uterine aspiration, as well as the resolution of complex medical and psychosocial presentations.

3. Mandatory attendance and submission of clinical cases and reviews in monthly SRH video conferences transmitted to all the centers associated with the GCA.

4. Of the three required scientific papers for graduation, one must be on an SRH topic.

31.2.2 Assessing Competence in SRH and Family Planning Skills through Milestones

The acquisition of knowledge, skills and attitudes must be achieved in the context of a necessary balance between learning by doing and reflecting on what has been learned. Social, cultural, legislative and health changes strongly impact training plans. For example, the legal change in relation to abortion generated the need for training in aspects of VTP. The emergence of gender-based violence in the country as a public health problem also determined the need to train health teams in the detection and timely management of these situations.

As a result of the process of decentralization of the teaching of post-graduate gynecology, the training is carried out in different health-care centers, as well as in different scenarios and medical care areas. For example, in the past the resident's training was almost exclusively in university hospitals in Montevideo. There was no training at the first level of attention or inside the country. Currently, the residency takes place in Montevideo and the interior of the country, at public and private health facilities in areas of hospitalization, emergency and primary care. Unified training criteria serve as a guide for both the student and the teachers and faculty in charge to guide and ensure the training to competence.

The acquisition of knowledge and hands-on practice is not always an orderly, sequential process. Adding SRH to the different care levels and training scenarios requires standardization to define what is expected in each year of postgraduate training in each area of the specialty and at each stage.

Competence is described in levels of autonomy that must be reached in each clinical event. These levels of autonomy are also intended to define the responsibilities that post-graduates *can* and *cannot* assume at each moment and level of training.

For this purpose, we define autonomy as the ability to act according to one's own professional judgment, regardless of the opinion or desire of others. These levels of autonomy include the following:

Level 1: The resident must be able to apply the skills acquired independently, without direct supervision, although always with the availabilty of faculty backup.
Level 2: The resident, although he/she has the right knowledge, has not yet developed enough experience to practice independently, needing supervision.
Level 3: The resident has knowledge, has seen, has participated in certain medical acts, but has no experience of his/her own. This corresponds to activities observed or assisted by the graduate while they are developed by the specialist.

In the area of SRH, the learning scenarios include the following:

1. The SRH services and the polyclinics of gynecology, focusing on the process of VTP and contraception.
2. The hospital emergency rooms, for cases of consultation for abortion in progress, incomplete abortion, complications of abortion, emergency contraception or sexual violence.
3. The areas of hospitalization, for cases of hospitalization due to VTP, post-abortion complications or tubal sterilizations.

The competences according to autonomy levels for the SRH area are listed in Table 31.1.

31.2.3 Teaching and Mentorship of Medical Students in Family Planning

Within the School of Medicine of the University of the Republic, ob-gyn is taught in the Gynecology-Neonatology Curricular Unit in the second triennium, in the fourth year.

Within the learning objectives of this unit, the issues of SRH are clearly specified, including aspects related to unwanted pregnancy and VTP (Table 31.2).

How these issues are approached and taught depends on the focus of each gynecological clinic. The GCA proposes an approach to these issues both from the theoretical point of view and in the form of workshops and seminars. During the Curricular Unit, all the students who attend the GCA participate in the following activities:

a. Theoretical class: Sexual and Reproductive Rights and SRH.
b. Seminar for small groups: Bioethics and Confidentiality in Gynecological Practice. This seminar is given by the head professor of the clinic. Different clinical cases are discussed, including the issue of unwanted pregnancy and VTP.
c. Seminar for small groups: Approaches in the medical consultation of situations of gender-based violence (GBV). The importance of considering unwanted pregnancy as one of the consequences of violence and abuse, and the role of the VTP law in these contexts is highlighted.
d. Theoretical class on contraception and discussion workshops.

The GCA also offers electives aimed at students in the second triennium of their medical education:

a. Optional subject on Humanism and Medical Professionalism in Gynecology and Obstetrics. It presents a theoretical and practical thirty-

Table 31.1 Clinical competences in SRH area according to autonomy levels for residents in Gynecology and Obstetrics.

	First year resident: At the end of the first year the resident will be able to:	Second year resident: At the end of the second year the resident will be able to	Third year resident: At the end of the third year the resident will be able to:
Level of autonomy 1	• Address consultations in general, and SRH in particular, respecting the principles of bioethics and sexual and reproductive rights and ensuring the confidentiality of consultations • Complete the history and advice in a contraceptive consultation, including: knowledge of natural and pharmacological methods; indications and contraindications of hormonal methods and intrauterine devices; indications and prescription of emergency contraception • Obtaining informed consent upon insertion of intrauterine devices (IUDs), implants and tubal sterilization • Subcutaneous implant insertion • Know and apply the legislation and regulations on SRH • Present clinical cases related to the subject of SRH in clinical meetings • Integrate the detection of gender-based violence in the usual gynecological consultation	• Make insertions of different IUDs in non-nulliparous women • Perform subcutaneous implant removal • Manage side effects of contraceptive methods • Perform contraception counseling in special situations (diseases, post obstetric event) • Participate in VTP 2 interdisciplinary consultations • Participate in VTP 3 consultations and correctly indicate medications for VTP • Conduct VTP 4 consultation and manage incomplete abortion treatment: medical treatment, vacuum uterine aspiration and manual vacuum aspiration (MVA). • Perform incomplete abortion uterine aspirations • Conduct guidance on gender-based violence once detected, coordinating specific actions: articulation with other technicians, coordination with reference team, identification of life-threatening situations	• Make insertions of different IUDs in nulliparous women. • Conduct the VTP 3 consultation and correctly indicate medications for VTP (although as stipulated in Law 18987, VTP 2 and 3 consultations must be performed by gynecologists). • Advise on the diagnosis of serious fetal malformations, and coordinate the actions proposed by the Law before the woman's request for voluntary termination of pregnancy. • Diagnose and treat complications after VTP • Perform tubal sterilizations by laparoscopic route. • Address the sexuality consultation, incorporating the subject in the interview in an empathetic and effective way • Perform a correct history and semiology of sexual disorders, referring the specialist in a timely manner. • Initial approach to the consultation for rape / sexual violence at the emergency door, with empathy, integrity and confidentiality. It includes actions for prevention of STI, emergency contraception and biological sampling if necessary.

Level of autonomy 2		
• Make insertions of different IUDs in non-nulliparous women • Subcutaneous implant removal. • Manage side effects of contraceptive methods • Perform contraception counseling in special situations (diseases, post-obstetric event) • Participate in VTP 2 interdisciplinary consultations • Participate in VTP 3 consultations and correctly indicate medications for VTP	• Perform insertions of different IUDs in nulliparous women. • Perform the VTP 3 consultation and correctly indicate medications for VTP • Advise on the diagnosis of serious fetal malformations, and coordinate the actions proposed by the law before the woman's request for VTP • Diagnose and treat complications after VTP • Perform laparoscopic tubal sterilizations • Address the sexuality consultation, incorporating the subject in the interview in an empathetic and effective way • Perform a correct history and semiology of sexual disorders, referring the specialist in a timely manner • Initial approach to the consultation for sexual violence at the emergency door, with empathy, integrity and confidentiality. It includes actions for prevention of sexually transmitted infection (STI), emergency contraception and biological sampling if necessary.	• Perform intrauterine evacuations by VTP in the first trimester. • Guide women and men in the initial resolution of sexual disorders. Indicate basic pharmacological physiotherapy treatments. • Perform intrauterine evacuations by VTP in the second trimester.
Level of autonomy 3		
• Observer in laparoscopic tubal sterilizations.	• Participate as an observer in intrauterine evacuations due to VTP in the first trimester	• Perform intrauterine evacuations due to VTP in the second trimester.

Table 31.2 Learning objectives in sexual and reproductive health for medical students, extracted from the Gynecology-Neonatology Curricular Unit Program

Thematic contents
Sexual and reproductive health and rights: comprehensive management and application in clinical consultation
Regarding the approach to unwanted pregnancy and VTP, the student should know: – Current national legislation, unsafe abortion and its complications   – Different stages of VTP consultation according to the law   – Role of the general practitioner in the VTP process, normal and alarm symptoms in the abortion process, main risks, pre- and post-abortion advice   – Abortion methods, generalities and risks, post-abortion contraception   – Recognize and act against problems posed in the exercise of the right to VTP
To achieve this, the student must be able to: – Integrate and apply bioethical principles, respect and maintain confidentiality in the consultation, integrate and coordinate actions with other services to solve problems, not impose personal beliefs   – Apply the laws in force regarding the health care of women, pregnant women and adolescents

hour workload and sixteen hours of home activity.

The general objective of the course is to support students in reflecting on how their beliefs, experiences and emotions can influence the care of their patients. Considering unwanted pregnancy, abortion and VTP, the topics covered include conscientious objection and conscience commitment, current legal framework, medical secrecy and confidentiality.

b. Summer internships: Comprehensive approach to women's health. This is included in the Optional Summer Internship Program of the School of Medicine. It includes sixty-four hours per month of face-to-face practice and forty hours per month outside of clinic. The general objectives of the internship are to provide medical students the experience of the specialty of ob-gyn and the opportunities to participate in caring for women at different stages of their lives and at different levels of care. The topic of VTP is addressed during internships by the SRH service in the company of a teacher tutor in charge.

31.3 Overcoming the Barriers of Conscientious Objection and Centralization of Medical Care

The implementation of the VTP law has faced several challenges since its approval, and these are also manifested in the training challenges.

One of the barriers to the implementation of the law is conscientious objection, which is more clearly seen in the interior of the country as a real obstacle in practice [15,16].

To overcome this barrier, it is essential to have gynecologists trained in the technical and legal aspects of the law, with conscientious commitment, who can carry out the implementation of the VTP law and lead SRH teams around the country.

Health professionals' right to conscientious objection is protected by law 18987 of VTP. Although at the time of passage of the VTP law, there was a significant number of gynecologists who were already applying the risk and harm reduction model due to unsafe abortion, conscientious objection appeared as a problem in some parts of the country.

While the exact data are difficult to specify, in June 2013, at a press conference, the Uruguayan Ministry of Health presented a preliminary overview of the application of VTP, at which it estimated that 30% of the gynecologists declared themselves to be conscientious objectors. The largest group of gynecologists claiming conscientious objection worked in the country's hinterland (outside of Montevideo), which includes 50% of the national population. This caused problems for certain inland departments where conscientious objection was more or less generalized. For instance, in the department of Salto (400 kilometeres from Montevideo), all the gynecologists alleged conscientious objection and initiated legal and administrative action against the law and its application [15].

In this regard, the extension of the training across the country is critical. The decentralization of training in ob-gyn has been one of the pillars of the post-graduate training plan of the GCA, and has become a key strategy to overcoming barriers in women's access to VTP. Classically, ob-gyn residents were trained in Montevideo, the capital of the country, in the two teaching hospitals where the clinics are located (Clinics Hospital and Pereira Rossell Hospital).

The GCA has committed to the objectives of national health reform in relation to post-graduate training, tending to the comprehensive training of specialists prepared to adequately meet the needs of the National Integrated Health System, also committing to the decentralization of the teaching-learning scenarios, with the objective of having fully trained specialists throughout the country [17].

In 2010, this decentralization process began. In the 2010–2018 period, ten Associated Teaching Centers were incorporated into the GCA, nine of which are located in the interior of the country. The Associated Teaching Centers are public or private health institutions that are committed to receiving gynecology residents. They must comply with an accreditation process, endorsed by the Graduate School of the School of Medicine, and must be associated with one of the three Gynecological Clinics, which have academic responsibility. The decentralization has succeeded in increasing the number of residents graduated, contributing to continuous medical training and facilitating and strengthening assistance at the local level, with the expectation of promoting the establishment of specialists in the interior of the country. An example of this process is what happened in the department of Salto, which initially had 100% of its gynecologists claim conscientious objection. Currently, there are several gynecologists based in that department who carry out VTP activities, all of them graduated from the GCA.

31.4 The Effect of Training on Professionalism, Knowledge, Attitudes and Practice

Since the approval and implementation of the VTP law in Uruguay, the GCA has been responsible for the training of most ob-gyn residents.

During the 2013–2018 period, 42.7% (56/131) of the resident graduates were trained by the GCA, having developed their clinical activity at the Women's Hospital of Pereira Rossell Hospital in Montevideo, and in the 10 Associated Teaching Centers dependent on the GCA in 8 departments of the country.

Starting from the hypothesis that training influences professional practice, a study was carried out with the objective of assessing the impact of the curriculum on SRH of the GCA on: training, professional activity and commitment of conscience, of clinic ob-gyn graduates since the passage of the VTP law (2013–2018).

An anonymous online survey was designed, using Google Forms technology, which was sent electronically to all post-graduate students of the GCA who had graduated from the gynecology residency after VTP law 18.987 had come into force. The survey contained eight main questions on sex, graduation year, place of practice (Montevideo or in the country's interior, in hospital or private health centers), SRH training, current professional activity, current geographic residence, VTP provision, and if not providing VTP, the reason(s) why.

This survey was sent to the 56 residents graduated in 6 generations from 2013 to 2018. A total of 53 responses were obtained. Of respondents, 75% (40/53) were residents at Pereira Rossell Hospital, and 25% (13/53), at other Associated Teaching Centers in Montevideo and the interior of the country. The distribution of post-graduates by year of graduation and the training center is shown in Figure 31.1. As a result of the decentralization process carried out by the GCA, in recent years the number of graduates from Associated Teaching Centers increased.

When analyzing the training according to whether it was carried out in Montevideo or the interior of the country, the same evolution is seen (Figure 31.2). This is very important, since it factors into where graduates will subsequently develop their professional activity.

Regarding their training during residency, 89% (47/53) of respondents reported having rotated for SRH services in their respective Associated Teaching Centers. Regarding their professional activity at the time of the survey, 83% performed VTPs in their usual practice (44/53). Of these, 57% resided in Montevideo and 26% in the interior of the country. The absolute

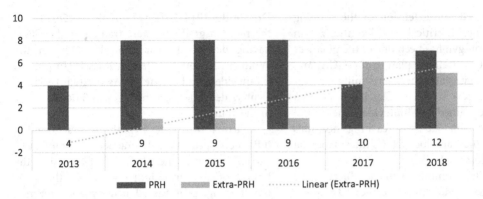

Figure 31.1 Number of post-graduate trainees (vertical axis) according to year of graduation and Training center (Pereira Rossell Hospital [PRH and extra-PRH], Uruguay, 2013–2018)

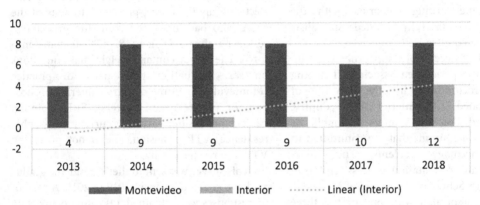

Figure 31.2 Number of post-graduate trainees (vertical axis) by year of graduation (horizontal axis) and place of training (Montevideo and interior of the country), Uruguay, 2013–2018

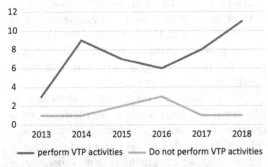

Figure 31.3 Number of post-graduate trainees (vertical axis) terminating pregnancies in their usual clinical practice by year (horizontal axis), Uruguay, 2013–2018

number of residents graduated from the GCA who carry out VTP activities has been increasing since 2013, as shown in Figure 31.3.

Eleven of these gynecologists (25%) held regular positions in SRH services. Seventeen percent of respondents (9/53) reported not making VTP consultations in their usual clinical practice: only 5 of the respondents declared conscientious objection (9%).

It is important to analyze separately the professional activity of gynecologists who develop their practice in the interior of the country: 32% (17/53) of respondents lived in the interior of the country. Of these, the vast majority, 82% (14/17), conducted VTP consultations in their clinical practice. Almost half of them, 43% (6/14), had regular positions in SRH services. Of those who did not perform VTP, 2 declared conscientious objection.

This study allowed us to verify that training influences professional practice. The majority of the residents trained in the GCA were trained in SRH and abortion, and at the time of the recent survey provided VTP care in their professional practice. Only 9% declared conscientious objection, which is a much lower percentage of the estimated 30% in the interior of the country.

In addition, 32% of graduates were located in the interior of the country, and the majority carried out VTP activities. This is essential since in the interior of the country one of the barriers to the implementation of VTP was the lack of professionals and conscientious objection.

31.5 The Effects of Training on Maternal Mortality

Uruguay has seen a drastic decrease in maternal mortality in the past twenty-five years, and, according to data from the Pan American Health Organization/World Health Organization, has the second lowest mortality in the Americas [18].

In Uruguay, all cases of maternal death require mandatory reporting (including monthly reports with zero maternal deaths). An intentional search for maternal deaths is performed by reviewing death certificates for all women between fifteen and forty-five years. All cases are analyzed by the National Commission for the Reduction of Mortality of Obstetric Cause.

An analysis of the evolution of maternal mortality from 1999 to 2018 was performed according to the data requested and obtained directly from the Division of Vital Statistics of the Ministry of Health. The temporal association of changes in maternal mortality with the implementation of different health and legal policies was analyzed. Thus, three great periods were defined:

Penalized abortion (1999–2004). There were no health policies in this regard, other than criminalization throughout the formal system and the promotion of secrecy.

Risk and harm reduction policy (2004–2012). Although the legal status remained unchanged, the risk and harm reduction strategy was formally implemented in the health system through ordinance 369/04. This period was also characterized by health reform and the inclusion of SRH Services.

Decriminalized abortion (2012 to date). VTP is a benefit within the National Integrated Health System. SRH services are consolidated and SRH is included in university curricula.

We emphasize that, with the low numbers of births in Uruguay (40,139 births in 2018), the maternal mortality ratio (MMR) can have important variations with very low numbers, the reason comparing periods is more accurate. The maternal mortality ratio in 2018 was 14.9. In Table 31.3 we can see the number of maternal deaths and the proportion of deaths due to abortion for each of the specified periods. The reduction of the global MMR stands out, as does the reduction of the proportion of deaths due to abortion.

We can therefore conclude that maternal mortality in Uruguay in the past twenty years has been declining. But the joint analysis with abortion mortality also allows us to visualize that the global reduction has undoubtedly been seen as a consequence of the decrease in abortion deaths [18].

We also highlight that since the implementation of the provision of VTP in the National Integrated Health System, there was only 1 case of maternal death related to the legal process of VTP in 54,990 procedures. This establishes a procedure mortality of 0.18 per 1,000 VTP procedures.

Table 31.3 Maternal mortality and deaths by abortion by period.

Period	Births (n)	MM (n)	MMR	Maternal deaths due to abortion (n)	(%)	Legal framework
1999–2004	311008	71	22,83	20	28,2	Penalized abortion
2005–2012	379150	71	18,73	8	11,3	Risk and harm reduction model
2013–2018	276236	51	18,46	4	7,8	Decriminalized abortion

Source: Ministry of Health Uruguay
MM: maternal deaths; MMR: maternal mortality ratio; %: proportion of deaths due to abortion

References

1. Poder Legislativo. Ley 18.987 Interrupción Voluntaria del Embarazo. Montevideo https://parlamento.gub.uy/documentosyleyes/ficha-asunto/107885

2. Briozzo L, et al. A risk reduction strategy to prevent maternal death associated with unsafe abortion. *Int J Obstet Gynecol.* 2006;**95**(2):221–226.

3. Briozzo L (ed.). *Iniciativas Sanitarias contra el Aborto Provocado en Condiciones de Riesgo. (Health Initiatives against induced abortion under unsafe conditions).* Montevideo, Uruguay: ARENA; 2007:21–44.

4. Briozzo L et al. From risk and harm reduction to decriminalizing abortion: the Uruguayan model for women's rights. *Int J Gynecol Obstet.* 2016;**134**(Suppl 1):S3–S6.

5. Briozzo L. Aborto provocado: un problema humano. Perspectivas para su análisis-Estrategias para su reducción. *Rev Med Urug.* 2003;**19**:188–200.

6. Labandera A, Gorgoroso M, Briozzo L. The implementation of the risk and harm reduction strategy against unsafe abortion in Uruguay: from a university hospital to the entire country. *Int J Gynecol Obstet.* 2016;**134**(Suppl. 1):S7–S11.

7. Lalonde AB, Grellier R. FIGO saving mothers and newborns initiative 2006–2011. *Int J Gynecol Obstet.* 2012;**119** (Suppl. 1):S18–21.

8. Briozzo L, Faúndes A. The medical profession and the defense and promotion of sexual and reproductive rights. *Int J Gynecol Obstet.* 2008;**100** (3):291–4.

9. Dickens BM, Cook RJ. Conscientious commitment to women's health. *Int J Gynecol Obstet.* 2011;**113**(2):163–6.

10. Poder Legislativo: Ley de Defensa del Derecho a la Salud Sexual y Reproductiva. https://parlamento.gub.uy/documentosyleyes/ficha-asunto/29685

11. Fiol V, Rieppi L, Aguirre, R, et al. The role of medical abortion in the implementation of the law on voluntary termination of pregnancy in Uruguay. *Int J Gynecol Obstet.* 2016;**134**(S1):S12–S15

12. Government of Uruguay. Ministry of Public Health. *Guía técnica para la interrupcion voluntaria del embarazo (IVE).* Montevideo, Uruguay: MSP; 2012.

13. Nozar F, et al. *Programa de formación del postgrado de la Clínica Ginecotocológica A.* 1st ed. Montevideo: Oficina del Libro-Fundación de Ediciones de la Facultad de Medicina/Universidad de la República Oriental del Uruguay; 2011.

14. F Coppola et al. Objeción de conciencia como barrera para implementar la Interrupción voluntaria del embarazo en el Uruguay: variaciones en la actitud y comportamiento de los ginecólogos. *Int J Gynecol Obstet.* 2016; **134**:S16–S19

15. MYSU. *Estado de situación de los servicios de salud sexual y reproductiva y aborto legal en 10 de los 19 departamentos del país. Sistematización de resultados Estudios Observatorio MYSU 2013–2017.* Montevideo: MYSU; 2017.

16. Nozar F, Briozzo L, Gallino V, et al. Descentralización de los escenarios de enseñanza-aprendizaje de los posgrados de Ginecotocología. Experiencia de la Clínica Ginecotocológica A. *Rev Méd Urug.* 2019;**35** (3):218–223. doi:10.29193/RMU.35.3.9

17. PAHO, WHO. *Health Situation in the Americas: Basic Indicators*; 2015. [Internet]. www.paho.org/hq/index.php?option=com_content&view=article&id=2470%3Adata-statistics&catid=1900%3Adata-statistics-home&Itemid=2003&lang=pt.

18. Briozzo L, Gómez Ponce de León R, Tomasso G, Faúndes A. Overall and abortion related maternal mortality rates in Uruguay over the past 25 years and their association with policies and actions aimed at protecting women's rights. *Int J Gynecol Obstet.* 2016;**134** (Suppl. 1):S20–23.

Chapter

32

Abortion Training and Integration of Legal Services in the Public Health System of Mexico City

Raffaela Schiavon and Patricio Sanhueza

32.1 Introduction: Where Abortion Is Illegal, It Is Usually Unsafe

Abortion is a frequent event in the reproductive lives of women, both spontaneous and induced. However, in many countries, laws completely or severely restrict access to safely and legally induced termination of pregnancy (TOP). Legal restrictions directly and indirectly affect availability of services and providers, limit access to technologies and medications and increase severe morbidity and mortality, with rising costs of hospital care for the health system, as well as costs for women and their families. Additionally, restricted legislation causes stigma among providers and toward women who seek medical care, who may also be subjected to overt criminalization. All these consequences are not equally distributed among socio-economic conditions: both morbidity/mortality as well as prison sentences differentially affect younger and poorer women, who have little access to education and information, to economic resources and to close networks to access safe services. In sum, legal restrictions represent a profound gender, health and social discrimination

mechanism, which causes multiple, unnecessary and preventable sufferings (Figure 32.1).

Where TOP is not permitted by the law, health professionals are not usually educated or trained in the theory and practice of induced abortion and post-abortion care; medical undergraduate and even post-graduate curricula are old-fashioned and extremely deficient. Theoretical contents describe concepts such as "criminal abortion" (that have no clinical relevance but are charged with stigma and discrimination), include old techniques (ie, dilation and sharp curettage [D&C] with general anesthesia) and ignore new evidence-based recommendations (manual or electrical vacuum aspiration [EVA/MVA]; medication abortion [MA]). Clinical practices are often empirical (self-taught) or based on superiors' or peers' limited experience, perpetuating malpractices and errors. As a consequence of the restrictive laws and the poor quality of abortion and post-abortion care, women suffer frequent and often severe rates of complications, and even deaths.

Consequently, health authorities and physicians perceive abortion as a risky and

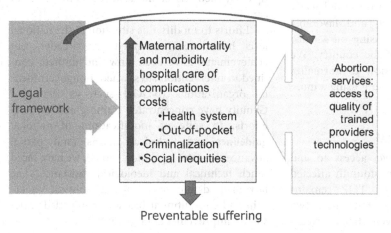

Figure 32.1 Conceptual framework of health impact of safe abortion

Legal framework → Maternal mortality and morbidity hospital care of complications costs
•Health system
•Out-of-pocket
•Criminalization
•Social inequities

Abortion services: access to quality of trained providers technologies

Preventable suffering

complicated procedure, generally reserved for specialized physicians, that requires secondary or even tertiary costly hospital care. Additionally, efforts to clinically improve quality of care and increase access to services for all women experiencing any type of abortion are frequently confused with advocacy to decriminalize TOP, and as such subtly or overtly ostracized.

These vicious cycles, which confound the clinical aspects of abortion with the effects of its clandestine quality and criminalization, prevent establishing good-quality care and normalizing its generalized provision within similar reproductive events (such as contraception and family planning, pregnancy and delivery). When performed in a legal context, induced abortion, particularly in the first trimester, is indeed the safest possible event a woman may face once she becomes pregnant, much safer than an ongoing pregnancy and term delivery [1].

32.2 Objective

This chapter analyzes efforts implemented to improve abortion care in Mexico, under diverse legal contexts, and particularly after legalization of first-trimester TOP in Mexico City. We describe strategies to train health professionals, to improve conditions of services, to disseminate new recommended technologies, to introduce and register medications and to generate updated guidelines and protocols. We also describe efforts undertaken to decentralize service delivery and expand health workers' cadres (task-sharing), with the objective of improving access, quality and safety of abortion services by increasing the number of sensitized and trained health professionals, including nonmedical providers. We finally present some recent data on how legality modified utilization of services and favorably affected abortion mortality, focusing on Mexico City compared to the rest of the country. We conclude with reflections on how to normalize and fully integrate abortion training using a more sustainable strategy.

32.3 Abortion in Mexico

In Mexico, as described above, access to and safety of abortion services are profoundly affected by the diverse legal contexts. TOP remains restricted by the law in thirty of its thirty-two states, and minimally applied even when allowed –

in the case of rape, when there is risk to a woman's life or severe risk to her health, in the case of serious fetal malformations and in very low socioeconomic conditions. At the national level, overall quality of care provided both in TOP and in post-abortion care (PAC: spontaneous, incomplete and unspecified abortions) is generally poor, in terms of human resources' technical and human skills, services, equipment and conditions. Overall, abortion care causes approximately one in ten maternal hospitalizations among women at reproductive age; however, legally induced TOP represents only 6.5% of all registered procedures at the national level, but less than 0.3% if we exclude Mexico City (author's analysis, data not shown). D&C is still the most often employed technology, usually carried out in maternity hospitals, in surgical theaters and under general anesthesia; post-abortion contraception is not routinely provided [2].

Rates of complications are high, although progressively declining in frequency and severity. Abortion-related deaths have consistently represented slightly more than 7% of all maternal losses in the country during the past three decades [3,4].

Mexican federal health authorities long considered abortion as a severe pathology of normal pregnancy, charged with clandestine, illegal and dangerous connotations that accordingly require costly care in higher-level facilities by specialized providers; therefore, few advances have been achieved to expand abortion services, whether it is for an uncomplicated spontaneous abortion, an incomplete abortion or a legally induced procedure, which should be provided by the widest range of trained health professionals, with simple and updated methods at the lowest possible level of care [5].

Efforts to modify this situation at the national level have been attempted for decades, but achievements have been slow and limited, confined to intervention sites, where nongovernmental organizations (NGOs) such as Ipas and Gynuity have concentrated training and capacity efforts. In spite of modifications of national guidelines and technical norms (and partial advances in states legal indications), we have faced much technical and ideological resistance. The lack of academic, technical and political leadership and commitment has so far impeded widespread improvements in quality of care.

32.4 Change of the Law in Mexico City and Implementation of Services

This impasse fortunately changed when, in April 2007, in Mexico City only, first-trimester TOP was decriminalized to be available at women's request [6]. The change of the law was immediately followed by the publication of local Ministry of Health (MOH) technical guidelines, and the legal termination of pregnancy (ILE in Spanish) program started operating in selected hospitals and clinics [7]. Thanks to the vast publicity generated by heated public debate, a sympathetic media environment and a vigorous activist movement, information rapidly spread in the capital city: women in need immediately presented at public hospitals asking for a legal abortion. The challenge for an ill-prepared health system was immediate and enormous. To overcome this challenge and to ensure the safe provision of these services, at the high expected volume, Mexico City MOH sought support to start an intensive, comprehensive, in-service training program, in collaboration with national and international NGOs, particularly those with technical experience in abortion care, such as Ipas and Gynuity. Services were rapidly initiated at fourteen sites, initially hospitals and highly specialized health centers. In preparation of creating the clinical space, an inspiring visit took place in 2015 with the Women's Options Center at the University of California's San Francisco General Hospital, consisting of a delegation that included the Minister of Health of Mexico City, the Vice Minister, the Reproductive Health Coordinator, and lead nurse responsible of the ILE program, as well as Dr. Schiavon, the Ipas country director at the time. The delegation found the newly remodeled Women's Options Center inspiring, particularly its architecture and furnishings specifically designed to create a welcoming, physically beautiful atmosphere to eliminate the stigma of abortion for women and staff alike. The new clinics in Mexico City were remodeled with the same intent and purpose: to offer an aesthetically pleasing and comforting environment.

32.5 In-Service Training

32.5.1 What, How and to Whom?

Immediately after the change in the law, a pervasive information and orientation program was begun in all the hospitals in the Mexico City health system to inform all personnel of the new legal guidelines and of their duty to inform and refer women requesting TOP to the selected sites.

At the same time, an intensive in-service training was initiated, with different teams in a rotation format, in the fourteen sites that were providing ILE services. Training teams included a certified obstetrician- gynecologist (ob-gyn), a nurse and a psychologist and/or social worker, all of them highly experienced in the provision of post-abortion/induced abortion care and post-abortion contraception. Training curricula and strategies were based on international and organizational recommendations (World Health Organization [WHO], Ipas, Gynuity, International Federation of Gynecology and Obstetrics [FIGO], Federación Latinoamerica de Sociedades de Obstetrica y Ginecologia [FLASOG]), adapted and reviewed for local conditions and regularly discussed with training teams [6,7].

In-service training took place for two to three weeks at each site; content included the new legal framework, values clarification and counseling, recommended new surgical techniques (such as MVA/EVA) and medical regimens and post-abortion contraception, among others. The entire health team was involved in the process, from physicians, nurses and midwives; social workers, psychologists (where available); to administrative personnel, such as receptionists and even police. Some core contents – with dynamic activities – were common to the whole team, particularly values clarification and attitudes transformation [8]. Intensive and dynamic sessions were also held on information, referral and pre-abortion counseling abilities to inform women where to go for ILE services, to inform and counsel them on available options in case of an unintended pregnancy ("balanced" counseling for TOP; adoption; acceptance – rare, but possible). Post-abortion counseling reinforced the importance of recognizing the normal progression of an abortion, potential warning signs, if and when to seek follow-up and health care. Counseling abilities of the different types of providers were also reinforced under one-to-one supervision.

Finally, a strong emphasis was placed on strengthening all providers' abilities to support women's free and informed decisions on post-abortion contraception, especially to strengthen immediate uptake of long-acting reversible contraceptive (LARC) methods. Providers became gradually competent to insert an intrauterine device (IUD) after a surgical procedure. However, post-MA, most contraceptives were initially short-term methods, because LARC provision was dependent on follow-up visits. Only after initiation of the "quick-start" protocol did providers' confidence improve and contraceptive implants insertion – immediately after the first dose of MA (mifepristone) – increase sharply. Post-abortion contraceptive counseling always insisted, however, on the centrality of women's informed consent and the importance of informing women about effective contraceptive methods but at the same time, ensuring they receive their method of choice [9]. Ethical concerns were particularly relevant because of multiple potential biases in favor of long- acting contraception, eventually receiving an overall government push at the national and local levels, stemming from incentives and the commercial interests of the pharmaceutical industry – and even from some sectors of the donors' community. Additional training content was

subsequently added for each type of health professional (see Table 32.1).

In the case of surgical abortion, the objective was to substitute D&C with modern and safer techniques: MVA and, in those areas with high TOP numbers, EVA. Intensive practice with pelvic models preceded hands-on training in women; inexperienced or unconfident providers were trained in the MVA technique for endometrial biopsy and incomplete abortion. Uterine evacuation procedures for induced abortion were initially carried on under a trainer's supervision, until proficiency was documented, usually after fifteen to twenty procedures. The high volume of TOP performed facilitated the rapid acquisition of surgical competencies and skills because initial guidelines and protocols restricted provision of services to ob-gyns. Particular care was paid to train providers in simple but essential techniques to guarantee adequate pain management, assure prevention of infections ("no-touch" techniques) and confirm completeness of surgical procedures. This last includes the systematic revision of uterine contents and fetal parts after evacuation, which rules out extrauterine implantation,

Table 32.1 Abortion training contents for health professionals

	Ob-gyn specialists/ general physicians	Professional nurses/ midwives	Social workers	Administrative personnel
Core training and sensitizing contents				
Values clarification and attitude transformations	X	X	X	X
Information and referral on legal abortion	X	X	X	X
Counselling on pregnancy options	X	X	X	
Counselling on post-abortion contraception	X	X	X	
Adolescents' appropriate abortion care	X	X	X	
Specific training contents				
MVA/EVA training: theoretical; pelvic model; hands-on training (endometrial biopsy, incomplete abortion, induced abortion)	X	X		
Medication abortion: Misoprostol alone, mifepristone and -misoprostol; routes and doses, follow-up; warning signs	X	X		
USP training: Gestational age; site of trophoblast implantation (intrauterine, ectopic, cervical; uterine scar); completeness of medication abortion	X	X		

without the need for more complex – and costly – post-surgical confirmatory diagnostics.

Medication abortion provided a new opportunity for easier, highly acceptable, extremely safe methodologies, which require fewer surgical skills and no special equipment in facilities and allow a wider cadre of potential providers, from general physicians to nurses and midwives, once adequately trained. At the beginning of the program, misoprostol alone was used, and innovative clinical protocols were introduced to confirm efficacy and acceptability of new routes of administration (buccal route). Starting in 2011, after mifepristone obtained official registration and was included in the local Essential Drugs List, the combined regimen became the gold standard for medication abortion. As collective expertise and confidence grew in the ILE program, protocols and guidelines for home administration of misoprostol ensued [10]. While most research protocols in MA were designed and conducted by Gynuity, Ipas Mexico collaborated closely and introduced intensive training contents, toolkits and counseling materials, for providers and women alike, focused on correct regimens (doses, timing and routes of administration), normal symptoms and warning signs of potential complications.

Specific training in ultrasound was also designed, since, again, official guidelines requested echography for gestational age determination; to conform with this requirement, all ILE sites in the Mexico City program were outfitted with US equipment. Training materials from Planned Parenthood Federation of America (PPFA) were translated and adapted. Both physicians and non-medical personnel were extensively trained. This strategy built new knowledge and skills in early pregnancy diagnosis for ILE providers: gestational age determination; site of trophoblast implantation (intrauterine vs. extrauterine: in cervical canal; in uterine scar); completeness of procedures. This type of training was essential to build on the growing clinical confidence among providers of medication abortion, and enabled them to recognize the rarity of ongoing pregnancy and prevent many unnecessary surgical interventions. Additionally, such skills were to become key for preventing rare but fatal abortion complications and deaths. While we are aware of the ongoing debate on the usefulness of ultrasound (US) in abortion practice, we are convinced that its widespread use in the ILE program in Mexico City strongly contributed to the safety of the procedure: no maternal deaths were recorded among the more than 240,000 women who received a first-trimester legal abortion since the program's inception.

Youth-appropriate abortion care represented a frequent challenge and a specific need during a training experience [11,12]. Based on the evidence, we designed a training module focused on the reproductive health needs of adolescents, including the international and national legal frameworks, the technical norms and official protocols that support their right to sexual and reproductive care; the bioethical principles and the concepts of evolving maturity; the specific counseling needs; and the clinical aspects of abortion care in teens. These training materials were used with primary care health personnel, many of them nurses, to identify needs and to strengthen adolescents' referral to the secondary level of care, and to the Legal Abortion Program.

With the support of Ipas colleagues in the USA, we disseminated a series of systematic clinical reviews of abortion literature to guide and support evidence-based practices, lessons learned from expert providers globally and updated recommendations among the trainees [13].

This comprehensive training curriculum, described above, allowed participants to strengthen their skills in surgical technologies and medical regimens that were unfamiliar to them or not part of their standard education curricula, due to the previous restrictive legal setting. Trainees were initially concerned about the legal risks and the potential liability of performing legal abortion procedures, even under the new law. Doubts most commonly expressed were related to adolescent care, to parental consent and to contraceptive methods eligibility criteria in the case of teenagers. Participants' initial knowledge of sexual and reproductive rights was minimal; but once the topic was brought up and discussed, it rapidly sparked their interest. Values clarification helped change their rapport with the patient/woman, and providers experienced a significant change in their attitude, from being detached, impatient or even intolerant, to a more respectful and humanized attitude. They became able to clarify their legal, ideological, moral or religious doubts ("I don't like this; this is just not me; this goes against my personal beliefs");

training and support also helped to reduce abortion stigma toward women requesting abortion and the stigma and finger-pointing that providers initially suffered from colleagues.

32.6 Beyond In-service Training

While in-service training is a crucial step in implementing legal access to abortion and post-abortion contraception to ensure clinical competence and address the complex emotional aspects of abortion care, additional learning strategies were developed: to keep up to date on new developments, to promote supervision and mentoring through periodic visits, assessment of care, training of trainers, task sharing, expansion of services sites and correct record keeping.

32.6.1 Distance Education and Digital Learning Platform

Training of providers increasingly included, over time, virtual learning strategies, directed to already trained providers as well as to new trainees. The objective of such strategies was multiple: (1) to create a community of health professionals and colleagues (trainees network), similarly sensitized, and capable of generating reciprocal support and feedback, both technical and emotional; (2) to keep them posted about new recommendations and updates, in a timely and efficient manner; (3) to produce training material in the local language (Spanish), often based on international evidence-based guidelines or locally generated, that could be used and replicated by trainees themselves, in their ongoing teaching activities, as a significant proportion of them do carry on formal teaching and/or informal training of medical students, interns and residents. To this end, we developed a Continuing Medical Education (CME) online course, with the most user-friendly interface possible to increase registration and user satisfaction, promoting dynamic and interactive activities for our provider networks as well as for new health professionals. A particularly successful product is the tutorial MVA video, produced in Mexico but reviewed and supervised by colleagues at Ipas NC [14]. We believe this type of CME materials offers, in a cost-effective way, great potential to strengthen the clinical expertise and networking capabilities of trained providers.

32.6.2 Mentoring and Supervision

Additional strategies that were implemented after hands-on training and digital learning, included mentoring trainees: periodic supervisory visits and calls, monitoring their productivity and identifying potential barriers and bottlenecks to their continuous and good quality practice, both in legal abortion and in post-abortion care [15].

Some of the factors identified during such mentoring processes required correction/improvement: lack of clinical confidence, need for re-training and resolving or correcting specific doubts or poor practices. Other factors that post-training supervision could identify were insufficient volume of procedures at the site to maintain clinical competency; unavailability of products (aspirators, cannulae or medications); and change of working responsibility (moved to administrative sites, etc). The latter cannot be corrected with mentoring strategies: on the contrary, they usually signal the need for a careful pre-selection of the health professionals to be trained to assure that they will directly provide abortion services. They also identify the need to assure global support to clinics/hospitals and make sure that trained providers have the appropriate surgical and medical supplies, hence the administrative and financial support needed to provide services. In the introductory stages, donations and/or very competitive sales might be contemplated to support a site: supplies are not acquired when there are no trained providers; but trained professionals cannot provide services without the adequate supplies.

32.6.3 Training of Trainers (TOT)

After a thorough process of training, supervising and monitoring the health site and guaranteeing their sustainability and quality and productivity, "trained sites" may become in turn "training sites," and provide the ideal setting for replicating in-service capacity for other health teams, in other states and even for other countries. We arranged exchange visits and short-term training (one week) with selected health teams from Chile and Argentina, preparing them for future changes in their laws and implementation of services, in a way that sums up technical, administrative, managerial and overall visioning of legal abortion care.

32.6.4 Task Sharing in Abortion

In Mexico City, technical guidelines for the ILE program shifted over time, from the initial hospital-based care provided by specialist physicians (ob-gyns or surgeons) to a first level of care provided by general practitioners. Clinical protocols establish preferential use of medical regimens up to nine or ten gestational weeks, with home administration of misoprostol [16]. In this model of care, assessing clinical eligibility such as gestational age, prescribing drugs (mifepristone, misoprostol and analgesics) and performing MVA are still formally reserved to physicians. Ultrasound is also a physician's task, but extensive training has been conducted among nurses. Nurses do play an essential role and oversee different functions, from pre-procedure counseling to post-abortion family planning provision. However, no advance has been achieved to formally strengthen tasks and functions of non-physician health professionals in this process of care. A last attempt to update ILE technical guidelines to include "trained midlevel providers" into the cadre of authorized health professionals in 2018 was unsuccessful [5].

32.6.5 Migration of Services: From Hospitals to First Level of Care Service

Due to increasing providers' clinical expertise and confidence, the implementation of medication abortion protocols, the high proportion of women seeking TOP in very early gestational ages and according to international evidence-based recommendations, the ILE program steadily moved outside the hospital setting to a first level of care, in basically equipped health clinics. In 2018, slightly more than seven out of ten legal abortions were provided in health clinics (Figure 32.2). This, however, implied re-training, supervision and evaluation of services to assure safety of procedure and continued quality of care for entire health teams.

32.6.6 Record Keeping

Ipas has consistently worked on the importance of strengthening correct registration and use of data for all maternal and reproductive health procedures, using International Classifications of Diseases (ICD) codes and national health registration systems. Ipas designed and conducted

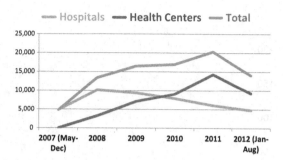

Figure 32.2 Legal abortions by provider type, Mexico City, 2007–2012

innovative training workshops, bringing together statisticians and clinicians alike, creating and providing support materials to improve the correct registration of abortion procedures, both for types of abortion (ICD-10 code) and for types of therapeutic procedures treatment (ICD-9 code).

32.7 Results

During the first 5 years of the training program, 174 training courses were offered, for a total of 2,616 hours of training, orientation and values clarification. The number of participants totaled more than 5,500, of which 216 were physicians directly performing uterine evacuations (UE). In the subsequent 3 years of the program, nearly 2,600 additional health-care professionals were reached, 341 of whom directly performed UE. We also provided mentoring, supervision and follow-up support to 333 direct UE providers via in-person visits, videoconferencing, phone calls, and electronic messages. More than 250 health professionals subscribed to the CME online course, which was completed by 151 providers. Through our work with the Federal District MOH and the Legal Abortion Program in Mexico City, we helped develop the capacity of the Federal District MOH to sustain and improve its services in multiple ways, allowing them to assume full responsibility for the program.

While in the first year of the ILE program, approximately one third of legal abortions were still performed with D&C, most of them in hospitals, this obsolete technique was, week by week, substituted for by safer surgical methods (MVA/EVA) and by medication regimens. Capacity, efficiency and quality of care in the program improved rapidly (Figure 32.3).

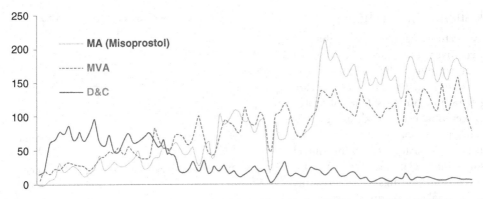

Figure 32.3 Number of legal abortions (vertical axis) by method, Mexico City, by week, 2007 and 2008 (horizontal axis)

Over the following years, the MOH issued new ILE guidelines and expanded services, from hospital-only to highly equipped health centers, for a total of 14 hospitals/clinics in Mexico City [16]. By the end of September 2019, a total of 216,755 women had been served in ILE public services: 77.4% of procedures were performed with medication abortion and 21.2% with MVA or EVA; D&C had completely disappeared. The large shift toward medication abortion played a major role in meeting women's high demand, simplifying the procedure and reducing the risk of complications. This shift was also possible because 86% of women requested the services within the first 9 weeks [17]. Contraceptive uptake immediately after TOP has increased, particularly of hormonal LARCs (subdermal implants); better registration and follow-up, are however, needed to support these data. No maternal death occurred among these legal abortion procedures in the public health system, and all abortion-related mortality rates have significantly declined in Mexico City, as well as (but less so) in the rest of the country [4].

32.8 Challenges, Lessons Learned and Some Recommendations

Thanks to many years of sustained work with health authorities in Mexico, we built on the successful case story of the ILE program in Mexico City, where the change of the law was coupled with access to and quality of services. Comprehensive, in-service multidisciplinary training in public health MOH facilities has been a key element for the implementation of legal abortion services and women's right to decide. These examples of success are a result of long-term, coordinated efforts with public health and hospital authorities to provide continuous technical assistance to update technical norms and guidelines; improvement and fine-tuning of in-service training strategy; and growing expertise in data use to strengthen the enabling environment and improve service delivery. Better supervision and evaluation post-training helped to analyze and then tailor intervention strategy to best meet the needs of each state and facility. Accordingly, we learned to couple training of human resources with strategic donations to intervention facilities as well as individual providers, to ensure that they have the necessary supplies and equipment to provide the highest quality of care.

Among the lessons learned, we like to share the following:

- Coordination with health authorities, both at the central level and at each facility level, is essential.
- Clinical and technical training must always be accompanied by sensibilization and values clarification dynamics, and the whole health team must be involved.
- Training must be sustained in terms of numbers of trained providers and in terms of time, to assure a critical mass of human resources ideologically committed, clinically prepared and able to change abortion standards of care from one generation of health professionals to the next.
- Training providers must go hand in hand with ensuring the availability of equipment and medications.
- Training strategies must be coupled with continuous technical assistance to improve

regulatory and normative frameworks to ensure up-to-date, evidence-based provision of services.

The main challenges we envision after this experience are:

- Facing the economic costs of such an in-service training strategy was possible only thanks to private donors' and foundations' support. However, such training costs would not be sustainable by a usually impoverished public health system.
- The path toward inclusion of mid-level providers into abortion care is still long and complex.
- Providing ample access to first-trimester abortion does not eliminate the need for later procedures [18,19]. Training challenges remain and are even greater for second-trimester abortions.
- In spite of impressive achievements in legal abortion provision in Mexico City, quality of care in PAC services has not improved in the rest of the country. The low rate of appropriate technology for PAC services in Mexico has been an ongoing challenge, with a national average of only 26%, with the exception of specific health facilities in some states, where we have developed sustained interventions over several years. But the challenge of scaling-up remains [20].

Some final recommendations based on our experience include the following:

- Abortion Care and Family Planning should be systematically included in pre-service and in-services curricula, for all types of health providers – physicians, nurses and professional midwives – to make it sustainable overtime.
- Health Science and Medical Curricula should be closely related to health needs and updated to changing practice environments, through Continuous Medical Education [21].
- Updated technical recommendations for abortion care should be implemented in all types of abortion procedures, from legally induced to incomplete abortion to miscarriage, to prevent stigma among providers and women.
- Medical societies and colleges should assume a strong academic leadership to adopt and disseminate continuously updated abortion guidelines among their members.

32.9 Final Remarks

The achievement of good quality legal abortion public services in Mexico City has been a gradual process in which health personnel's training played a central role in the implementation of women's right to decide. As one member of the training team expressed: "We are changing a chapter in these women's lives, we are changing the scenario for them from here on, I don't know how many times we have to repeat that scene, because this is another story, but I'm definitely satisfied with that."

References

1. Raymond EG, Grimes DA. The comparative safety of legal induced abortion and childbirth in the United States. *Obstet Gynecol*. 2012;**119**(2 Pt 1):215–219.

2. Schiavon R, Troncoso E, Polo G. Use of health system data to study morbidity related to pregnancy loss. In S Singh, L Remez, A Tartaglione (Eds.), *Methodologies for Estimating Abortion Incidence and Abortion-Related Morbidity and Mortality: A Review*. New York and Paris: Guttmacher Institute, IUSSP; 2010:147–163. www.guttmacher.org/pubs/

compilations/IUSSP/IUSSP-Chapter11.pdf

3. Schiavon R, Troncoso E, Polo G. Analysis of maternal and abortion-related mortality in Mexico in the last two decades, 1990–2008. *Int J Obst Gynecol*. 2012;**118**(Suppl 2): S78–86.

4. Darney BG, Fuentes-Rivera E, Polo G, Saavedra-Avendaño B, Alexander LT, Schiavon R. Con la ley y sin la ley/With and without the law: utilization of abortion services and case fatality in Mexico, 2000–2016. *Int J Gynecol Obstet*. 2020;**148** (3):369–374. doi:10.1002/ ijgo.13077

5. Schiavon R, Troncoso E. Inequalities in access to and quality of abortion services in Mexico: can task-sharing be an opportunity to increase legal and safe abortion care? *Int J Gynecol Obstet*. 2020;(Suppl). doi:10.1002/ijgo.13002

6. WHO. *Clinical Practice Handbook for Safe Abortion*. Geneva: World Health Organization; 2014. www.who .int/reproductivehealth/ publications/unsafe_abortion/ clinical-practice-safe-abortion/ en/

7. Turner KL, Huber A. (Eds.). *Woman-Centered, Comprehensive Abortion Care:*

Reference Manual, 2nd ed, Chapel Hill, NC: Ipas; 2013. https://ipas.azureedge.net/files/ACREFE16-WomenCenteredCACReferenceManual.pdf

8. Turner KL, Page KC. *Abortion Attitude Transformation: A Values Clarification Toolkit for Global Audiences*. Chapel Hill, NC: Ipas.; 2008. https://ipas.azureedge.net/files/VALCLARE14-VCATAbortionAttitudeTransformation.pdf

9. Rogers C, Dantas JAR. Access to contraception and sexual and reproductive health information post-abortion: a systematic review of literature from low- and middle-income countries. *J Fam Plann Reprod Health Care*. 2017; **43** (4):309–318. doi:10.1136/jfprhc-2016-101469)

10. Official Diary of Federal District. Notice to Inform about the Second Update of Essential and Institutional Drug List of Federal District Ministry of Health; August 16, 2011 [in Spanish]. www.ordenjuridico.gob.mx/Documentos/Estatal/Distrito%20Federal/wo64068.pdf

11. Turner KL, Börjesson E, Huber A, Mulligan C. 2011. *Abortion Care for Young Women: A Training Toolkit*. Chapel Hill, NC: Ipas. www.ipas.org/resources/abortion-care-for-young-women-a-training-toolkit

12. Renner RM, de Guzman A, Brahmi D. Prestación de Servicios de Aborto Para Adolescentes y Jóvenes: Revisión Sistemática Ipas Bolivia; 2014.

13. Ipas NC. *The Clinical Updates in Reproductive Health*. www.ipas.org/clinical-updates/

14. Aspiración manual endouterina: ¡aprende el procedimiento! Online video clip. https://youtu.be/JOzVIc8G1T0 https://www.ipasmexico.org/recursos/

15. Turner KL, Huber A. *Clinical Mentoring and Provider Support for Abortion-Related Care*. Chapel Hill, NC: Ipas; 2014. www.ipas.org/resources/clinical-mentoring-and-provider-support-for-abortion-related-care

16. Becker D, Diaz-Olavarrieta C. Decriminalization of abortion in Mexico City: the effects on women's reproductive rights. *Am J Public Health*. 2013;**103** (4):590–593.

17. Mexico City Ministry of Health. Legal Termination of Pregnancy. Statistics April 2007–September 2019 [in Spanish]. http://ile.salud.cdmx.gob.mx/wp-content/uploads/Interrupcion-Legal-del-Embarazo-Estadisticas-2007-2017-26-de-septiembre-2019.pdf

18. Saavedra-Avendano B, Schiavon R, Sanhueza P, Rios-Polanco R, Garcia-Martinez L, Darney BG. Who presents past the gestational age limit for first trimester abortion in the public sector in Mexico City? *PLoS ONE*. 2018;13(2): e0192547. https://doi.org/10.1371/journal.pone.0192547

19. Alexander L., Fuentes E, Saavedra-Avendaño, B., et al. Utilisation of second-trimester spontaneous and induced abortion services in public hospitals in Mexico, 2007–2015. *BMJ Sex Reprod Health*. 2019;45:283–289. DOI:10.1136/bmjsrh-2018-200300

20. RamaRao S, Townsend JW, Diop N, Raifman S. Postabortion care: going to scale. *Int Perspect Sex Reprod Health*. 2011;37(1):40–44.

21. National Academies of Sciences, Engineering, and Medicine. *Strengthening the Connection between Health Professions Education and Practice: Proceedings of a Joint Workshop*. Washington, DC: The National Academies Press; 2019. doi.org/10.17226/25407

33

Abortion Training Models in Sweden

Kristina Gemzell-Danielsson and Amanda Cleeve

33.1 Introduction

The Swedish abortion law from 1974, which came into practice in 1975, aims to protect the right to safe abortion [1]. The Swedish Board of Health and Welfare (BoHW, www.socialstyrelsen.se/en/regulations-and-guidelines/national-guidelines/) is a government agency under the Ministry of Health and Social Affairs, which oversees health-care issues, medical latencies and specialist certifications, collects official statistics and interprets and regulates the current abortion law. Until gestational week 18+0, the decision to undergo an abortion is the woman's and no governmental approval is required. From week 18+1, an approval is needed from the BoHW, which can grant approvals for specific indications up to "viability of the fetus outside of the uterus." In practice, this limit is now 21+6 gestational weeks for healthy pregnancies. It is the responsibility of obstetrics and gynecological (ob-gyn) hospital departments to ensure that abortion is provided without delay and by a qualified professional. The national abortion law states that abortion has to be done in a health-care facility to protect the health and life of the woman. These are either public ob-gyn clinical departments, which are obliged to provide abortions, or outpatient ob-gyn clinics that have permission from the BoHW to provide first-trimester abortions. For medication abortions (mifepristone and misoprostol), the consensus is that an abortion is considered "done" when mifepristone has been taken. This means that all women have to take mifepristone in a health-care facility. In first-trimester medication abortions, women can then take the misoprostol in the comfort of their own home. All women seeking an abortion have the right to receive social counseling; however, it is not mandatory.

Since 2008, anyone can have an abortion in Sweden, and they do not need to be a Swedish citizen. When a pregnancy has to be interrupted to save the woman's life, this falls outside of the abortion law ("termination of pregnancy") and the aim is to save the woman's as well as the life of the fetus. In that case, no application/permission is needed for pregnancies beyond 18+0. Knowledge of the abortion law and abortion care is part of the curricula for medical students and obligatory for residents in obstetrics and gynaecology (ob-gyn) and midwifery students.

33.2 Past and Current Context

Under the old Swedish law, abortion and infanticide were illegal and punished with death. The punishment for abortion was altered in 1921, the same year that Swedish women earned the right to vote, to six months' to two years' imprisonment for those involved (woman and abortion provider). In 1938, abortion was still considered a criminal offense but could be granted for specific indications including medical (if the pregnancy meant a serious threat to the woman's life), humanitarian (incest and rape, underaged women/girls) and eugenic indications (for which the law changed in 1974 and the practice ended much earlier). In 1946, a socio-medical indication was added, meaning that abortion could be granted for women with many pregnancies and births and where another pregnancy would mean health risks. In 1963, a fetal indication was added, mainly as a consequence of the thalidomide catastrophe. In all of these cases, an abortion had to be approved by two doctors or by the BoHW.

In the 1930s, an estimated 20,000 illegal abortions were performed each year, causing many women to die or be permanently injured [2]. The number of safe and legal abortions increased over the years, and by 1974 an estimated 30,000 legal abortions were granted. The reduction in illegal and unsafe abortions was driven by a more liberal interpretation of the grounds on which abortion could be provided.

During the 1960s and 1970s, several major societal changes occurred in Sweden that paved the way for the new liberal abortion law. This period was characterized by protests in the labor movement, the women's movement and student groups, who were voicing demands for increased equality. Social reforms giving women equal rights in the home and the workplace followed. The liberalization of established social and moral attitudes to sex came to the fore in the late 1960s with the concepts of alternative family structures, contraception, and abortion becoming much more acceptable.

When the 1975 abortion law came into force, the work on prevention of unplanned pregnancy intensified, youth clinics opened, midwives achieved the right to prescribe contraceptives and contraceptive counseling became free of charge. The total numbers of abortions among adult women did not change instantly. However, there was a huge drop in teenage pregnancy, births and abortions during the decade that followed [3]. The legalization of abortion in 1975 followed by the introduction of medical abortion in the 1990s (in clinical trials from the mid-1980s and regulatory approval in 1992) led to a majority of abortions being done in the first trimester. In 2018, almost 36,000 abortions were done in Sweden, with an abortion rate of 19/1,000 women of reproductive ageand <10/1000 among those 15–19 years of age. The current average length of gestation at the time of an abortion is below 7 weeks, and 85% of abortions are done before 9 weeks. Fewer than 1% of pregnancies are conducted beyond 18 weeks of gestation, with the majority of these done for fetal indications.

33.3 Political and Legal Journey

In order to meet the legal requirement of providing safe and legal abortion on request and without delay, as stipulated by law, the training curricula for residents in ob-gyn had to change. To manage during the transition period and to protect women from delays due to conscientious objection (CO), the leaders of every ob-gyn clinical department were charged with employing trained abortion providers in sufficient numbers. Safe abortion provision became a part of the job description for all specialists in ob-gyn and was

subsequently introduced as part of the training curricula for ob-gyn residents. In 2015, it was made a mandatory requirement enforced and overseen by the BoHW.

In the 1970s and 1980s, when a large proportion of abortions were performed in the second trimester and prior to the introduction of medication abortion, abortion methods included extra amniotic installation techniques. These methods are now considered outdated by the World Health Organization (WHO). When prostaglandin analogs were created at Karolinska Institutet, one of the first clinical applications studied was induced abortion. When mifepristone was created at the French pharmaceutical company Rousell Uclaf in the mid-1980s, it was only moderately effective in inducing abortion. However, the research group at the WHO collaborating center at Karolinska Institutet (KI) discovered that a combination of mifepristone and a low-dose prostaglandin analog was highly effective to induce uterine contractions. This was subsequently developed into the combined method of mifepristone and a prostaglandin analog, now known as medical abortion and used worldwide.

In the years that followed, many clinical trials leading to the development of medication abortion were conducted. Following the regulatory approval of medication abortion in 1992 (up to 9 weeks and in 1994 including second-trimester abortion), the ob-gyn department at Karolinska University Hospital, integrated with the WHO collaborating center, provided theoretical training to all ob-gyn residents and developed training curricula and national guidelines under the Swedish Society for Obstetrics and Gynaecology (SFOG). Following the development of medication abortion, abortion care also became part of the job description for nurse-midwives [4].

33.4 Abortion Care Provision

Abortion care is currently offered in public and private hospitals as well as clinics with permission from the BoHW. All ob-gyn clinical departments in Sweden are legally obliged to provide abortion, as it is considered mainstream health care. Abortion is considered "care that cannot be postponed" (similar to emergency care, it can't be denied). Abortion care is delivered by physicians and midwives. In Stockholm and a few other larger cities, outpatient clinics operating outside of the hospitals have permission to provide abortion during the first trimester. A vast majority of these outpatient clinics are publicly funded and the cost for the patient is the same as for abortions provided in hospitals. Most outpatient clinics limit abortion to gestational ages below ten weeks and by medication abortion, while hospitals provide medication and surgical abortion during the first trimester, and medication abortion during the second trimester.

In Sweden and the other Nordic countries, surgical second-trimester abortion has been completely replaced by medication abortion for two reasons: (1) because the surgical method requires more training to be equally safe as medication abortion; (2) because there are too few second-trimester abortions performed per institution for personnel to allow training and to maintain required skills. Women have a choice to self-administer misoprostol at home or in the clinic. Counseling via telemedicine is currently investigated, as is allowing self-administration of abortion medications.

33.5 Abortion Training and Practice Integration

33.5.1 Medical Students

There are seven universities in Sweden with medical schools, and midwifery programs are offered at twelve universities or colleges. The curricula for medical students are similar at all universities, but the exact order of the individual courses varies. Students enter undergraduate medical school after finishing high school and spend eleven semesters in course work and core rotations followed by a twenty-two-month internship in which the student rotates in surgery, internal medicine, psychiatry and general medicine. Students then sit for an exam before a licence can be issued by the BoHW. Within the next few years, the present curricula will change to a six-year medical school program to adapt to EU regulations. Ob-gyn and pediatrics are taught during the tenth or eleventh semester of medical school and students usually spend eight weeks in ob-gyn. The learning objectives include abortion (all methods and gestational ages) with regard to legal, medical and ethical aspects. It is not mandatory to do a clinical rotation in the abortion clinic, although it is officially recommended. It is possible to opt out from the clinical rotation in the abortion clinic (although students rarely do so) but not from the obligatory seminars or from reaching the theoretical learning objectives.

33.5.2 Ob-Gyn Resident Training

The duration and content of residency training depend on the specialty, regulated by the BoHW, which issues the specialist certificate upon completion of learning objectives and obligatory courses. Specialization in ob-gyn can be achieved within approximately five years of training. In contrast to medical students, ob-gyn residents cannot opt out of abortion training [5]. Abortion has been part of the practical ob-gyn residency training since the current abortion law came into force. However, in the past decade, the theoretical, three- to four-day course in abortion and contraception, provided by SFOG, has been obligatory for all residents. Theoretical courses have to be documented and certificates submitted to the BoHW to obtain a specialist certificate. The curricula, including learning outcomes, basic and more advanced knowledge and skills for residents in ob-gyn, was created by SFOG and approved by the BoHW. Abortion care in Sweden is organized based on the size of the hospital and patient volume. Some hospitals have specialized abortion clinics, while other hospitals integrate abortion in their outpatient clinics. All residents take care of second-trimester abortion patients because these patients are treated in gynecological clinics. Each clinic has a director for resident training, and each resident has an appointed supervisor who certifies that the resident has met the expected skills acquisition including those in abortion care. Competence is not measured in time spent in learning, but in quality and performance. Time spent in abortion clinics and the number of abortions performed independently are not fixed but vary by resident competence and usually amount to several weeks spent providing abortion care.

33.5.3 Midwives in Abortion Care

Nurse-midwives in Sweden have a three-year-long university education to become nurses and then eighteen months of additional training to become midwives. Since 2016, the Swedish Association of Midwives is responsible for developing a description of core competencies for registered nurse-midwives and issues recommendations for their expected knowledge and skills level and professional approach. Abortion care is listed as a core competency in the latest edition of their core competencies, "Description of Required Competences for Registered Midwives," from 2018 and includes the ability to provide relevant information and counsel women, the ability to provide care during induced abortions and care for women experiencing a spontaneous abortion, the ability to identify complications and provide adequate care [6]. Although all midwives learn basic information about legal, medical and ethical aspects of abortion in their theoretical training, clinical experience in abortion care during midwifery training is often limited. Thus, in order to be able to provide abortion care, they must complete advanced training. An investigation by the BoHW in 2008 suggested that delegating abortion care to midwives was an effective way of increasing access to abortion. Subsequently, SFOG took on a mandate, suggested by BoHW, to develop a formal training program for abortion care certification for nurse-midwives.

Following pilot training of individual nurse-midwives, the first formal course for nurse-midwives in abortion care was created by the SFOG Reference Group for Reproductive Health (FARG) in collaboration with the WHO Collaborating Center for Research and Research Training in Human Reproduction at Karolinska Institutet (WHO collaborating center). The first course was held jointly in 2013 by SFOG and the Swedish Association of Midwives (SBF). The first nurse-midwife-operated abortion care unit opened in 2009 at Karolinska University Hospital, for healthy women up to 9 weeks with a clear intrauterine pregnancy who opt for a medication abortion. In 2012, there were 9 operating units, and by 2016 an estimated 50 operating units were nurse-midwife led out of approximately 130 clinics offering abortion care.

For a nurse-midwife to be admitted to the course run by SFOG, he or she needs to have clinical experience in abortion care. The first part of the course is a theoretical component (approximately one week) and includes legal, ethical and medical aspects and counseling on abortion and post-abortion contraception. The second part of the course is practical and includes hands-on training in ultrasound, using both simulators and patients. After having completed the courses and a written exam, each nurse-midwife keeps a logbook and continues the practical training

under the supervision of a local mentor at the home clinic. A minimum of fifty supervised and fifty independent scans should be documented. A sample of ultrasound images are sent to course leaders for a second opinion. The certificate requires completion of the theoretical and practical courses, a written exam and an approved logbook and sample of ultrasound scans. Supervision is provided by ob-gyns.

33.5.3.1 Challenges with Training

There are two major challenges with training. First, training residents in uterine aspiration skills has become challenging, as few abortions (<10%) are done using surgical methods. Second, while women's values and preferences are said to be of the utmost importance, women are now mainly offered medication abortion and are only offered surgical abortion in hospital settings. For example, the midwifery-led clinics in the Stockholm region only offer medication abortion.

33.5.3.2 Conscientious Objection

Sweden does not allow conscientious objection to abortion provision, because abortion care is part of the job description for ob-gyns and midwives. A study of this legal framework demonstrated that it guarantees adequate access to reproductive health-care services by reducing barriers and delays and causes no negative impacts on providers. According to studies that have evaluated perceptions of abortion care among Swedish providers, both gynecologists and midwives support the existing abortion legislature and do not hesitate to take part in abortion care even though they sometimes are presented with complex and difficult situations when providing this care. They sometimes experience this work as complex but also gratifying [7].

33.6 Conclusion

The past forty-five years have seen a transition from a restricted legal environment with high rates of unsafe abortion to a society in which abortion care is widely accessible and socially acceptable. Legalization of abortion, the development of medication abortion, the legal protection of access to abortion, allowing midwifery provision, the implementation of research into clinical practice and mainstreaming of abortion care have all contributed to reduction in stigma and training of a cadre of abortion providers who are proud of their work. These changes have had and continue to have a significant impact on women's health and lives.

References

1. The Swedish Abortion Act (1974:595) www.riksdagen.se/sv/Dokument-Lagar/Lagar/Svenskforfattningssamling/Abortlag-1974595_sfs-1974-595/

2. SOU SOU. Abort i Sverige-Betänkande av Utredningen om utländska aborter. https://www.regeringen.se/49b6ab/contentassets/22f47f54bdc1451d8ad4d7c08e501de7/abort-i-sverige-del-1-missiv-kap.-6. 2005.

3. The Swedish official abortion statistics. www.socialstyrelsen.se/statistik/statistikefteramne/aborter

4. Kopp Kallner H, Gomperts R, Salomonsson E, Johansson M, Marions L, Gemzell-Danielsson K. The efficacy, safety and acceptability of medical termination of pregnancy provided by standard care by doctors or by nurse-midwives: a randomised controlled equivalence trial. *BJOG*. 2015 Mar;**122**(4):510–517.

5. Fiala C, Gemzell Danielsson K, Heikinheimo O, Guethmundsson JA, Arthur J. Yes we can! Successful examples of disallowing 'conscientious objection' in reproductive health care. *European J Contracept Reprod Health*. 2016 Jun;**21**(3):201–206.

6. The Swedish Association of Midwives. Description of core competencies for registered midwives; 2018. https://storage.googleapis.com/barnmorskeforbundet-se/uploads/2018/05/Kompetensbeskrivning-for-legitimerad-barnmorska-Svenska-Barnmorskeforbundet-2018.pdf

7. Andersson IM, Gemzell-Danielsson K, Christensson K. Caring for women undergoing second-trimester medical termination of pregnancy. *Contraception*. 2014 May;**89**(5):460–465. doi:10.1016/j.contraception.2014.01.012

Chapter

34

Abortion Training and Integration in the United Kingdom

Patricia A. Lohr and Lesley Regan

34.1 Introduction

In the United Kingdom,[1] the 1861 Offences Against the Person Act (OAPA) made having or providing an abortion a crime with a potential life sentence. The Abortion Act, passed in 1967 [1], did not replace the OAPA or decriminalize abortion. Rather, it defined the circumstances in which an abortion could be performed without the risk of prosecution. These include having two doctors agree that a woman meets one of five grounds (Table 34.1). In cases where an abortion is necessary to save a woman's life or prevent grave permanent injury, only one doctor's authorization is required. Most abortions are undertaken under clause C, which relates to the preservation of mental and physical health. When considering these clauses, doctors may apply the World Health Organization definition of health, which emphasizes the presence of well-being and not just the absence of disease. Doctors may also consider the impact of a pregnancy in a woman's foreseeable future.

The Abortion Act 1967 extended only to England, Scotland and Wales, leaving the OAPA as the governing statute in Northern Ireland. As a result, only rarely have lawful abortions been undertaken there. The OAPA was repealed in Northern Ireland in October 2019 but, at the time of writing this chapter, a framework for service delivery is not yet in place. Almost all women in Northern Ireland who need an abortion are forced to travel to Britain or another country to access services, or obtain abortifacient medications online [2], placing them at risk of criminal prosecution.

---

[1] The United Kingdom of Great Britain and Northern Ireland, or UK, is made up of four countries; England, Scotland, Wales and Northern Ireland. Britain or Great Britain refers to the landmass of England, Scotland and Wales.

Table 34.1 Statutory grounds for legal abortion in Britain

A	The continuance of the pregnancy would involve risk to the life of the pregnant woman than if the pregnancy were terminated.
B	The termination is necessary to prevent grave permanent injury to the physical or mental health of the pregnant woman.
C	The pregnancy has NOT exceeded its 24th week and that the continuance of the pregnancy would involve risk, greater than if the pregnancy were terminated, of injury to the physical or mental health of the pregnant woman.
D	The pregnancy has NOT exceeded its 24th week and that the continuance of the pregnancy would involve risk, greater than if the pregnancy were terminated, of injury to the physical or mental health of any existing child(ren) of the family of the pregnant woman.
E	There is a substantial risk that if the child were born it would suffer from such physical or mental abnormalities as to be seriously handicapped.

By law, only doctors may perform abortions, but it is permitted to share some responsibilities with other members of a health-care team. Nurses and midwives, for example, commonly undertake pre-abortion assessments and manage most aspects of medication abortion [3]. However, they may not authorize an abortion, prescribe abortifacient drugs or provide a termination of pregnancy service alone without a doctor retaining overall responsibility [4]. It is often assumed that only doctors can perform surgical abortions, although a legal analysis of the 1967 Act published in 2017 concluded that it would be lawful for appropriately trained nurses or midwives, to carry out uterine aspirations when acting as part of a multidisciplinary team [5].

The Abortion Act also stipulates that abortions may only be performed in National Health Service (NHS) hospitals or places approved by the Secretary of State for Health. Until 2018, when "home" was approved as a place where women could take their prescribed misoprostol as part of an early medication abortion regimen [6], the other places were mainly regulated abortion clinics in the independent sector and private hospitals.

34.2 Past and Current Context for Abortion Care

The Abortion Act received royal assent in October 1967 and came into force in Britain six months later. Eight months of data were collected in 1968, and 23,641 abortions were recorded for England and Wales [7] and 1,500 in Scotland [8]. Numbers increased sharply in the first 3 years after the Act and generally continued to rise until the early 2000s. Since then, numbers have slightly fluctuated, but remained around 200,000 per year. In 2018, there were 218,581 abortions reported across Britain [7].

Abortion after legalization was undertaken mainly in NHS hospitals [9]. Within individual hospitals, whether and for whom abortion was available depended on the opinions of senior gynecologists. For example, some services restricted abortion to married women or those who already had children, and some imposed tight catchment areas or applied gestational limits lower than those permitted by the Act [10]. This led to considerable geographical disparity in service delivery, with many women being forced to travel long distances to access care, or to pay private providers for abortions they should have been able to obtain at no additional cost through the NHS [9,10].

In those hospitals where the clinicians were committed to facilitating abortion care, terminations of pregnancy were recognized as a crucial component of women's health care and became a standard part of a gynecologist's day-to-day practice. First-trimester abortions were undertaken surgically with uterine aspiration and those in the second trimester by medication induction using instillation of prostaglandins [11]. Importantly, medical student exposure to abortions in these settings was routine because abortion procedures were included in most elective surgical lists. However, for young ob-gyns training in hospitals where abortion was not provided, trying to develop these important skills was difficult and required special arrangements for clinical placements or rotations elsewhere. Sadly, this meant that all too often these trainees – the next generation of consultant gynecologists – missed out on gaining the vital practical experience they needed to ensure that they could look after their patients' needs in the future.

In the fifty years since the Act was passed, there have been several attempts to change the law, but only one has been successful. In 1990, an amendment to the Human Fertilization and Embryology Act reduced the upper gestational age limit for abortion for grounds C and D from twenty-eight to twenty-four weeks. In general, however, social attitudes in Britain have become more liberal, and the practice of clinical medicine, including abortion care, has shifted from a paternalistic approach toward one that respects people's autonomy and decisions [12]. Although the requirement for two doctors to authorize an abortion remains in place, the health-related grounds for abortion are now interpreted very broadly by most doctors and present few barriers to care [13].

Another particularly important aspect of abortion care that has changed in the UK since the passage of the 1967 Act is the location of provision. As the number of abortions increased in Britain, NHS hospitals failed to increase capacity to meet demand and were slow to adopt outpatient models of care [9,14]. In England, during the 1970s and 1980s this led to a large proportion of abortions being undertaken in private clinics at great cost to women. In an attempt to address these shortfalls, the NHS subcontracted much of their abortion workload to non-profit independent-sector abortion clinics in the 1990s, which resulted in a dramatic decline in the number of women needing to pay for private care and did improve access to abortion [14]. Today, 98% of abortions in the UK are funded by the NHS and are therefore free for women at the point of delivery [7]. Since June 2017, funding has also been available for women residents in Northern Ireland to enable them to travel from there to Britain to obtain abortion care. Some service constraints persist, particularly for those needing abortion care in a hospital [15], but most women in the UK are now able to access funded care that is close to home.

Almost three quarters of abortions in England and Wales are now provided by independent-sector organizations on behalf of the NHS [7]. They may operate from freestanding clinics or may be delivered from, but not integrated into, NHS hospitals or GP practices. In Scotland, abortions are only provided by the NHS, either from hospitals or community sexual and reproductive health clinics. Services in Scotland are limited to about eighteen weeks of gestation for clauses C and D. After this point in pregnancy, women must travel from Scotland to England to access a termination, mainly in the independent sector.

Ninety percent of abortions are performed at less than thirteen weeks of gestation [7]. In England and Wales, over 80% of abortions in the first ten weeks of pregnancy are undertaken medically but after that gestational age 66 to 87% of abortions are performed surgically [7]. In Scotland, medication abortion predominates at all gestations, and dilation and evacuation (D&E) as a method of second-trimester abortion is not available.

Although the Act stipulates that only a "registered medical practitioner," meaning a doctor, may terminate a pregnancy, nurses and midwives have played an integral role in the delivery of abortion care since legalization. In the late 1960s, nurses and midwives were responsible for most second-trimester abortions, which were induced by instilling prostaglandins into or around the amniotic sac. The doctor's involvement in these cases was often limited to inserting the catheter through which the medicine was administered. A nurse or midwife would attach the catheter to a pump, add the necessary infusion, turn on the pump, adjust the flow of prostaglandins as necessary and oversee the labor and delivery [4]. The legality of this degree of delegation was clarified in a case brought by the Royal College of Nursing (RCN) in 1981 [5]. The majority decision was that a doctor "should accept responsibility" for all stages of treatment, but did not necessarily need to carry out specific actions him- or herself [5]. Mifepristone was registered for medication abortion in the UK in 1991 and is now used in combination with misoprostol for most abortions up to ten weeks' gestation and has superseded instillation techniques in the second trimester. The role of nurses and midwives in the delivery of this method of abortion has grown with its increasing use.

Nurses and midwives now plan, lead and manage a significant proportion of care for women undergoing medication abortion at all gestations, with doctors responsible largely for legal authorizations and prescription of medications [4].

34.3 Training and Education in Abortion Care

Undergraduate and post-graduate curricula in obstetrics and gynecology (ob-gyn) and sexual and reproductive health include learning objectives in abortion care, but these are implemented inconsistently. Over time, the number of abortions performed in NHS hospitals, which is where undergraduate and post-graduate training occurs, has declined significantly. This has reduced the opportunities for skills acquisition, role-modeling and mentorship in abortion care. There is limited formal training available for nurses and midwives, although they provide most of the medication abortion care in Britain.

The Royal College of Obstetricians and Gynaecologists (RCOG) has published a national undergraduate curriculum in ob-gyn that promotes standards for educational content in medical schools and is designed to provide medical students with the relevant competencies needed to practice as a foundation year[2] doctor [16]. A key learning outcome in the module on sexual and reproductive health is that students should understand and demonstrate appropriate knowledge, skills and attitudes in relation to abortion. This includes demonstrating the ability to take a history related to unplanned pregnancy and knowledge criteria on termination of pregnancy including mode of action and efficacy, methods, indications, contraindications and complications. The RCOG acknowledges that some students may hold a conscientious objection to the acquisition of knowledge and skills related to abortion. However, it believes and states that it is important

---

[2] Following graduation from medical school, trainees enter into a two-year foundation program prior to entering specialty training. The first year is aimed at attaining competence in essential clinical skills, communication and teamwork. In the second year, trainees have increasing responsibility for patient management decisions, learning about clinical effectiveness and leadership. www .foundationprogramme.nhs.uk

that undergraduates be familiar with the issues and with the management options. It also emphasizes that undergraduates and trainees must be aware of and able to recognize complications of abortion and trainees must be fully competent to provide appropriate emergency care during their career.

A new RCOG core curriculum for postgraduate training in ob-gyn was released in 2019 [17]. There are several specific knowledge requirements for abortion including the law, preprocedure assessment, methods (medication and surgical), identification of complications and aftercare. Other issues related to high-quality abortion care are also included, such as appreciating the issues of confidentiality, marginalized and vulnerable patient groups, service organizations and the importance of networks and multi-agency working. In regions of the UK where abortion is restricted, such as Northern Ireland, trainees remain responsible for having knowledge regarding abortion and managing a person presenting with an unplanned pregnancy. They are expected to gain full experience and competency in the practical procedures of medical management of miscarriage and surgical management of miscarriage (up to twelve weeks' gestation). These procedural skills are identical and therefore transferable for medication termination of pregnancy and surgical termination of pregnancy (up to twelve weeks' gestation).

In the last two years of training in ob-gyn, all trainees undertake at least two Advanced Training Skills Modules (ATSMs) to develop the skills in their specialist areas of interest. Since 2007, 5,284 trainees have registered for and 3,614 have successfully completed 1 of 20 ATSMs, which include subjects such as advanced labor ward, colposcopy and subfertility. An ATSM in Abortion Care has been available during this period, but only 33 trainees had completed it, in part due to a lack of available training sites within the NHS and a loss of focus by gynecologists on this skill as a key aspect of the specialty. The module was revamped and re-launched in 2018 as an Advanced Skills Module (ASM) in The Safe Practice in Abortion Care. It can be taken as an optional module of the Acute Gynecology & Early Pregnancy ATSM or a stand-alone module and is open to trainees as well as consultants that want to expand their skill set. Unlike the previous ATSM, surgical skills may be developed to one of three gestational ages up to

twenty-four weeks and there is a greater focus on management of complex cases. It is anticipated that the revised module will lead to improved uptake and facilitate the organization of appropriate placement into training centers, including the independent sector.

The Faculty of Sexual and Reproductive Healthcare (FSRH) includes unplanned pregnancy and abortion care in its specialty training in community sexual and reproductive health (CSRH). Previously, the training pathway in the UK in Sexual and Reproductive Healthcare was through Obstetrics and Gynecology as a subspecialty. In 2009, the UK Parliament recognized SRH as an independent specialty. Specialty training in CSRH is a six-year run-through program which includes three years of basic obstetrics, gynecology and sexual and reproductive health, followed by two intermediate years that include abortion care, and a final advanced training year to prepare for a role as a consultant. The knowledge and skills for abortion care for CSRH trainees are like ob-gyn, but with a lower gestational age limit for surgical skills acquisition (fourteen weeks' gestation). The FSRH aims to provide trainees with the knowledge, skills and attitudes to lead or establish an abortion service. The FSRH also have a Special Skills Module (SSM) in Abortion Care, which combines theoretical and practical components and is aimed at doctors, nurses, midwives and others who regularly work in sexual and reproductive health care and wish to expand or revise their knowledge and skills.

Formal education in abortion care is not integrated into nursing or midwifery pre-registration education, although midwives may be involved in co-management of medication terminations of pregnancy for fetal anomaly or pregnancy loss. A specific curriculum exists for the role of Clinical Nurse Specialist in Early Pregnancy Care, including miscarriage management up to twenty-four weeks of gestation. Nurses who have specialized in this area learn ultrasound skills and undertake medication and surgical management of early miscarriage. The Royal College of Nursing is engaged in an ongoing discussion about the need to extend nursing skills in abortion care. The SSM modules on consultation and early medication abortion may be taken by nurses and midwives, but most obtain "on the job" training when engaged to work in an abortion service.

As doctors progress through training, they collect evidence that demonstrates their development and acquisition of the key skills, procedures and knowledge. Examples include completion of e-learning or other courses, reflective practice accounts, and objective structured assessment of technical skills (OSATs), which are validated assessment tools that assess technical competency in a technique. Formative OSATS, which are supervised learning events, permit the trainee to practice and get feedback for a given procedure. Summative OSATS, which are an assessment of performance, are used to demonstrate competence in a procedure and progress in training. Evidence is reviewed by the trainee's Educational Supervisor who makes a global assessment of the progress against learning outcomes with the goal of demonstrating the ability to undertake activities independently.

Nurses or midwives who undertake the FSRH SSM modules similarly collect evidence to demonstrate competency in consultations and early medication abortion. Work-based training in the independent sector follows a similar model but is not nationally recognized or assessed against quality standards by regulatory or training bodies.

34.4 Conscientious Objection in Law and Training

There is a conscientious objection clause within the Abortion Act. This gives health-care professionals the legal right to opt out of participating in treatment except when an abortion is necessary to save the woman's life or prevent grave permanent injury. The General Medical Council [18] has guidance on how doctors with a conscientious objection must act. They are obliged to make sure a woman has enough information to arrange to see another doctor who does not object or, if it's not practical for a woman to arrange to see another doctor herself, the doctor must provide or facilitate a prompt referral. Professional standards and guidance on the limited application of the clause as it relates to nurses and midwives are also available [4,19].

The core curriculum in ob-gyn includes guidance for those whose personal beliefs conflict with the provision of abortion [17]. Trainees considering a career in ob-gyn are encouraged to discuss concerns with program directors or heads of schools before embarking on training. If issues

arise once training has commenced, trainees are encouraged to meet with their Educational Supervisor for support to find a solution. The FSRH has similar guidance [20] and will award qualifications to those who fulfill all training requirements and are willing to show that they will put patient care first, regardless of their personal beliefs [21].

To achieve qualifications in ob-gyn and CSRH, a doctor must be willing to participate in the provision of all forms of care excepting that which is defined as protected by conscientious objection in the 1967 Abortion Act. In addition, any part of the curriculum may be assessed in examinations. This can include knowledge and practical assessment of the provision of contraception (all methods including emergency contraception) and abortion care but will not include the demonstration of the skills to perform an abortion procedure. Competencies not attempted because of conscientious objections should be clearly recorded and signed by the trainer.

34.5 Challenges

In 2008, a joint RCOG/FSRH study day was held to identify what is not working in the delivery of abortion care in the UK, how it should be addressed and by whom. A consensus report [22] identified insufficient and variable educational opportunities in abortion care as a significant contributor to inadequate service provision. This was viewed as problematic not only for skills acquisition but also for the ability of students and trainees to gain an understanding of women's views and experiences of abortion and the significance of abortion to their future practice. The meeting participants also noted that specialty trainees in ob-gyn often failed to participate in abortion services during their training years. This was attributed to a lack of interest or competition with other specialty or core requirements, rather than a confirmed conscientious objection. The deficiency of clinical provision in training hospitals in areas where some or all provision was contracted out to the independent sector was also highlighted.

A survey of UK medical schools conducted in 2019 showed that, in practice, it remains the case that undergraduate medical education on abortion varies widely and is subject to a range of barriers (Jayne Kavanagh, personal communication). The number of hours allocated to teaching and the range of topics covered were not consistent, with most medical schools spending fewer than two hours teaching the clinical aspects of abortion and 15% having no compulsory clinical teaching at all. Respondents cited lack of curriculum time and willing staff to teach, difficulty in accessing clinical placements and the perception of abortion as a sensitive topic as impeding their ability to provide comprehensive abortion education. Most respondents requested further guidance on teaching from institutions such as the Institute for Medical Ethics, RCOG and FSRH. These findings were supported by a letter to the editor and two rapid responses published in the *BMJ* where medical education in abortion care at three schools was described as lacking in clinical content and exposure to direct patient care [23].

These problems also persist in post-graduate training despite improvements in written curricula. As a result, services – whether in hospital or not – struggle to hire staff or may only be able to hire individuals with limited skills requiring lengthy periods of workplace-based training. It has also led to a crisis in hospital-based abortion services where the management of women who have medical or other comorbidities and cannot be managed in freestanding independent sector clinics is seriously compromised [15]. Even where hospitals do provide care, it is often limited to the first trimester. Where second-trimester care is provided, gestational age limits or indications (eg, terminations only for fetal anomaly but not so-called social reasons) are imposed, and methods may be limited to medication induction.

Post-graduate training in the UK is modular and therefore may be provided at several hospitals and under different educational supervisors. The approach to training has the potential for trainees to discuss their status with regard to conscientious objection across training years, but there is no formal process defined for this to occur. Partial participation is not a model of education in abortion care that has been adopted formally and programs typically take an "opt-in" approach. In most cases, trainees have inconsistent and limited exposure to clinical abortion services, women who need or want an abortion, and to senior clinicians who integrate abortion regularly into their practice or lead termination services. There are currently no clear pathways to training

in the independent sector for those who are motivated to obtain these skills despite the limitations of the hospitals in which they are training. This has impacted core as well as advanced training in abortion care, with very few trainees either taking up the advanced module or only being able to complete first-trimester and perhaps early second-trimester competencies. Only rarely have trainees, either in ob-gyn or community and sexual and reproductive health care, succeeded in gaining support to train out of service in the independent sector, or to gain second-trimester surgical abortions skills.

For nurses and midwives, the absence of specific abortion-related training in their pre-registration years means most obtain skills while already in practice. While the FSRH has opened their SSM to registered and practicing nurses and midwives, most struggle to take time away from work to complete the competencies. Very few have therefore engaged with this formal training pathway. Since the SSM began in 2006, fifty-two individuals have competed it and of these, five were nurses.

34.6 Looking to the Future

Abortion is recognized as an essential component of comprehensive reproductive health care in the UK. It is funded by the National Health Service in almost all cases and most women can access the care they need without delay and close to home. Recent changes to the law governing abortion in Northern Ireland will result in the availability of legal abortion there when training and services can be established.

Guidance from the National Institute for Health and Care Excellence (NICE) released in 2019 [24] made specific recommendations to improve education and training in abortion. It recognized the important role of nurses and midwives, advocating for their involvement to be "maximized." In addition, it recommended that trainee health-care professionals and students who may care for women who request an abortion (eg, nurses, midwives and GPs) should have the chance to gain experience in termination services. Specialties that include abortion in the core curriculum were recommended to ensure training was provided on an opt-out (rather than opt-in) basis and include practical experience of abortion services and procedures in the curriculum. The guidance also recommended that trainees should be able to gain experience with whoever is providing abortion care in their area (ie, either in the NHS or in the independent sector).

Medical, nursing and midwifery colleges throughout the UK are actively working on improving the status of education in abortion care. A webinar organized by the British Society of Abortion Care Providers set out what effective undergraduate medical education might look like, and work is currently being undertaken to develop guidance on how to provide teaching that equips junior doctors to do abortions or treat complications in a clinically, legally, professionally and ethically robust way. The RCOG established an Abortion Task Force in 2017 to improve abortion services and training, and the Royal College of Nursing has published a report with recommendations for further work on career pathways, progression and skills development for nurses in abortion care [25].

It is anticipated that these various streams of concerted work on abortion education supported by the NICE guideline recommendations, will improve the status of abortion education in the UK and therefore, contribute to the creation of equitable service delivery.

References

1. Abortion Act 1967. https://www.legislation.gov.uk/ukpga/1967/87/contents

2. Aiken ARA, Gomperts R, Trussell J. Experiences and characteristics of women seeking and completing at-home medical termination of pregnancy through online telemedicine in Ireland and Northern Ireland: a population-based analysis. *BJOG*. 2017;**124**(8):1208–1215.

3. Berer M. Provision of abortion by mid-level providers: international policy, practice and perspectives. *Bull World Health Organ*. 2009;**87**(1):58–63.

4. Royal College of Nursing. *Termination of Pregnancy: An RCN Nursing Framework*. London: RCN; 2013.

5. Sheldon S, Fletcher J. Vacuum aspiration for induced abortion could be safely and legally performed by nurses and midwives. *J Fam Plan Reprod Heal Care*. 2017;**43**(4):260–264.

6. Royal College of Obstetricians & Gynaecologists, FSRH, BSACP. *Clinical Guidelines for Early Medical Abortion at Home - England*. RCOG/BSACP Home Use Misoprostol Guidance; 2018.

7. DHSC. *Abortion Statistics for England and Wales: 2018.*

London: Department of Health and Social Care; 2019; last update 2020. www.gov.uk/government/statistics/abortion-statistics-for-england-and-wales-2018

8. ISD. *Termination of Pregnancy Statistics: Year Ending December 2016*. Information Services Division Publication Report. NHS, National Services Scotland; 2017.

9. Lewis TLT. Legal abortion in England and Wales 1968–78. *BMJ*. 1980;**280**(6210):295–296.

10. Davis G, O'Neill J, Parker C, Sheldon S. All aboard the "Abortion Express": geographic variability, domestic travel and the 1967 Abortion Act. In S Sethna, G Davis (Eds.), *Abortion across Borders: Transnational Travel and Access to Abortion Services*. Baltimore: Johns Hopkins University Press; 2019.

11. Munday D, Francome C, Savage W. Twenty one years of legal abortion. *BMJ*. 1989;**298** (6682):1231–1234.

12. Lee E, Sheldon S, Macvarish J. The 1967 Abortion Act fifty years on: abortion, medical authority and the law revisited. *Soc Sci Med*. 2018;**212**:26–32.

13. Küng SA, Darney BG, Saavedra-Avendaño B, Lohr PA, Gil L. Access to abortion under the heath exception: a

comparative analysis in three countries. *Reprod Health*. 2018;**15**(1):107.

14. Paintin D. *Abortion Law Reform in Britain 1964–2003: A Personal Account*. Stratford upon Avon: British Pregnancy Advisory Service; 2015.

15. British Pregnancy Advisory Service. *Medically Complex Women and Abortion Care*. London: BPAS; 2018.

16. RCOG. *National Undergraduate Curriculum in Obstetrics and Gynaecology*; n. d. www.rcog.org.uk/globalassets/documents/careers-and-training/undergraduate-curriculum/undergraduatecurriculum_og.pdf

17. Royal College of Obstetricians and Gynaecologists. *Core Curriculum for Obstetrics & Gynaecology*; 2019.

18. General Medical Council. *Personal Beliefs and Medical Practice*. London: GMC; 2013. www.gmc-uk.org/guidance.

19. Nursing and Midwifery Council. *The Code: Professional Standards of Practice and Behaviour for Nurses, Midwives and Nursing Associates*. London; 2018. https://www.nmc.org.uk/standards/code/

20. Guidance for those undertaking or recertifying FSRH qualifications whose

personal beliefs conflict with the provision of abortion or any method of contraception London: Faculty of Sexual and Reproductive Healthcare. www .fsrh.org/documents/guidance-for-those-undertaking-or-recertifying-fsrh/

21. Kasliwal A, Hatfield J. Conscientious objection in sexual and reproductive health – a guideline that respects diverse views but emphasises patients' rights. *BMJ Sex Reprod Health.* 2018;**44**(1):5–6.

22. RCOG/FSRH. Abortion Care Study Day, 28 April 2008 – Consensus Statement. 2008.

23. Burton R. UK medical students should be taught how to manage unwanted pregnancy. *BMJ.* 2018;362:k3800. doi:10.1136/gmj.k3800

24. National Institute for Health and Care Excellence. NICE guideline: Abortion care (NG 140); 2019. www.nice.org.uk/ guidance/ng140

25. Royal College of Nursing. *Nursing Education in Termination of Pregnancy Services.* London: RCN; 2019. www.rcn.org.uk/professional-development/publications/ pub-007959

Chapter

35

Abortion Training and Integration in Ireland

Mary Higgins, Cliona Murphy and Maeve Eogan

35.1 Introduction

A 2018 referendum in the Republic of Ireland supported, by a significant majority, the introduction of more liberal provision of abortion care. Prior to this, abortions could only be legally provided when there was a "real and substantial risk to the life of the mother," thus restricting abortion care to limited and often high-risk emergency care. The legal barrier to abortion was based on an amendment to the constitution of Ireland (the eighth amendment), which provided a constitutional protection to the life of the unborn child. By January 2019, women living in the Republic could have access to abortion care that was "free, safe and legal." The development and integration of this service, the education of care providers and the challenge to the interpretation of the legal framework in the context of care provision have been challenging.

This chapter reviews the current system for provision of abortion care under the four legal sections – to pregnant people under twelve weeks' gestation, those with physical or mental health issues, those carrying pregnancies affected by a fetal anomaly and those with an emergency issue in the pregnancy. Educational programs that were provided prior to the introduction of the service and continue to be provided are described. Challenges, both anticipated and unanticipated, are discussed.

35.2 Past and Current Context

35.2.1 History

Abortion was first legally prohibited in Ireland by the Offences against the Person Act of 1861. A referendum in 1983 added the "eighth amendment" to the Irish Constitution that provided protection to fetal life stating that the "State acknowledges the right to life of the unborn, and with due regard to the equal right to life of the mother, guarantees in its laws to respect, and, as far as is practicable, by its laws to defend that right." This amendment to the constitution was passed by a large majority. Several legal cases challenged this, and all were initially upheld due to the need for another constitutional amendment.

35.2.2 The Political and Legal Journey

It became increasingly clear that there was a need for another referendum to put the option of an extended abortion service to the vote in Ireland. Three significant steps preceded this:

1. A "Citizens Assembly" allowed one hundred "ordinary" Irish citizens, representative of the population at large, to debate the topic of abortion provision. The Citizens Assembly heard from national and international experts as well as people who had been directly affected by the legal situation. The Assembly voted overwhelmingly in support of an extended abortion provision.

2. A committee of elected parliamentary representatives reviewed the findings and recommendations of the Citizens Assembly. The committee also made further "ancillary" recommendations, including universal access to routine antenatal ultrasound, extensive education for children and teenagers on sexual health and contraception and government-funded contraception.

3. A draft Bill on Termination of Pregnancy was prepared to inform the electorate on the proposed legal framework.

The 2018 referendum resulted in two thirds of the voting population supporting repeal of the constitution. The proposed Bill was passed into law [1], and it was announced that provision of care would start on January 1, 2019. This resulted in an extensive multidisciplinary national project to provide education, develop care pathways and write guidance prior to the start date.

35.2.3 How Abortion Care Is Provided in the Republic of Ireland

While official numbers are not yet available, the impression is that most abortions are early medication abortions (EMAs) provided in community care under nine weeks' gestation. Between nine and twelve weeks' gestation, referral to hospital occurs. Up to twelve weeks' gestation (defined as twelve weeks plus zero days), a person does not have to disclose the reason why they are requesting termination of pregnancy. After twelve weeks' gestation, an abortion can only be provided if there is a severe fetal anomaly or significant risk to the pregnant person's life or severe risk to their health. Clinical Guidance Documents were prepared and disseminated by the relevant post-graduate training bodies to assist clinical staff with care provision and certification and notification obligations (Figure 35.1).

Information on abortion care is freely available via a website provided by the Health Service Executive (www.myoptions.ie) and supported by a national free telephone line. The website provides links to further information and support and access to extensive information booklets on both medication and surgical abortion.

The national free telephone line provides the following:

- How to access the abortion service
- Counseling
- Nurse-midwife-provided information on complications post abortion care

Both the information and counseling services are largely provided within daytime hours; nurse-provided information on possible post-abortion complications is available on a 24/7 basis.

35.2.3.1 Abortion Care under Twelve Weeks' Gestation [2]

Pregnant women have the option of early medication (EMA, provided in the community and within hospitals) or surgical abortion (hospital only). Unlike other jurisdictions, there are no stand-alone abortion clinics. At under nine weeks' gestation, most pregnant women access abortion care in the community unless they have a contra-indication to medication abortion. Between nine and twelve weeks' gestation, care is provided in a hospital setting.

Prior to initiation of service, there was much discussion about the appropriate model of care. Some community doctors were concerned that there was insufficient capacity and knowledge within primary care. Within secondary and tertiary care (stand-alone maternity hospitals and general hospitals with an obstetrics and gynaecology [ob-gyn] department), some suggested abortion clinics were the best option, separate from other care. These suggestions were resisted, as they risked stigmatization and silo working. In reality, integrating care within these clinical services has allowed those attending to maintain privacy and confidentiality and has enabled provision of a respectful patient-centered approach to care.

There is a legally mandated three-day wait period between certification of a pregnancy being less than twelve weeks and commencement of the abortion process (surgical termination or administration of mifepristone). Therefore, (non-emergency) termination of pregnancy will always require at least two consultations. Medical advocates argued, however, that this wait was not medically indicated or evidence based.

At the first community visit, the doctor confirms that the pregnancy is less than nine weeks' gestation. If an ultrasound is required, a referral is made to a funded national ultrasound service. It is the person's own decision whether they wish to view the images or listen to the fetal heartbeat.

A significant advantage of community provision of EMA below nine week's gestation is that following administration of mifepristone, the person is given the appropriate dose of misoprostol to administer at home. A low-sensitivity pregnancy test is also provided to use two weeks following the abortion.

There is an option for a post-abortion follow-up visit to discuss further issues including provision of contraception if it was not possible to provide this at the time of the abortion. As in other countries, the attendance rate for follow-up is low.

Above nine weeks' gestation, a comparable process occurs (but within a hospital setting), an ultrasound is performed and the option of medication or surgical abortion will depend on the wishes of the pregnant person, their gestational age, medical background and local factors.

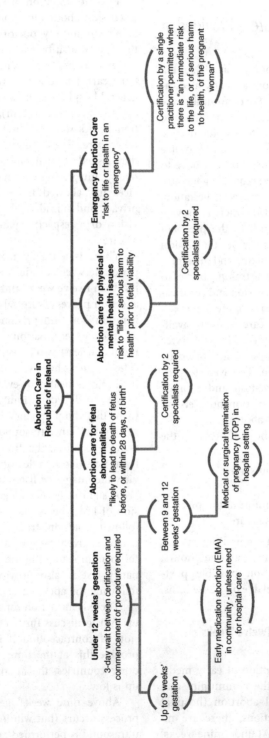

Figure 35.1 Abortion care algorithm

Medication termination has easier access than surgical at present in many centers.

Unfortunately, as the ancillary recommendation for free contraception has not yet been implemented, options for contraception are dependent on the financial means of the patient. Multiple advocacy groups, including medical advocates, continue to call for provision of funded contraception.

For those with a Rhesus-negative blood group, immunoglobulin is offered over seven weeks' gestation. This recommendation acknowledges the low risk of sensitization at this gestation but was based on extensive review of international guidelines and evidence. It is hoped that further research will clarify the quantum of this risk and inform future guidelines regarding prophylaxis. At present, those over seven weeks will have their blood group checked, and if negative they must be referred to a hospital for immunoglobulin administration. However, this additional visit is a barrier for some people. Antibiotics are prescribed for those undergoing surgical abortion.

35.2.3.2 Abortion Care for Fetal Abnormalities [3]

Abortion for fetal abnormalities is legally permitted if two specialists (one obstetrician and one "medical professional of a relevant speciality," eg, a neonatologist, fetal cardiologist or fetal medicine specialist) are of the reasonable opinion formed in good faith that there is a fetal condition "likely to lead to the death of the foetus either before, or within 28 days of, birth." This definition therefore excludes non-fatal conditions, even if there is a significant risk of severe disability.

Conditions such as anencephaly, bilateral renal agenesis, thanatophoric dysplasia and triploidy are fatal fetal abnormalities / severe life-limiting conditions in which the diagnosis and prognosis are unequivocal. It is more challenging to provide a definitive opinion where there is a potential fatal abnormality but the prognosis is not clear during the pregnancy and becomes clear after birth. As with other areas of medicine, if there is a difficulty in achieving consensus, then a multidisciplinary team opinion is sought so that the most appropriate advice is provided.

A significant challenge in the provision of care for fetal abnormalities is the lack of a routine antenatal ultrasound service across the country. Of the nineteen antenatal units within the Republic, only one third provide routine universal anatomy ultrasound between eighteen and twenty-two weeks' gestation [4]. Those wishing to undergo first-trimester screening for aneuploidy must "opt in" and will pay individually for this service. This has been highlighted as a barrier to provision of high-quality antenatal care, and a recommendation was made that there should be universal first- and second-trimester ultrasound assessment, independent of geographic location.

Following a diagnosis of a significant fetal abnormality, referral is generally made to a fetal medicine specialist for confirmation of the anomaly, further assessment and investigation and discussion of options.

Those with a significant abnormality have three main options:

1. To continue in the pregnancy, with postnatal options of therapeutic care or palliative care as appropriate
2. If the anomaly meets the legal criteria, to undergo an abortion within the Republic of Ireland
3. If the anomaly does not meet the legal criteria, and the parent(s) do not wish to continue with the pregnancy, to travel to another jurisdiction for an abortion

There is currently minimal experience with second-trimester surgical abortion care within the clinical community in the Republic of Ireland and medication abortion is therefore usually the option for second-trimester fetal anomalies. It is acknowledged that surgical second-trimester abortion is the preference for some pregnant people, and this expertise needs to be developed. It is also acknowledged that feticide, though potentially emotionally challenging for clinical staff and for patients, is an appropriate part of abortion care for many close to viability. Neither feticide nor second-trimester surgical abortions are curricular requirements for general ob-gyn training but will need to be integrated in subspecialist education programs. Colleagues in the United Kingdom have offered to support training in this area.

Following termination of pregnancy for fetal abnormalities, families are offered a package of care like that provided for intrauterine deaths. As an example, access to specialist bereavement midwives or nurses, input from appropriate chaplaincy or religious support groups and referral to counseling services are provided. "Memory-making" activities (taking footprints, professional photography, keeping the baby in the mother's room and allowing family to visit) are available for those who want them. While there is a limited perinatal postmortem service nationally, there is an option to have an examination if this may be useful to guide advice for future pregnancies or give a definitive diagnosis.

35.2.3.3 Abortion Care for Maternal Medical or Mental Health Issues [5]

Abortion for maternal physical or mental health issues is legally permitted if two specialists (one obstetrician and one "appropriate medical professional") agree there is a "risk to the life or of serious harm to the health of the pregnant women," the "fetus has not reached viability" and it is "appropriate to carry out the termination in order to avert the risk" to the life or health of the pregnant person.

Like the fetal criteria, the expertise of the second medical professional depends on the clinical condition (eg, nephrology, oncology).

What is immediately obvious is that the definition of "severe harm to health" is an objective one. If there is a difference in opinion, it is possible to obtain a second opinion via a review process or to seek a wider multidisciplinary input. Multidisciplinary involvement is also important in planning and advising care regardless of whether the woman continues the pregnancy or decides to seek an abortion.

35.3 Abortion Training and Practice Integration

Education on abortion care was challenging, as this was a new area of practice for most clinicians. Clinicians had familiarity with abortion care in lifesaving emergencies (eg, chorioamnionitis), and several clinicians working in the Republic of Ireland completed training abroad and gained experience in abortion in that context. Furthermore, nearly all clinicians had familiarity with the provision of post-abortion care after women had accessed abortions abroad (or had taken medications at home) and developed post-abortion complications.

Even though a huge number of doctors publicly supported the referendum to repeal the eighth amendment and saw the overwhelming referendum result as a significant mandate to introduce a world-class responsive women's health service, there was much discussion in both community and hospital services on implementing a new service in the context of underfunding of primary care, maternity and gynecology services. Gynecology waiting lists are extensive, many maternity units are providing care in overburdened and infrastructurally outdated clinical sites and studies have reported low morale among doctors, with burnout at an all-time high [6,7]. There was concern about the rush to implement the service, with political expediency seeming to outweigh practical issues and areas of concern. As data on the number of women from Ireland accessing termination of pregnancy prior to 2019 were only estimates, there were concerns that general practice (GP) and hospital-based providers would be overwhelmed by the numbers of women requesting termination of pregnancy, and unable to safely deliver care, once it was available in this jurisdiction.

35.3.1 Background Skill Set

A significant advantage in the introduction of abortion care was the extensive preexisting knowledge of clinicians in the care of women undergoing a miscarriage and intrauterine death.

In the Republic of Ireland, clinicians enter Family Practice (called General Practice) following structured post-graduate training four or five years after graduation from medical school; ob-gyn a nine- to ten-year program post–medical school. Most general practitioners (GPs) complete a four-month rotation through ob-gyn in hospital, and have additional exposure in community practice. A GP is trained to provide community care for miscarriage, and would have defined pathways of care for women requiring hospital care and additional supports following a miscarriage.

In ob-gyn, following completion of structured post-graduate training, most consultants (Attendings) continue to practice both ob-gyn. Even most of those in subspecialized positions still have familiarity with early pregnancy complications, mid-trimester pregnancy loss and intrauterine death. Clinicians working in ob-gyn are competent in the use of mifepristone, misoprostol and first-trimester uterine evacuation of retained pregnancy tissue (ERPC). Two areas in which the speciality identified a competency gap were the provision of feticide and second-trimester dilation and evacuation (D&E).

While the initial training priority was to ensure that sufficient GPs and trained obstetricians and gynecologists had the requisite competencies to deliver abortion care from early 2019 on, doctors in training also required education. While conscientious objection exempts a trainee from actively providing termination of pregnancy care (unless it is an emergency), it does not exempt a trainee from referring onward as appropriate, providing ancillary care and fulfilling curricular requirements including attending any mandatory courses. The training year commences in July every year, and abortion care has been included on the ob-gyn training curriculum starting in July 2019.

Essentially, this means that the expectation for trainees is that the theory of abortion care, and a course on values clarification, will be a mandatory component of their training program. Practical provision is an optional component of training, where trainees will be permitted to "opt out" based on moral or ethical grounds. To date, many of the senior trainees have opted in to provision of care under close consultant supervision, often due to conscientious provision and/or a practical appreciation that training in abortion care may be a desirable feature for permanent posts. Given the small numbers of abortions within a hospital setting, trainees do not currently have dedicated rotations in abortion care but instead integrate the practice into a general ob-gyn training year. Those undergoing a fellowship in maternal–fetal medicine will also have the option of training in more specialized counseling (for maternal and fetal cases) or in practical procedures such as feticide. Some recent graduates have opted for training in second-trimester surgical abortion as part of their training abroad.

It will be an option that trainees may complete basic and more advanced research in this area. For peer-reviewed publications, ethics applications often require detailed discussion of issues and extensive commentary on protection of data under the European Union data protection regulations (General Data Protection Regulation, GDPR) that may be too complex for trainee-level research unless linked to a full-time research year.

Medical schools will also need to adjust their curriculums and learning outcomes to reflect current clinical practice – a survey of the six medical schools in Ireland in 2017 revealed that only two provided training on termination of pregnancy [8].

The Irish Medical Council guidelines [9] recommended that while a doctor could have a conscientious objection to provision of care, this objection could not apply to referral or emergency situations. Some doctors strongly objected and advised that they were not willing to refer people for further care; a new version of the guidelines has been published and recommends that any doctor who objects to referral must provide the person with sufficient information to be able to attend another clinician who will provide a service. These guidelines apply to all doctors working within the Republic of Ireland. Breach of these guidelines may result in a Fitness to Practice review, though this has not yet been tested.

35.3.2 Technical Skills

As the time frame for implementation of service was short, the development and dissemination of relevant clinical guidance and models of care as well as service planning, multidisciplinary liaison and education had to happen concurrently. While there was a significant political and societal imperative to introduce this service promptly, which included a commitment to fund training and implementation, health-care professionals (obstetricians, GPs, nurses and midwives), hospital managers and post-graduate training bodies had to drive implementation prior to actual receipt of funding.

Contemporaneously, the bill was still passing through the requisite legal stages with various amendments and suggestions being tabled at parliamentary debates – indeed, the legislation was only signed into law on December 20, 2018, only a few working days prior to January 1, 2019, when clinical service was mandated to commence. In the final weeks of 2018, many formal and informal meetings and working groups were required to prepare best practice recommendations, ensure appropriate clinical interpretation of legislation and ensure that medical professionals were informed on all relevant aspects of this new service. The legislation includes the provision that "it shall be an offence for a person ... to intentionally end the life of a foetus otherwise than in accordance with the provisions of this Act," which heightened clinicians' anxiety in terms of ensuring that they fully understood all aspects of the legislation [1].

A wealth of information about best practice abortion care was accrued through visits to established clinical sites in the UK and Scandinavia, and experienced UK colleagues provided formal training on medication and surgical termination of pregnancy (including manual uterine vacuum aspiration, MVA). The formal training days also provided opportunities for (anonymous) case-based discussion and management of complications.

Visits to established clinical sites also informed local service development – international colleagues shared their experience of clinic structure, organization and design including provision of clinic-based MVA, surgical care (eg, integration of surgical termination with general ob-gyn operating room lists versus provision of care on "separate" operating room or day case schedules). International models for provision of funded contraception impressed us greatly; while our health service has publicly acknowledged a motivation to fund contraception in the context of abortion care, this has yet to materialize and was not within the scope of initial service development. Nevertheless, training on post-abortion contraception including long-acting reversible contraception (LARC) was included in the pre-implementation education. Education of community providers (GPs and family planning doctors) was also provided by the Irish College of General Practitioners (www.icgp.ie) and, in several geographic sites, by the START group (www.startireland.ie), a group of committed GP providers of abortion care.

35.3.3 Non-technical Skills

Every medical practitioner is aware that non-technical skills are a crucial part of patient care, hard to teach and easy to get wrong. With the introduction of more extensive abortion care, clinicians were keen to provide person-focused, kind, compassionate and appropriate clinical care. The use of appropriate language was highlighted as an area of educational need. Prior to 2018, "abortion" was a highly politicized word and clinicians preferred to use the abbreviation TOP (termination of pregnancy); following the advice of focus groups prior to implementation, clinicians learned to say "abortion," "pregnant person" and "unplanned pregnancy" (rather than "crisis pregnancy").

35.3.4 Values Clarification

Reform of Irish abortion law followed many years of societal debate, with strongly held, frequently polarized, opinions. Furthermore, in contrast to other aspects of care provision, this was a new departure – practitioners cannot "refuse" to attend an antenatal clinic or operating room, but doctors and nurse-midwives may refuse to participate in direct aspects of termination of pregnancy (unless the situation is an emergency). In tandem with this, however, health-care providers are expected to fulfill fiduciary duties – that is, to put the needs of their patients first, ahead of their own [10] – and practitioners who find themselves unable to deliver medically indicated care to their patients for reasons of their personal conscience still bear ethical responsibilities for them. The International Federation of Gynecology and Obstetrics (FIGO) addresses both sides of conscience regarding delivery of termination of pregnancy care in their "Ethical Guidelines on Conscientious Objection": "practitioners have the right to respect for their conscientious convictions in respect both not to undertake, and to undertake, the delivery of lawful procedures" [11].

It was clear, therefore, that clinical sites needed to offer health-care providers opportunities to discuss stigma, myths and concerns and indeed forums to differentiate their own personal beliefs and attitudes from the needs of women seeking termination of pregnancy. We were supported in doing this by colleagues from the Sexual and Reproductive Health division of the World Health Organization (WHO), who had also provided much support in informing the debate prior to legislative reform [12]. In the first instance, eight of these workshops occurred in a variety of geographic locations around the country, each accommodating about twenty multidisciplinary participants (medical, nursing, midwifery, medical social work etc). These were facilitated by colleagues from the WHO, who also supported local health-care providers to develop the skills to run these workshops again by "training the trainers." The workshops addressed a range of topics, including lessons learned from countries with liberal legislation but poor implementation, interventions that delay or limit access and potential consequences for health and human rights and the potential impact of both refusal and conscientious commitment to provide safe abortion care. They included group exercises on exploring personal values and professional responsibilities, and there was a commitment given that discussions would be respectful, solution focused and confidential.

35.3.5 Supporting Each Other

Abortion work is considered by some to be stigmatizing. Individual success in deflecting stigma is bolstered by three factors – a liberal political environment, support from family and friends and the strength of the clinical community [13]. While the Republic of Ireland was traditionally considered a very conservative community – and therefore with a high risk of stigma toward those providing abortion care – the overwhelming mandate provided by the population in voting for repeal suggested this had changed.

During the first few months of provision of care, there was an intense media interest in the service; it was common to have front page stories covering the implementation. This added to the pressure on clinicians providing abortion care.

Working closely together, joining international organizations such as the British Society of Abortion Care Providers and discussing difficult cases or new challenges as a group of providers have all helped to support each other and strengthen the community. One of the most valuable outcomes of the implementation of services are closer links between General Practice and Obstetrics and Gynaecology, links that we hope to continue with integration of training.

35.3.6 Challenges

The journey has started, but is by no means complete. At the time of writing, there continues to be significant geographic inequity in terms of access to hospital-based care for termination of pregnancy (except in an emergency). While most of the nineteen maternity units are providing ancillary supports (eg, blood group, Rhesus prophylaxis, ultrasound), medication and surgical termination of pregnancy is not being undertaken in all units.

A request to the health service executive (HSE) for a clinical lead to support ongoing training in abortion care remains unfunded. It is anticipated that appointment of this role could provide necessary knowledge, skills and support for clinicians who currently feel they lack the necessary competencies. Development of online training specific to the situation in Ireland is also crucial to maintain and further develop education among those providing and wishing to provide the service.

Some clinical sites are not offering service for reasons of conscientious objection. In a publicly funded health service, institutions must strive to deliver legally permitted care per their patients' needs. Despite this, no medical practitioner, nurse or midwife is obliged to carry out a procedure to which they have a consciences objection, and a service cannot be offered if none of the medical staff will deliver abortion care. Experience has shown that education on abortion can result in health-care staff being more willing to participate in the service. A coordinated nationwide program is required to ensure equity of access.

Additional legislation and service developments remain outstanding – legislation around safe access zones is required, as antiabortion protests have been more frequently seen at community clinics and GP practices than at hospital sites. Funding for post-abortion contraception is also imperative and is likely to be cost saving. Inaccessibility and high cost of contraception may be significant barriers to uptake; incorporating funded contraception into the abortion care package has been widely endorsed but remains outstanding.

Commitment to undertake ongoing audit, guideline and model of care review and legislative reform are important to ensure that we build on the immense body of work that has been done to date. Holistic abortion care in Ireland is already so much better than it was prior to 2019, but service user, institutional and clinician feedback must be integrated into ongoing developments to ensure optimal, equitable and responsive access to care.

It is important that we remain ambitious in building our services. Even though the initial role out was time pressured, we now can look at service and knowledge gaps and ensure these are remedied. Access to specialist components of care (eg, feticide and second-trimester surgical abortion) is required, and ongoing training of a group of providers in these areas of practice will be needed. Ideally, subspecialist training in sexual and reproductive health would ensure quality abortion care for future cohorts.

Despite the challenges and outstanding issues, the significant proportion of abortion care being provided by general practice and family planning doctors must be acknowledged. No hospital site has been numerically overwhelmed by the demand for medication or surgical abortion – women are choosing to attend community practitioners, and are doing so sufficiently early in pregnancy that the care can be completed in the community. This is a model of care we should be proud of, and a cohort of colleagues we must thank – community-based, early medication abortion means that hospital services can be reserved for women at later gestations, women with complications, fetal abnormalities or significant comorbidities.

35.4 Acknowledgment of International Support

As wider provision of abortion care was only recently introduced into the Republic of Ireland, this chapter reflects the very early stages of education and provision. With the imminent introduction of legal abortion, an extensive educational program was provided by both the Irish College of General Practitioners and the START doctors group, the Institute of Obstetricians and Gynaecologists, including the development of interim guidance documents, pathways of care and clinical updates.

We wish to sincerely thank several colleagues for their significant input in this educational process. Clinicians were welcomed to visit clinics in Scotland, England, Wales, Norway and other countries; colleagues in the WHO provided experience, evidence and support, emails and telephone calls crossed to Canada, the USA and Australia. People were generous with their time and expertise to help start the service only days after legislation was passed. Without this support and collegiality this would not have been possible. As some of the advocates for people accessing the service, in their names we thank everyone who helped and continues to help.

References

1. Health (Termination of Pregnancy) Act 2018, Government of Ireland. www.irishstatutebook.ie/eli/2018/act/31/enacted/en/html. Accessed May 8, 2019.

2. Institute of Obstetricians and Gynaecologists. *Interim Clinical Guidance. Termination of Pregnancy under 12 weeks.* Dublin: Institute of Obstetricians and Gynaecologists, Royal College of Physicians of Ireland; 2108. https://rcpi-live-cdn.s3.amazonaws.com/wp-content/uploads/2018/12/FINAL-INTERIM-CLINICAL-GUIDANCE-TOP-12WEEKS.pdf. Accessed May 8, 2019.

3. Institute of Obstetricians and Gynaecologists.*Interim Clinical Guidance. Pathway for Management of Fatal Fetal Abnormalities and/or Life Limiting Conditions Diagnosed during Pregnancy – Termination of Pregnancy.* Dublin: Institute of Obstetricians and Gynaecologists, Royal College of Physicians of Ireland; 2109. https://rcpi-live-cdn.s3.amazonaws.com/wp-content/uploads/2019/01/IOG-TOPFA-PATHWAY-FINAL-180119.pdf. Accessed May 8, 2019.

4. Hayes-Ryan D, McNamara K, Russell N, Kenny L, O'Donoghue K. Maternity ultrasound in the Republic of Ireland 2016; a review. *Ir Med J.* 2017; **110**(7): 598.

5. Institute of Obstetricians and Gynaecologists. *Interim Clinical Guidance. Risk to Life or Health of a Pregnant Woman in relation to Termination of Pregnancy.* Dublin: Institute of Obstetricians and Gynaecologists, Royal College of Physicians of Ireland; 2019. https://rcpi-live-cdn.s3.amazonaws.com/wp-content/uploads/2019/05/FINAL-DRAFT-TOP-GUIDANCE-RISK-TO-LIFE-OR-HEALTH-OF-A-PREGNANT-WOMAN-220519-FOR-CIRCULATION.pdf. Accessed July 5, 2019.

6. O'Connor P, Lydon S, O'Dea A, et al. A longitudinal and multicentre study of burnout and error in Irish junior doctors. *Postgrad Med J.* 2017; **93**(1105):660–664.

7. Hayes B, Prihodova L, Walsh G, Doyle F, Doherty S. Doctors don't Do-little: a national cross-sectional study of workplace well-being of hospital doctors in Ireland. *BMJ Open.* 2019;**9**:e025433.

8. Nuzum D, Higgins MF, Cotter R, O'Donoghue K. Learning from each other and working together with families in mind-perinatal bereavement education for medical and midwifery students in the Republic of Ireland. Presented as an abstract to the International Stillbirth Alliance meeting, Scotland, 2018.

9. Irish Medical Council. *Guide to Professional Conduct and Ethics for Registered Medical*

Practitioners, 8th ed. Dublin: Irish Medical Council; 2016.

10. Chavkin W, Abu-Odeh D, Clune-Taylor C, et al. Balancing freedom of conscience and equitable access. *Am J Public Health*. 2018;**108**:(11) 1487–1488.

11. FIGO Committee for the Ethical Aspects of Human Reproduction and Women's Health.Ethical guidance on conscientious objection. *Int J Gynecol Obstet*. 2006;**92**:333–334.

12. *Safe Abortion: Technical and Policy Guidance for Health Systems*, 2nd ed. Geneva: World Health Organisation, Department of Reproductive Health and Research; 2012.

13. O'Donnell J, Weitz TA, Freedman LR. Resistance and vulnerability to stigmatization in abortion. *Soc Sci & Med*. 2011;7(9):1357–1364.

Index

Printed in the United States
by Baker & Taylor Publisher Services